INTRACORONARY DIAGNOSTIC TECHNIQUES

F. ALFONSO, MD, PhD, FESC

Interventional Cardiology Department
Cardiovascular Institute
«San Carlos» University Hospital
Madrid, Spain

J. BOTAS, MD, PhD, FESC

Interventional Cardiology Unit
Cardiology Department
«Gregorio Marañón» University Hospital
Madrid, Spain

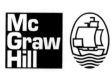

McGRAW-HiLL · iNTERAMERiCANA

MADRID · BUENOS AIRES · CARACAS · GUATEMALA · LISBOA · MEXICO
NUEVA YORK · PANAMA · SAN JUAN · SANTAFE DE BOGOTA · SANTIAGO · SÃO PAULO
AUCKLAND · HAMBURGO · LONDRES · MILAN · MONTREAL · NUEVA DELHI · PARIS
SAN FRANCISCO · SYDNEY · SINGAPUR · ST. LOUIS · TOKIO · TORONTO

INTRACORONARY DIAGNOSTIC TECHNIQUES

McGRAW-HILL/INTERAMERICANA DE ESPAÑA, S. A. U.
Edificio Valrealty
Basauri, 17, 1.ª planta
28023 Aravaca (Madrid)

ISBN: 84-486-0486-5
Depósito legal: M. 19.559-2003

Phototypesetting: MonoComp, S. A. Cartagena, 43. 28028 Madrid
Printed in EDIGRAFOS, S. A. Volta, 2. Pol. Industrial San Marcos.
28906 Getafe (Madrid)

Impreso en España - Printed in Spain

EDITORS

FERNANDO ALFONSO, MD, PhD, FESC
Interventional Cardiology Department
Cardiovascular Institute
«San Carlos» University Hospital
Madrid, Spain

JAVIER BOTAS, MD, PhD, FESC
Interventional Cardiology Unit
Cardiology Department
«Gregorio Marañón», University Hospital
Madrid, Spain

CONTRIBUTORS

WILBERT AARNOUDSE, MD
Cardiovascular Center Aalst,
Belgium

FLAVIO AIROLDI, MD
Columbus Clinic and San Raffaele Hospital
Milan, Italy

PALOMA ARAGONCILLO, MD
Department of Pathology
Cardiovascular Institute
«San Carlos» University Hospital
Madrid, Spain

JUAN JOSÉ BADIMON, PhD
Cardiovascular Biology Research Laboratory
Cardiovascular Institute
Mount Sinai School of Medicine
New York, USA

DIETRICH BAUMGART, MD
Department of Cardiology
University Clinic Essen
Germany

CLEMENS VON BIRGELEN, MD, PhD
Department of Cardiology
University Clinic Essen
Germany

CEEST-JOOST BOTMAN, MD
Catharina Hospital, Eindhoven,
The Netherlands

ROBERTO CORTI, MD
Cardiovascular Biology Research Laboratory
Cardiovascular Institute
Mount Sinai School of Medicine
New York, USA

BERNARD DE BRUYNE, MD, PhD
Cardiovascular Center Aalst
OLV Hospital
Belgium

CARLO DI MARIO, MD
Columbus Clinic and San Raffaele Hospital
Milan, Italy

JOUKE DIJKSTRA, PhD
Leiden University Medical Center
Division of Image Processing
Section Intravascular Ultrasound
Leiden, The Netherlands

HOLGER EGGEBRECHT, MD
Department of Cardiology
University Clinic Essen
Germany

JAIME ELÍZAGA, MD, PhD
Interventional Cardiology Unit
Cardiology Department
«Gregorio Marañón», University Hospital
Madrid, Spain

RAIMUND ERBEL, MD, FACC, FESC, FAHA
Department of Cardiology
University Clinic Essen
Germany

JAVIER ESCANED, MD, PhD, FESC
Interventional Cardiology Department
Cardiovascular Institute
«San Carlos» University Hospital
Madrid, Spain

ERLING FALK, MD, PhD
Department of Cardiology
Research Unit
Aarhus University Hospital
Skejby, Denmark

WILLIAM F. FEARON, MD
Cardiovascular Medicine
Stanford University
CA, USA

PIM. J. DE FEYTER, MD, FESC
Cardiology Department
University Hospital Rotterdam
Dijkzigt Heart Center
Rotterdam, The Netherlands

PETER J. FITZGERALD, MD, PhD
Center for Research in Cardiovascular Interventions
Stanford University
Stanford, CA, USA

JUNBO GE, MD
Department of Cardiology
University Clinic Essen
Germany

MICHAEL HAUDE, MD
Department of Cardiology
University Clinic Essen
Germany

SAMIR R. KAPADIA, MD
University of Washington
Seattle, Washington, USA

MORTON J. KERN, MD
Gerard Mudd Cardiac Catheterization Laboratory
St. Louis University Health Sciences Center
St. Louis, MO, USA

JURGEN LIGTHART, MD
Cardiology Department
University Hospital Rotterdam
Dijkzigt Heart Center
Rotterdam, The Netherlands

JORGE LUNA, MD
Interventional Cardiology
Division of Cardiovascular Medicine
Stanford University School of Medicine
Stanford, California, USA

CARLOS MACAYA, MD
Interventional Cardiology Department
Cardiovascular Institute
«San Carlos» University Hospital
Madrid, Spain

JACOB MARSVIN LAURBERG, MD
Department of Cardiology
Aarhus University Hospital
Skejby, Denmark

JAVIER MORENO, MD
Interventional Cardiology Department
Cardiovascular Institute
«San Carlos» University Hospital
Madrid, Spain

HARALD MUDRA, MD
2. Medizinische Abteilung
Krakenhaus München Neuperlach
Chefarzt, Kardiologie.
München, Germany

JULIO I. OSENDE, MD
Cardiovascular Biology Research Laboratory
Cardiovascular Institute
Mount Sinai School of Medicine
New York, USA

NICASIO PÉREZ CASTELLANO, MD
Interventional Cardiology Department
Cardiovascular Institute
«San Carlos» University Hospital
Madrid, Spain

NICO H. J. PIJLS, MD, PhD
Department of Cardiology
Catharina Hospital, Eindhoven
The Netherlands

GELA PIMENTEL, MD
Interventional Cardiology Department
Cardiovascular Institute
«San Carlos» University Hospital
Madrid, Spain

FAUSTO J. PINTO, MD, PhD, FESC, FACC
University Hospital Sta. Maria
Division of Cardiology
Lisbon University Medical School
Lisbon, Portugal

MANEL SABATÉ, MD, PhD
Interventional Cardiology Department
Cardiovascular Institute
«San Carlos» University Hospital
Madrid, Spain

JAVIER SORIANO, PhD, FESC
Interventional Cardiology Unit
Cardiology Department
«Gregorio Marañón», University Hospital
Madrid, Spain

CHRISTODOULOS STEFANADIS, MD, FACC,
FESC
University of Athens
Department of Cardiology
Hippokration Hospital
Athens, Greece

KENGO TANABE, MD
Cardiology Department
University Hospital Rotterdam
Dijkzigt Heart Center
Rotterdam, The Netherlands

KOSTANTINOS TOUTOUZAS, MD
Hippokration University Hospital
Athens, Greece

PAVLOS TOUTOUZAS, MD, FACC, FESC
University of Athens
Department of Cardiology
Hippokration Hospital
Athens, Greece

E. MURAT TUZCU, MD
The Cleveland Clinic Foundation
Cleveland, Ohio, USA

MANOLIS VAVURANAKIS, MD, FACC
Department of Cardiology
Hippokration Hospital
Athens, Greece

JULIÁN VILLACASTÍN, MD
Interventional Cardiology Department
Cardiovascular Institute
«San Carlos» University Hospital
Madrid, Spain

ALAN C. YEUNG, MD
Division of Cardiovascular Medicine
Stanford University School of Medicine
Stanford, California, USA

Content

SECTION I
General Considerations on Atherosclerosis. Pathologic Aspects. Coronary Physiology. Need for New Intracoronary Diagnostic Modalities

SECTION II
Intracoronary Ultrasound

SECTION III
Intracardiac and Great Vessels Ultrasound

SECTION IV
Coronary Angioscopy

SECTION V
Intracoronary Doppler

SECTION VI
Pressure Wire

SECTION VII
Other Diagnostic Modalities

Preface

Atherosclerotic coronary artery disease remains the leading cause of morbidity and mortality in the Western world. During the last four decades, the information obtained by coronary angiography has significantly changed our understanding of coronary artery disease. Since the first percutaneous coronary intervention performed in 1977 by Andreas Gruentzig, the field of interventional cardiology has developed exponentially, producing unprecedented advances in diagnosis and therapy. These advances, in turn, have challenged old paradigms in coronary artery disease. Although coronary angiography has endured over the years as the «gold stardard» for diagnosing coronary artery disease and guiding percutaneous interventions, the inherent limitations of this technique have been clearly recognized in the last decade. An alternative technique free of the constraints of angiography in terms of diagnostic accuracy and interventional guidance remains to be found. However, several new *intracoronary diagnostic techniques* have flourished, providing unique and complementary information to the luminogram obtained by angiography. Nowadays, these *intracoronary diagnostic techniques* are widely used either for clinical decision-making or research purposes. In light of the rapid advances in this field, this book was written to explore with the reader the fundamental uses of *intracoronary diagnostic techniques* for diagnostic and research purposes, from a multidisciplinary approach. Technical pearls and pitfalls will merge together with evidence-based-medicine findings from recent clinical trials to provide a comprehensive and up-to-date overview of these exciting techniques.

The first section of the book reviews the often forgotten histopathology of coronary artery disease, including a chapter by Falk on the pathology of acute coronary syndromes, a review of the basic concepts of coronary physiology by Kern, and a review of the limitations of coronary angiography. This is followed by several chapters which constitute the focus of the book that exhaustively review intracoronary ultrasound, a technique that has reached maturity after only a decade of use in clinical practice. Intracoronary ultrasound is reviewed in depth, from the basics of image interpretation to speculation about the future of this tool by Fitzgerald, one of the *gurus* of the technique. The importance of vascular remodeling is addressed in a specific chapter by Erbel, and the use of the technique for diagnostic purposes in several chapters, including one by Tuzcu on transplant vasculopathy, one of the earlier uses of this technique. Advances in three-dimensional ultrasound are summarized by von Birgelen. The use of intracoronary ultrasound during coronary interventions is addressed in specific chapters by leading experts in the field, such as Pinto, Yeung, and Mudra. Likewise, intravascular ultrasound of the great vessels (in a chapter by Erbel) and intracardiac ultrasound are reviewed in detail. Although coronary angioscopy is no longer available in certain regions of the world, De Feyter addresses its value during coronary interventions in a specific chapter. At this point, the focus on the detailed analysis of coronary anatomy shifts to physiology. Two chapters are dedicated to reviewing the use of Doppler ultrasound to study coronary circulation, including its usefulness as a guide in percutaneous interventions, in the chapter by Di Mario. The next three chapters target the attractive new concept of fractional flow reserve as obtained with the pressure wire. The technique is comprehensively reviewed by its developers, Pijls and De Bruyne. Emerging techniques, such as thermography and magnetic resonance imaging, are discussed by experts in the technique, such as Stefanidis and Corti who reviewed the experience that has accrued in Mount Sinai. Finally, the experience of our two Madrid groups is presented in several chapters of the book, which were designed to minimize gaps and smooth out the inconsistencies that sometimes affect books with various authors.

We feel indebted to the authors and proud to have brought together an outstanding group of professional colleagues and friends for the development of this book. We are grateful to them for sharing this endeavor.

We sincerely hope that this book will be a practical tool for the medical community and that it will help fellows in-training, clinical cardiologists, interventional cardiologists, and researchers to keep up with new developments in the field. Better yet, we hope that it will help to generate challenging new ideas for clinical or research applications that will bring us closer to reaching our common goal of increasing knowledge and improving patient care.

Fernando Alfonso MD, PhD, FESC
Javier Botas MD, PhD, FESC

ACKNOWLEDGEMENTS

We are indebted to all the medical staff and nurses of the catheterization laboratories at «Hospital Universitario Clínico San Carlos» and «Hospital Universitario Gregorio Marañon», both in Madrid, who gave their best during each intervention for decision-making, continuous research, and patient care. We would also like to thank McGraw-Hill publishers for their professionalism in bringing this book to press and their commitment to excellence.

SECTION I

General Considerations on Atherosclerosis. Pathologic Aspects. Coronary Physiology. Need for New Intracoronary Diagnostic Modalities

Pathology of Coronary Atherosclerosis

PALOMA ARAGONCILLO, MD

Morphology of subepicardial coronary arteries. Coronary atherosclerosis. References.

MORPHOLOGY OF SUBEPICARDIAL CORONARY ARTERIES

The coronary arteries are muscular and comprise three layers: the intima, media, and adventitia. The internal elastic lamina marks the limit between the intima and media, although there are areas where these layers are poorly delimited, as in the case of bifurcations, side branches, or curved areas. The limit between the media and adventitia is marked by the external elastic lamina. The luminal cross-section of the proximal coronary arteries has been related to the weight of the heart and the patient's age and sex. Thus, larger luminal areas have been described in hearts with a larger left ventricular mass.[1] The purpose of this increased areas would be to increase blood flow into the myocardium. In the absence of heart disease, younger people and women tend to have smaller luminal areas than men or older subjects. The process of increasing the arterial areas is called remodeling and is a normal arterial response that is designed to ensure blood flow and wall tension.[2] Mulvany et al.[3] attribute the changes in vessel caliber to a redistribution of arterial wall components, rather than to cell proliferation.

In postmortem studies of newborns and children, differences have been noted in the constitution of the walls of the coronary arteries as compared with other muscular arteries. These differences lie mainly in the intima. In the coronary arteries, the intima varies in thickness from a very thin layer to a thickness similar to that of the media. Where it is thinnest, the intima comprises the endothelium, basement membrane, and subendothelial layer, which consists of elastin, collagen, proteoglycans, and scattered smooth muscle cells.

In the areas where the intima is thicker, it presents two layers separated by an elastic lamina, the external elastic muscle layer. This layer is made up of longitudinally aligned elastic fibers and smooth muscle cells that originate in the medial layer and internal elastic lamina. The innermost layer, the subendothelial layer, consists of elastic fibers, proteoglycans, smooth muscle cells, and a few macrophages.

Intimal thickening may be eccentric or diffuse, or it may affect the entire vessel circumference.[4] Diffuse affectation is not common and is found in no specific location. Eccentric thickening, however, is found in specific locations such as areas of bifurcation or side branches, which are areas with a certain predisposition to atherosclerotic lesions. The most striking location is the bifurcation of the coronary trunk, at the origin of the left anterior descending and circumflex coronary arteries.

Intimal thickening is considered to be a phenomenon of vessel adaptation to mechanical stress secondary to variations in flow and/or wall tension and maturity. No differences in intimal composition have been found in relation to race or gender, but differences have been observed in the extension of intimal thickening.

In a study of coronary artery structure in different ethnic groups, Vlodaver et al.[5] observed that intimal thickening is more extended among Ashkenazi Jews than among Bedouins, and among Ashkenazi boys than girls.

Researchers have reported the presence of activated T cells, dendritic cells, some mast cells, and scant B lymphocytes in areas of intimal thickening in children and young adults.[6] There have been recent references[8] to the presence of a network of dendritic cells in the intima of children, which is denser in the areas of bifurcation and more dispersed on the rest of the arterial wall. The role of the dendritic network in atherogenesis has yet to be clarified, although it has been suggested that it may be related with this process since it is denser in the areas most predisposed to atherosclerosis.

As has been seen, intimal thickness varies. It is usually described in relation to the thickness of the media. Ratios of 0.1 to 1, or more, are cited as normal[4]. Sims et al.[8] described a gradual, age-related increase in intimal thickness up to a value of 4.1 times the thickness of the media layer in persons 50 to 60 years old. This increase in the intima is more marked in males than in females at any age.

The media is approximately 100 microns thick and basically consists of compact bunches of smooth-muscle cells arranged in a circle, with an occasional helicoidal bunch.

Elastic fibers and collagen fibers are interspersed among the muscle cells.

The adventitia is made up of elastic fibers, collagen fibers, and fibroblasts. Vasa vasorum and nerve fibers can be seen. The vasa vasorum irrigate the adventitia and the outer two-thirds of the media. The inner third of the media and intima are nourished directly by diffusion from the vessel lumen.

CORONARY ATHEROSCLEROSIS

Atherosclerotic lesions are more frequently observed in certain sites on the coronary tree. The left coronary artery has a higher incidence of atherosclerotic lesions in the area where the trunk bifurcates, proximal to the left anterior descending and circumflex coronary arteries. The right coronary artery shows a preponderance of atherosclerotic lesions in the proximal and middle segments.[9] Stary[10] maintains that advanced atheromatous plaques are located in areas of eccentric thickening in normal coronaries. Atherosclerotic lesions are designated in accordance with their morphology. The World Health Organization (1958)[11] defines four characteristic lesions: *fatty streak, fibrous plaque, atheroma, and complicated plaque.* Most of the literature describes three lesions,[12, 13] *fatty streak, fibrolipid plaque, and complicated plaque.* The fibrolipid plaque is considered complicated when hemorrhage, calcification, rupture, erosion, or thrombosis are present.

In order to unify the clinical and pathological criteria of coronary sclerosis, the Committee on Vascular Lesions of the Council on Atherosclerosis of the American Heart Association[14, 15] has drawn up a 6-part histological classification of the morphology of atherosclerotic lesions and their progression. The first three types are considered precursors of an established lesion[10] and are seen in the first decades of life. Types IV-VI are classified as advanced atherosclerotic lesions.

Virmani et al.[16] proposed a seven-category morphological classification of atherosclerotic lesions based on lipid accumulation and its relation with the formation of the fibrous capsule. The seven types proposed are grouped first into non-atherosclerotic intimal lesions: intimal thickening and intimal xanthoma or the «fatty streak,» and then into progressive atherosclerotic lesions: pathological intimal thickening, fibrous capsule atheroma, thin fibrous capsule atheroma, calcified nodule, and fibrocalcific plaque. Atheromas with a fibrous capsule and pathological intimal thickening, atheromas with a thin capsule and a fibrous, calcified plaque, and calcified nodules may rupture, erode, and originate thrombosis.

In this chapter we will be following the classification (I to VI) of the Committee on Vascular Lesions of the Council on Atherosclerosis of the American Heart Association (Table 1-1).

Type I, the initial lesion, is characterized by the presence of small clumps of fat-laden macrophages on the innermost layer of the intima, mainly in areas of intimal thickening.

Type II corresponds to the fatty streak (Fig. 1-1). The fatty streak is the first lesion that can be identified with the naked eye and stained with specific fat-soluble dyes, such as Sudan III or Sudan IV. It is a yellowish, flat, or slightly raised intimal lesion in the form of streaks (or possibly a rounded lesion), which is generally located where the artery branches.

Foam cells can also be seen in the intima, largely located beneath the endothelium. Most are fat-laden macrophages and monocytes with a phagocytic function. The monocytes pass through the endothelium and capture low-density, oxidized lipoproteins, thus becoming foam macrophages.[17] Smooth muscle cells containing lipids can also be detected in deep layers, close to the internal elastic lamina, but are not numerous in the lipid streak. The smooth muscle cells are activated by scavenger receptors[18] and low-density lipoprotein receptor-related protein.[19] Very few extracellular lipids are visible and collagen and elastin fibers are fragmented. MacGill et al.[20] have described three types of lipid streaks that are differentiated by lipid content and time of onset. «Juvenile» streaks

Table 1-1. Classification of Coronary Atherosclerosis

TYPE I:	Initial lesion. Small groups of fat-laden macrophages.
TYPE II:	Fatty streak. First lesion that can be recognized by the naked eye. (Lipids remain intracellular).
TYPE III:	Pre-atheromatous lesion. (Presence of extracellular lipids).
TYPE IV:	Fibrolipid and atheromatous plaque (Soft plaques: including a defined capsule and lipid core).
TYPE V:	Hard plaque. (Mainly consisting of collagen and smooth muscle cells): a) Intimal collagenation. b) Predominantly calcified (or TYPE VII). c) Predominantly formed by connective tissue (or TYPE VIII).
TYPE VI:	Complicated lesion: a) Type IV or V lesion with superficial disruption (plaque rupture). b) Type IV or V lesion with superficial bruising/bleeding (plaque erosion/intraplaque hemorrhage). c) Type IV or V lesions that present superficial thrombosis. abc) Type IV or V lesion with findings of all three complications.

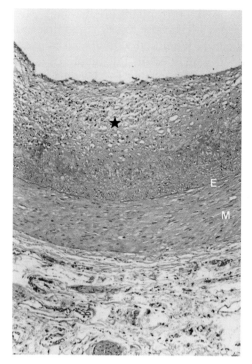

Figure 1-1. Lipid streak. The intima is thickened and foam cells can be seen, mainly underneath the endothelium (star). The internal elastic lamina (E) is conserved, as is the media layer (M).

are found in children and adolescents and are characterized by the presence of lipids that are basically intracellular, with very little connective tissue formation; this lesion is considered reversible and does not progress to atheroma. The fatty streak in young adults, in which extracellular lipids and connective tissue formation can be seen, is thought to be a potential precursor of atheromatous plaque. Finally, the lipid streak is characteristically found in the elderly, and has diffuse lipid infiltration, few extracellular lipids, and little cellularity; it does not seem to progress to more severe lesions.

A type III pre-atheromatous lesion would be an intermediate stage between type II and type IV. It is characterized by the presence of extracellular lipids forming numerous small cores. In a recent article, MacGill et al.[21] describe an association between the extension of streaks and risk factors or age, and thus consider type III lesions as a transition towards an established lesion.

Fibrolipid plaques are the characteristic lesions in atherosclerosis, with a morphology that varies depending on the relative proportions of its components.[22, 23] They are pearly-white lesions of the intima that protrude into the lumen and may be yellow or whitish-colored on section, depending on their lipid content. Plaques may be concentric or eccentric, depending on whether the entire circumference, or only part, is affected. Eccentric plaques are the most frequent ones, with slight intimal thickening of the wall opposite the lesion. Concentric plaques tend to contain more fibrous components and are only slightly cellular.

Fibrolipid plaques, atheromatous plaques, soft plaques, or type IV lesions exhibit a disorganized intima with a well-defined lipid nucleus located in the deepest area of the intima, which is surrounded by connective tissue and separated from the lumen by a capsule.

The lipid core is made up of necrotic remains, crystals of free cholesterol, cholesterol esters, lipoproteins, and phospholipids. It is generally avascular and has few cells. Collagen destruction by metalloproteinases[24] and lipoproteins released in the course of foam cell necrosis or apoptosis are the initiators of the lipid core, the size of which increases as a result of similar mechanisms in the foam cells surrounding the core.[25] Lipid core rigidity is temperature-dependent, i.e., the higher the temperature (as in the case of inflammation), the softer the core.[26]

Fibrous capsules vary in thickness from very thin (Fig. 1-2) to thick and well-defined (Fig. 1-3), with an inverse relationship between capsular thickness and the lipid core.[27] Thin capsules have less collagen, abundant macrophages,[28] T lymphocytes, and mast

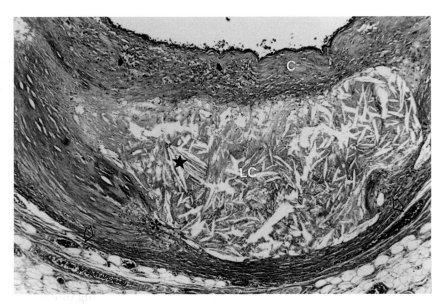

Figure 1-2. Fibrolipid plaque with fine fibrous capsule (C) less than 150 microns thick, containing foam cells and inflammatory elements (black arrows). Acellular lipid core (LC) with cholesterol crystals (star), and macrophages on the periphery (asterisk). Marked atrophy of the media layer (space open between two arrows).

cells.[29] There are few, if any, smooth muscle cells. This loss of smooth muscle cells may be a consequence of apoptosis.[30] This composition is characteristically found in the area known as the «shoulder» of the plaque, where the plaque joins the unaffected part of the artery.

Thick capsules (Fig. 1-3) have an extracellular matrix, but very few cells. The few cells they have are mostly smooth muscle cells. The variations in capsular thickness may be determined by the macrophages, which may secrete metalloproteinases that cause connective tissue degradation. Thicker capsules may contain abundant collagen produced by the smooth muscle cells. Libby et al.[31] contend that the capsule is not a static structure, but undergoes constant changes in composition. These changes are controlled by inflammatory mediators, which underlines the importance of inflammation in plaque stability and its therapeutic implications.[32]

Most patients present more than one kind of plaque, although small groups of patients

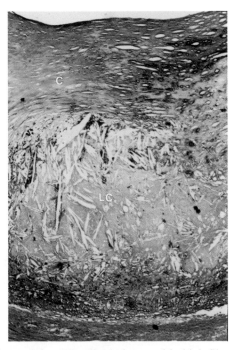

Figure 1-3. Fibrolipid plaque with thick fibrous capsule (C), showing abundant collagen. Lipid core (LC) with characteristics similar to those in Figure 1-2.

have been described with a single type of lesion. All plaques are soft or fibrous.[22]

Plaques with a large lipid core and a thin capsule measuring less than 150 μ thick with abundant macrophages, T lymphocytes, and few smooth muscle cells are considered vulnerable. That means that they are highly likely to rupture,[28] a likelihood that is totally unrelated to plaque size or the degree of stenosis.[33]

Type V or hard plaque (Fig. 1-4) is fibrocellular, and consists mainly of collagen and smooth muscle cells. A very small amount of lipids can be observed, and there is no evident lipid core. Type V is divided into three subtypes: a, b, and c. Type Va shows intimal collagenation around the lipid core, with abundant myocytes rich in rough endoplasmic reticulum, and the proliferation and growth of capillaries. In type Vb, the plaque contains more connective tissue and calcification, whereas in type Vc, the lesion is largely made up of connective tissue, with little or no lipids. In a recent publi-

cation, Stary[34] replaced types Vb and Vc with the types VII and VIII. Type VII lesions would be predominantly calcified and type VIII would be largely fibrous. Both types would result from the regression or changes in the lipids found in type IV and V lesions.

Both fibrolipid and fibrocellular plaques appear stratified. In some lesions, multiple lipid layers are observed, with lipid cores separated by connective tissue. In others, connective tissue alternates with smooth muscle cells and proteoglycans. This stratification has been interpreted as the result of repair of thrombosis or erosions.[16]

Small vessels, (Fig. 1-4) consisting solely of endothelium or a media with a few smooth muscle cells, are seen in atheromatous plaques; these vessels are fragile and bleed easily. The origin of these vessels has yet to be determined and several hypotheses have been proposed: vasa vasorum, de novo formation from the arterial lumen, or formation from organized thromboses that are incorpor-

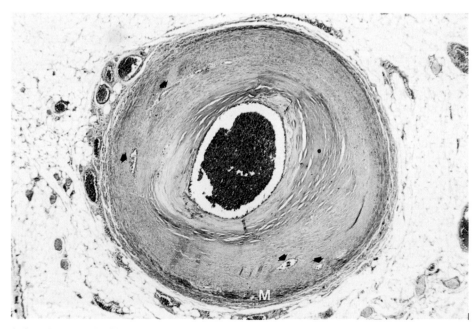

Figure 1-4. Concentric fibrous plaque comprising collagen and scant smooth muscle cells. Vasa vasorum (arrows) can be seen inside the plaque. The media (M) is retained in the entire arterial circumference.

ated by the atheromatous plaque. The purpose of this angiogenesis is not fully understood, although it is generally thought to be a response of the vessel to ischemia. It has been suggested that these vessels may influence the evolution and complications of the atheromatous plaque: thrombosis might promote smooth muscle cell emigration and proliferation, rupture might lead to bleeding within the plaque and produce a sudden increase in the size of the lesion. O'Brien et al.[35] suggest that these blood vessels may be involved in controlling the development and progress of the atheromatous plaque and arterial restenosis. JK Williams[36] has speculated on their role in plaque rupture and thrombosis. In experiments, it has been observed that a reduction in lipids reduces neovascularization, thereby limiting plaque progression and stabilizing the plaque.[37]

Calcium deposits can be observed in both the lipid core and capsule as either small granules or extensive deposits. Calcification is found in severe lesions and in those with little luminal narrowing. The amount of cal-

cium is directly related to the degree of stenosis (Fig. 1-5). These calcium deposits increase with age[38] and in the presence of chronic renal failure and hypercalcemia.[39] The Virmani classification offers a description of a lesion called calcium nodules, which are characterized by the presence of large subcapsular calcium deposits encroaching on the vascular lumen and possibly leading to rupture of the capsule and luminal thrombosis (Fig. 1-6).

In the area of the plaque, the internal elastic lamina shows duplication, fragmentation, and may even disappear entirely (Fig. 1-7). In areas occupied by fibrolipid plaques, the media is thin and disorganized, or even atrophic. The adventitia is thick and fibrotic, has an increased vasa vasorum network, and mast cell infiltrates.

Glagov et al.[40] have described enlargement of the coronary arteries in connection with the plaque area. Consequently, the luminal section, which is the area bordered by the internal elastic lamina in the absence of intimal thickening, or the potential luminal

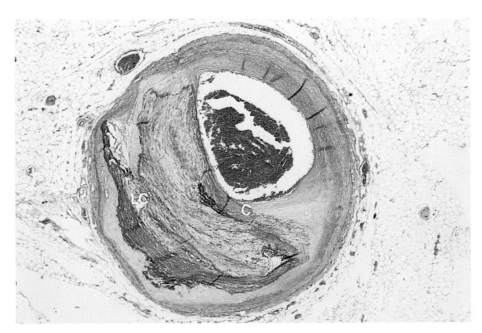

Figure 1-5. Eccentric plaque revealing extensive calcium deposits affecting both the capsule (C) and lipid core (LC).

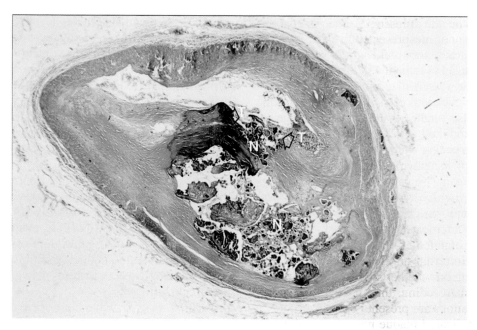

Figure 1-6.   Fibrous plaque with calcium nodule (N) extending into the arterial lumen. Rupture of the capsule (between arrows) with luminal thrombosis (T).

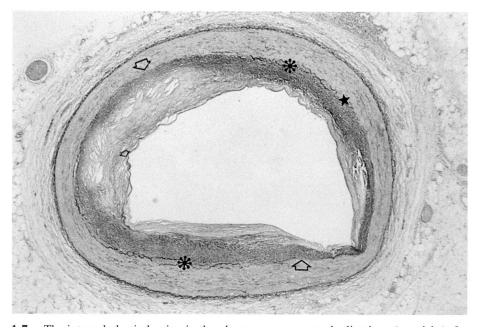

Figure 1-7.   The internal elastic lamina in the plaque area presents duplications (asterisks), fragmentation (stars), and may even disappear (arrows).

section in the presence of atheromatous plaques, does not present significant stenosis until the lesion occupies more than 40% of the internal elastic lamina. In addition, not only has positive arterial remodeling been described in the presence of atherosclerotic lesions, but also a negative remodeling causing arterial narrowing that would accelerate luminal stenosis.[41-42] Both types of remodeling may be observed in the same artery and it is not clear why one type or another takes place. Davies et al.[43] believe that arteries with severe stenoses or fast-growing plaques experience a remodeling failure.

The complicated, or type VI, lesion is divided into four subtypes, a, b, c, and abc, depending on whether superficial disruption, hematoma/bleeding, thrombosis, or all three complications are present. The substratum of the complicated plaque may be a type IV or type V lesion and the complication may ap-

pear in patients with any degree of stenosis.[33] Atheromatous plaques with large lipid cores and thin capsules show a greater risk of rupture (Fig. 1-8).[25] The rupture may affect the capsule and reach the lipid core, producing intraplaque bleeding. In the area of the crack or rupture, luminal thrombosis occurs and, on occasions, the thrombus contains components of the plaque. When the substrate is a type V lesion, the plaque normally breaks in the area where the capsule shows an accumulation of macrophages and inflammatory cells, even if it is only a small area (Fig. 1-9).

Erosion of the atheromatous plaque is characterized by the fact that it involves only the surface of the plaque, without producing ruptures or cracks in the plaque. The substrate of the erosion may be a thin capsule with macrophages and inflammatory cells and a well-constituted lipid core, or a fibrocellular plaque without a lipid core (Fig. 1-10)[44].

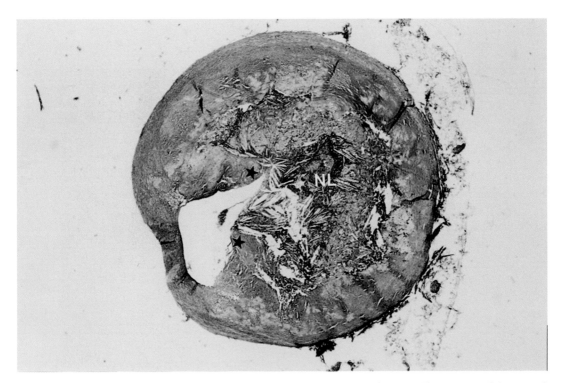

Figure 1-8. Complicated fibrolipid plaque, revealing a large lipid core (NL). The rupture of the capsule corresponds to the space between the two stars.

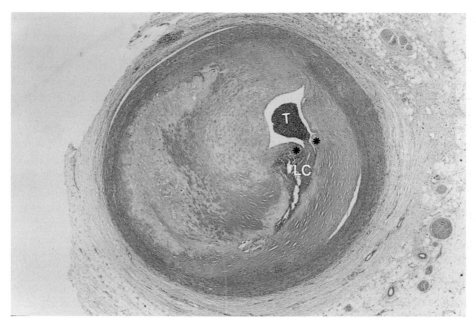

Figure 1-9. Type V plaque, with a small lipid core (LC) located below the capsule, revealing a crack in the capsule (space between the two asterisks) with intraplaque hemorrhage and luminal thrombosis (T).

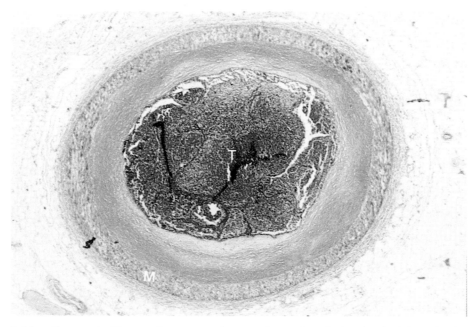

Figure 1-10. Concentric fibrous plaque, revealing erosion and occlusive luminal thrombosis (T). The media (M) is conserved throughout the vessel circumference.

REFERENCES

1. Roberts CS, Roberts WC. Cross-sectional area of the proximal portions of the three major epicardial coronary arteries in 98 necropsy patients with different coronary events. Relationship to heart weight, age and sex. *Circulation* 1980; 62:953-959.
2. Jamal A, Bendeck M, Langille BL. Structural changes and recovery of function after arterial injury. *Arterioscler Thromb* 1992; 12:307-317.
3. Mulvany MJ. Determinants of vascular structure. *J Cardiovasc Pharmacol* 1992; 19 (Suppl 5):S1-S6.
4. Stary HC. Macrophages, macrophage foam cells, and eccentric intimal thickening in coronary arteries of young children. *Atherosclerosis* 1987; 64:91-108.
5. Vlodaver Z, Kahn HA, Neufeld HN. The coronary arteries in early life in three different ethnic groups. *Circulation* 1969, 39: 541-550.
6. Wick G, Romen M, Amberger A, et al. Atherosclerosis, autoimmunity, and vascular-associated lymphoid tissue. *FASEB J.* 1997; 11:1199-1207.
7. Millonig G, Niederegger H, Rabl W, et al. Network of vascular-associated dendritic cells in intima of healthy young individuals. *Arterioscler Thromb Vasc Biol* 2001; 21:503-508.
8. Sims FH, Gavin JB, Vanderwee MA. The intima of human coronary arteries. *Am Heart J* 1989; 118-132.
9. Montenegro MR, Eggen DA. Topography of atherosclerosis in the coronary arteries. *Lab Invest* 1968; 18:586-593.
10. Stary HC. Evolution and progression of atherosclerotic lesions in coronary arteries of children and young adults. *Atherosclerosis* 1989; 9(supp 1):I-19-I-32.
11. World Health Organization. Classification of atherosclerotic lesions. Report of a study group. *WHO Techn Rep Ser* 1958; 143:1-20.
12. Crawford T. Atherosclerosis in the pathogenesis of ischaemic heart disease. In Crawford T (ed). Pathology of ischaemic heart disease. London. *Butterworths & Co.* 1977:28-46.
13. Woolf N. The morphology of atherosclerotic lesions. In Wolf N, (ed). Pathology of atherosclerosis. London. *Butterworths & Co.* 1982:47-82.
14. Stary HC, Chandler AB, Glagov S, et al. A definition of initial, fatty streak, and intermediate lesions of atherosclerosis. A report from the Committee on Vascular Lesions of the Council on Atherosclerosis, American Heart Association. *Circulation* 1994; 89: 2462-2478.
15. Stary HC, Chandler AB, Dinsmore RE, et al. A definition of advanced types of atherosclerotic lesions and histological classifications of atherosclerosis. A report from the Committee on Vascular Lesions of the Council on Atherosclerosis, American Heart Association. *Arterioscler Thromb* 1995; 15:1512-1531.
16. Virmani R, Kolodgie FD, Burke AP, Farb A, Schwartz SM. Lessons from sudden coronary death. A compressive morphological classification scheme for atherosclerotic lesions. *Arterioscler Thromb Vasc Biol* 2000; 20:1262-1275.
17. Brown MS, Goldstein JL. Lipoprotein metabolism in the macrophage: implications for cholesterol deposition in atherosclerosis. *Annu Rev Biochem* 1983; 52:223-261.
18. Vijayagopal P, Glancy L. Macrophages stimulate cholesteryl ester accumulation in cocultured smooth muscle cells incubated with lipoprotein-proteoglycan complex. *Atheroscler Thromb Vasc Biol* 1996; 16: 1112-1121.
19. Martinez-Gonzalez J, Llorente-Cortes V, Badimon L. Cellular and molecular biology of atherosclerotic lesions. *Rev Esp Cardiol* 2001; 54:218-231.
20. McGill HC. The lesion. In: Schettler G and Weizel A (eds). Atherosclerosis III. Proceedings of the Triad International Symposium. Berlin. *Springer-Verlag.* 1974:27-38.
21. McGill HC, McMahan CA, Zieske AW, et al. Association of coronary heart disease risk factors with the intermediate lesion of atherosclerosis in youth. The pathobiological determinants of atherosclerosis in youth (PDAY) research group. *Arterioscler Thromb Vasc Biol.* 2000; 20:1998-2004.
22. Hangartner JRW, Charleston AJ, Davies MJ, Thomas AC. Morphological characteristics of clinically significant coronary stenosis in stable angina. *Br Heart J* 1986; 56:501-508.

23. Kragel AH, Reddy SG, Wittes JT, Roberts WC. Morphometric analysis of the composition of atherosclerotic plaques in the four major epicardial coronary arteries in acute myocardial infarction and in sudden coronary death. *Circulation* 1989; 80:1747-1756.

24. Davies MJ. Stability and in stability: two faces of coronary atherosclerosis. *Circulation* 1996; 94:2013-2020.

25. Falk E, Shah PK, Fuster V. Coronary plaque disruption. *Circulation* 1995; 92:657-671.

26. Lunderberg B. Chemical composition and physical state of lipid deposits in atherosclerosis. *Atherosclerosis* 1985; 56:93-110.

27. Felton CV, Crook D, Davies MJ, Olivier MF. Relation of plaque lipid composition and morphology to the stability of human aortic plaques. *Atheroscler Thromb &infiltration in acute Vasc Dis* 1997; 17:1337-1345.

28. Moreno Pr, Falk E, Palacios IF, Newell JB, Fuster V, Fallon JT. Macrophage infiltration in acute coronary syndromes: implications for plaque rupture. *Circulation* 1994; 90: 775-778.

29. Kaartinen M, Penttila A, Kovanen PT. Accumulation of activated mast cell in the shoulder region of human coronary atheroma, the predilection site of atheromatous rupture. *Circulation* 1994; 90:1669-1678.

30. Taylor AJ, Farb AA, Angello DA, Burwell, Virmani R. Proliferative activity in coronary atherectomy tissue: clinical, histopathologic, and immunohistochemical correlates. *Chest* 1995; 108:815-820.

31. Libby P. The molecular bases of the acute coronary syndromes. *Circulation* 1995; 91: 2844-2850.

32. Libby P. Current concepts of the pathogenesis of the acute coronary syndromes. *Circulation* 2001; 104:365-372.

33. Mann JM, Davies MJ,. Vulnerable plaque. Relation of characteristics to degree of stenosis in human coronary arteries. *Circulation* 1996; 94:928-931.

34. Stary HC. Natural history and histological classification of atherosclerotic lesions. An update. *Arterioscler Thromb Vasc Biol.* 2000; 20:1177-1178.

35. O'Brien ER, Garvin MR, Dev R, et al. Angiogenesis in human coronary atherosclerotic plaques. *Am J Pathol* 1994; 145:883-894.

36. Williams JK, Heista DD. The vasa vasorum of the arteries. *J Mal Vasc* 1996; 21 (Suppl C): 266-269.

37. Moulton KS, Séller E, Konerding MA, et al. Angiogenesis inhibitors endostatin or TNP-470 reduce intimal neovascularization and plaque growth in apolipoprotein E-deficient mice. *Circulation* 1999; 99:1726-1732.

38. Waller BF, Roberts WC. Cardiovascular disease in the very elderly. Analysis of 40 necropsy patients aged 90 years or over. *Am J Cardiol* 1983; 51:403-421.

39. Roberts WC, Waller BF. Effect of chronic hypercalcemia on the heart. *Am J Med 1981;* 71:371-384.

40. Glagov S, Weisenberg E, Zarins CK, Stankunavicius R, Kolettis GJ. Compensatory enlargement of human atherosclerotic coronary arteries. *N Engl J Med* 1987; 316:1371-1375.

41. Pasterkamp G, Wensing PJW, Post MJ, Mali WPTM, Borst C. Paradoxical arterial wall shrinkage contributes to luminal narrowing of human atherosclerotic femoral arteries. *Circulation* 1995; 91:1444-1449.

42. Pasterkamp G, Schoneveld AH, Van Wolferen W, et al. The impact of atherosclerotic arterial remodeling on percentage of luminal stenosis varies widely within the arterial system. A postmortem study. *Arterioscler Thromb Vasc Biol* 1997; 17:3057-3063.

43. Davies MJ. Coronary artery remodeling and the assessment of stenosis by pathologists. *Histopathology* 1998; 33:497-500.

44. Van der Wal AC, Becker AE, Van der Loos CM, Das PK. Site of intimal rupture or erosion of thrombosed coronary atherosclerotic plaques is characterized by an inflammatory process irrespective of the dominant plaque morphology. *Circulation* 1994; 89:36-44.

2

Pathophysiology of Acute Coronary Syndromes: Plaque Evolution and Vascular Remodeling

JACOB MARSVIN LAURBERG, MD
ERLING FALK, MD

Pathophysiology of acute coronary syndromes: Plaque evolution and vascular remodeling. Initiation of atherosclerosis: endothelial activation and dysfunction. Regional differences. Lipid accumulation. Atheroma growth. Remodeling. Coronary calcification. Plaque instability. Extrinsic factors. Intrinsic factors. Plaque cap degradation. Plaque rupture. Vasoconstriction. Visualization of atherosclerosis. Clinical manifestations. Acknowledgment. References.

PATHOPHYSIOLOGY OF ACUTE CORONARY SYNDROMES: PLAQUE EVOLUTION AND VASCULAR REMODELING

Despite numerous advances in the understanding and treatment of cardiovascular diseases, they still are a major clinical problem. In the United States as well as in Europe and many other parts of the world, cardiovascular diseases remain by far the most common cause of death in both men and women of all ethnic groups. Just as importantly, they also lead to disability, prompting the World Health Organization to place coronary heart disease (CHD) at the top of the list of expected leading causes of disability by the year 2020, and stroke, another atherosclerosis-related disease, in fourth place. Although genetic factors play an important role in the development of atherosclerosis, the vast majority of atherosclerosis-related diseases, including CHD, are predominantly acquired.

Coronary atherosclerosis has two different manifestations: stable angina pectoris and acute coronary syndrome. Stable angina pectoris is generally a benign, chronic disease characterized by a slowly progressive narrowing of one or more coronary arteries. It has a relatively low mortality rate and, in most patients, angina symptoms can be eliminated by medication, coronary angioplasty, or coronary artery bypass grafting. The acute coronary syndrome, on the other hand, is characterized by acute thrombosis of a ruptured or eroded atherosclerotic plaque leading to occlusion or sub-occlusion of a coronary artery. It has a high mortality rate and requires acute intervention, either invasive or non-invasive. In 1976, sudden coronary death was the first symptom of coronary heart disease in 10-14 % of patients[1] and there is no evidence that this has changed since. Based on these observations, it is clear that prophylaxis is as important, if not more, than actual treatment in the battle against coronary atherosclerosis and death.

INITIATION OF ATHEROSCLEROSIS: ENDOTHELIAL ACTIVATION AND DYSFUNCTION

Initially, atherosclerosis evolves under an intact, but activated and dysfunctional, endothelium. It takes place primarily in atherosclerosis-prone areas with pre-existing intimal thickening. The endothelium here is characterized by hyper-adhesiveness for monocytes due to over-expression of adhesion molecules, among them *vascular cell adhesion molecule-1* (VCAM-1), enhanced permeability to plasma proteins, and functional imbalances in local pro- and antithrombotic factors, growth stimulators and inhibitors, and vasoactive substances.[2] There is also increased transcytosis and intimal retention of lipoproteins. The collective term for these changes in the endothelium is *endothelial activation.* Inflammation and immune responses play a pivotal part in this process from the very beginning.[3,4] The enhanced permeability to lipoproteins, including *low-density lipoprotein* (LDL), enables them to enter the arterial intima. In the arterial intima, oxidized LDL may reduce the bioavailability of nitric oxide and activate pro-inflammatory signaling pathways such as that of nuclear factor kappa B.[4] This further enhances the expression of VCAM-1 and the recruitment of macrophages, further increasing inflammation and endothelial activation and effectively establishing a vicious circle.[4]

In the clinical situation, endothelial dysfunction is measured as an impaired response to stimuli that should lead to vasodilation of the normal artery. This clinical measure is thought to reflect endothelial activation and has been shown to have a strong relation to atherosclerotic disease.[5] It also has a strong relation to most of the known risk factors for atherosclerotic heart disease, including hypercholesterolemia, hypertension, smoking, diabetes mellitus, and aging.[6] It has yet to be determined if endothelial dysfunction is a cause or an effect of atherosclerosis.

REGIONAL DIFFERENCES

There is great variety in the extent of atherosclerotic changes in different parts of the arterial tree. The coronary arteries, carotid arteries, and arteries of the lower limbs are often involved in the atherosclerotic process, whereas other arteries, like the internal mammary artery, are highly resistant. Even in the same vascular bed, the extent of atherosclerosis can vary considerably. Regardless of atherogenic stimuli, non-obstructive intimal thickening is present at constant locations in everybody from birth, particularly at branch points on the opposite side of the flow divider, and downstream from stenoses, where disturbances in laminar flow result in re-circulation eddies, flow separation, and oscillatory flows.[7] Intimal thickening progresses with time.

LIPID ACCUMULATION

The initial step in the formation of the atherosclerotic plaque itself is the influx of lipoproteins into the subendothelial space. This transendothelial flux is facilitated by hypercholesterolemia and increased endothelial permeability. In the intima, trapped LDL is probably oxidized by monocyte-derived, activated macrophages. Oxidized LDL, but not native LDL, is then avidly ingested through scavenger receptors of the macrophages, a process that packs the cytoplasm of these cells with droplets of cholesteryl esters. This leads to the formation of foam cells, macrophages with a «foamy» appearance due to the high lipid content of their cytoplasm.[8] The foam cell is the characteristic cell type in atherosclerotic plaques. Other inflammatory cells found in fatty streaks are T cells, but in much lower numbers, approximately one T cell for every 50 foam cells. The presence of both T cells and activated macrophages in abundance suggests that immunological reactions play an important role in the evolution of the atherosclerotic plaque.

The exact antigen(s) triggering this reaction have not yet been identified, but both endogenous (e.g. oxidized LDL)[9] and exogenous (*Chlamydia pneumoniae*) antigens have been suggested.[10]

Although immunoglobulins are found in abundance in atherosclerotic lesions, B cells and polymorphonuclear neutrophils are virtually absent. Plasma cells have been found in the adventitial inflammation surrounding atherosclerotic arteries.[11]

The accumulation of foam cells leads to the fatty streak. There is little or no extracellular lipid, the oxidized LDL being contained within the foam cells. Fatty streaks are present in the aorta of infants all over the world, irrespective of ethnicity, diet, or prevalence of ischemic heart disease in the population.[12] Fetuses present fatty streaks in their aorta, especially if they have hypercholesterolemic mothers.[13] In laboratory animals, fatty streaks are the easiest atherosclerotic lesions to induce, and usually regress completely with reduction of the dietary intake of cholesterol.

It is generally accepted that fatty streaks can progress to more advanced atherosclerotic lesions because they occur in the same anatomical sites and borderline lesions have been observed.[14] Fatty streaks superimposed on areas of pre-existing intimal thickening appear to have a particular tendency to progress into advanced, symptomatic lesions.[14] The mode of progression, however, and the factors controlling it remain unclear. Many conflicting observations have been made, suggesting that the progression of the fatty streak to more advanced, symptomatic, and, eventually, dangerous lesions is far from linear and inevitable.[12] Various endogenous and exogenous factors probably play a part.

High-density-lipoprotein (HDL) is not only a transport lipoprotein related to a low risk of cardiovascular disease.[4] It has a marked positive influence on endothelial function[15] and there is growing evidence that it can reverse the process of lipid accumulation in the arterial wall directly.[16]

ATHEROMA GROWTH

In contrast to the smooth, asymptomatic fatty streaks that do not protrude into the lumen and thus do not cause symptoms, advanced atherosclerotic lesions may indeed protrude into the lumen, causing narrowing, impaired blood flow, and symptoms. While fatty streaks are highly cellular lesions, the atheromatous core of a mature plaque is avascular, hypocellular, lipid-rich, mushy, and totally devoid of supporting collagen.[17] The size of the soft core is critical for plaque stability.

The transformation from simple fatty streak to advanced atherosclerotic lesion takes place when lipids start to accumulate extracellularly. Oxidized LDL is not found in the normal intima but is abundant in the atherosclerotic plaque. At least two processes may be involved in the extracellular accumulation of lipids: blood-derived atherogenic lipoproteins can be trapped in the proteoglycan-rich extracellular matrix and/or lipids may be released by macrophage foam cells following their death.[8] Lipids and other cell constituents released from dead macrophage foam cells contribute significantly to the formation and growth of the atheromatous core.[18] Macrophage death by apoptosis is seen in the advanced lesions, but not in the simple fatty streak.[19]

Besides the accumulation of extracellular lipids, other processes are associated with the progression beyond the asymptomatic fatty-streak stage. Connective tissue produced by smooth muscle cells accumulates within the lesion. This gives rise to a wide variety of plaque types. Some are lipid-rich whereas others have a low lipid content. Plaques of different composition may evolve adjacent to each other. Early in the progression of the lesion the endothelial surface is continuous. Denuded areas related to superficial foam-cell infiltration and inflammation, sometimes with adhered platelets, are seen over mature, advanced plaques.

Neovascularization is another prominent feature of the advanced atherosclerotic lesion. The neovascularization is comprised of a network of capillaries that arise from the adventitial vasa vasorum and extend into the base of the atherosclerotic lesions.[20] The new vessels are often expressing leukocyte adhesion molecules such as VCAM-1 and ICAM-1, facilitating further extravasation of macrophages and leading to further inflammation, thus promoting progression of the disease.[20] Extravasated erythrocytes are also commonly seen in these neovascularized areas.

REMODELING

Vascular remodeling is the ability of the vessel wall to reorganize its cellular and extracellular components in response to a chronic stimulus. In human atherosclerosis there is ample evidence of active remodeling during the early stages of disease, prior to the appearance of significant luminal stenosis. It was originally assumed that atherogenesis

was always associated with more or less compensatory dilation of coronary arteries during plaque growth,[21] but it is now known that this remodeling is bidirectional.[22] Plaques responsible for acute coronary syndromes are usually relatively large and associated with compensatory dilation. This tends to preserve a normal lumen despite the presence of significant, and potentially dangerous, vessel wall disease. In contrast, plaques responsible for stable angina pectoris are usually smaller but, nevertheless, may cause more severe luminal narrowing because of concomitant local shrinkage of the artery. Intravascular ultrasound examinations can provide images of arterial wall disease even with a non-stenotic lumen[23] (Fig. 2-1).

CORONARY CALCIFICATION

Focal calcification in atherosclerotic plaques is common and increases with age in both men and women. Both lipid-rich and

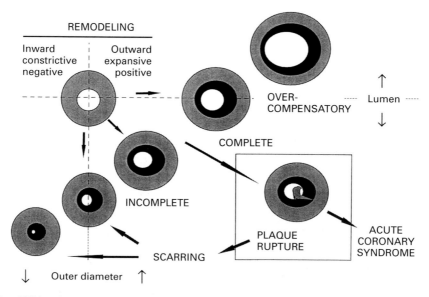

Figure 2-1. With atherosclerotic plaque growth, outward remodeling may preserve or even increase lumen size. However, necessary degradation of extracellular matrix by metalloproteinases may increase the risk of plaque rupture. Healing processes after plaque rupture may result in inward remodeling. Thus, the «lumenography» of coronary angiography is not an efficient way to evaluate vessel wall disease. The terminology of arterial remodeling is full of synonyms.

collagen-rich components may calcify and the process may be active and controlled, resembling calcification in bone, rather than passive and «dystrophic.»[12] Coronary calcification in adults is almost always atherosclerosis-related and intimal.[12] Both autopsy and clinical data indicate that coronary calcification is a marker for, and correlates closely with, the overall atherosclerotic plaque burden,[24] but calcification of a plaque does not correlate with its flow-limiting capacity (degree of stenosis)[24] or the risk of sudden occlusion (vulnerability). If anything, heavily calcified plaques appear to be more stable than non-calcified plaques.[24] The vascular remodeling phenomenon is the likely explanation for the poor correlation of plaque calcification with lumen narrowing and/or the severity of stenosis.[24] It appears that coronary calcification is not a marker of high risk of rupture for the individual plaque, but is a marker of the overall plaque burden and, consequently, the overall risk of a plaque rupture in the coronary arterial tree. The more plaques that are present, the greater the likelihood is that one of them will be vulnerable and prone to thrombosis.

PLAQUE INSTABILITY

A subgroup of advanced atherosclerotic lesions, *vulnerable plaques*, are particularly dangerous, because they are at high risk of being complicated by luminal thrombosis.[17,25] Rupture of these vulnerable plaques with subsequent superimposed thrombosis is the most frequent cause of *acute coronary syndrome* (ACS), which consists of myocardial infarction, unstable angina pectoris, and sudden coronary death.[17,26] Thrombosis superimposed on an advanced plaque is divided into two categories. The most frequent cause is *plaque rupture:*[27] the rupture of the fibrous cap separating the lumen from the atherosclerotic core, exposing the thrombogenic content to the circulating blood. In approximately 20 % of cases no plaque rupture can be found, and the thrombus is attributed to *plaque erosion.* The mechanisms of erosion and subsequent thrombosis are not clear, and the term may refer to more than one pathophysiological entity. It is possible that systemic pro-thrombotic properties play an even larger role in these thrombi than in thrombi caused by plaque rupture. Plaque rupture is thought to result from a dynamic interaction between intrinsic plaque vulnerability and extrinsic mechanical forces acting on the plaque (triggers).

EXTRINSIC FACTORS

Elevated sympathetic activity with high blood pressure and increased heart rate and blood flow might be extrinsic triggers of plaque rupture. This would explain why acute myocardial infarction is most frequent in the first hours after awakening, during physical exercise, sexual activity, fear, or anger.[28] However, the common nature of these triggers, along with the fact that they can be demonstrated in only 1 of 5 cases,[28] makes their clinical relevance questionable. On the other hand, β-blockers, which blunt sympathetic bursts, reduce the incidence of reinfarction in patients who have suffered an acute myocardial infarction by approximately 20 %.[29] This obviously suggests that high sympathetic activity plays a part, though other mechanisms might be responsible. Exercise stress testing, a test designed to impose maximal biomechanical stress on the cardiovascular system, very rarely triggers an acute coronary event,[30] even in patients with advanced atherosclerotic disease, suggesting that ultimately plaque vulnerability plays a more important role than triggers in plaque rupture.

INTRINSIC FACTORS

The risk of plaque rupture is more dependent on the type of plaque than on plaque size (Figs. 2-2 and 2-3). Soft, lipid-rich plaques

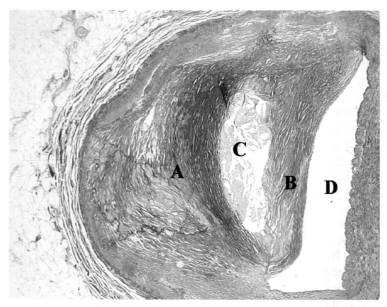

Figure 2-2.   A stable plaque with a large collagen-rich area (A) and a relatively thick fibrous cap (B) separating the rather small lipid core (C) from the lumen (D). Very little inflammation is present in the cap.

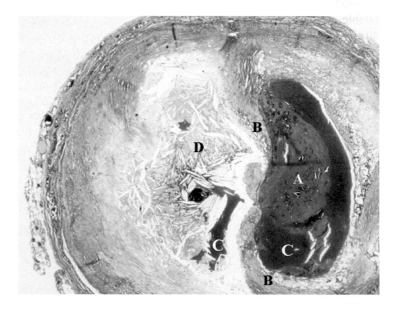

Figure 2-3.   A stenotic and ruptured plaque with a non-occlusive platelet-rich thrombus (A) superimposed. Intense inflammation with macrophage foam cells (B) is present in the cap. Contrast medium is injected postmortem (C). The plaque's lipid-rich core (D) is much larger than in the stable plaque in Figure 2-2, increasing the risk of rupture.

have a higher risk of rupture than collagen-rich plaques.[17] They also have a higher tissue-factor content and are thus more thrombogenic.[31] The risk of rupture is higher when the plaque cap does not contain smooth muscle cells. Obviously, the thickness and collagen content of the fibrous cap is very important for its strength and stability; the thinner the cap is, the weaker and more vulnerable to rupture the plaque will be.[27,32] Inflammation of the plaque is another factor that increases the risk of plaque rupture. In short, lipid accumulation, macrophage infiltration, and the absence of smooth muscle cells destabilize plaques, making them vulnerable to rupture. In contrast, smooth muscle cell-mediated healing and repair processes stabilize plaques, protecting them against rupture.[33] It is as yet unknown why smooth muscle cells are absent in sites of plaque rupture, but evidence suggests that apoptotic cell death might play an important role.[19] Plaque size and the severity of stenosis tell us nothing about a plaque's vulnerability.[34] Many vulnerable plaques are angiographically invisible due to their small size and compensatory vascular remodeling.

PLAQUE CAP DEGRADATION

Ruptured fibrous caps are usually heavily infiltrated by macrophage foam cells.[17,27] These rupture-related macrophages, as well as T cells in the area, are activated, indicating ongoing inflammation at the site of plaque rupture.[35] Further evidence of immune activation is the up-regulated expression of CD40-receptor and its ligand by all cell types present in advanced atherosclerotic lesions.[36]

Activated macrophages are capable of degrading extracellular matrix by phagocytosis or secretion of proteolytic enzymes, such as members of the matrix metalloproteinase family (MMPs) and others, which may weaken the fibrous cap predisposing it to rupture.[37] These proteinases have been identified in human plaques and implicated in plaque rupture, but

the actual enzymatic culprits have not yet been conclusively identified.[38] Collagen confers stability on plaques and human macrophages are, indeed, capable of degrading the old and mature collagen present in advanced aortic plaques.[39] Besides macrophages, a wide variety of cells may produce MMPs. Activated mast cells may secrete powerful proteolytic enzymes, such as tryptase and chymase, which can activate pro-MMPs secreted by other cells (e.g., macrophages). Mast cells are actually present in shoulder regions of mature plaques and at sites of rupture, although in very low density.[40] Neutrophils are also capable of destroying tissue by secreting proteolytic enzymes, but they are rarely seen in intact plaques.

It has been suggested that several infectious agents may play an active role in the development of cardiovascular diseases, most notably *Chlamydia pneumoniae*,[10] but also others such as herpesviruses (including cytomegalovirus) and *Helicobacter pylori*.[10] However, there is no consensus that lesions can be induced or accelerated experimentally in animals by the injection of these organisms, which brings their etiologic role in question.

Non-specific, but sensitive, blood markers of inflammation such as *C-reactive protein* (CRP) have been identified as strong risk factors for future cardiovascular events in apparently healthy persons,[41] patients with stable and unstable angina, and after myocardial infarction. No strong relation has been found between CRP and atherosclerosis, as measured by the ankle/brachial blood pressure index, suggesting that inflammation as measured by the CRP at best plays a small role in the atherosclerotic process. However, it could play a much larger role in the transformation of a stable into a vulnerable plaque.[42]

PLAQUE RUPTURE

Vulnerable plaques rupture frequently. Autopsy data indicate that 9% of previously healthy persons dying from non-coronary causes harbor ruptured plaques (without superimposed thrombosis) in their coronary arteries, a figure that increases to 22 % in persons with atherosclerosis-related diseases such as diabetes or hypertension.[49] In fatal coronary artery disease, more than one ruptured plaque, with or without superimposed thrombosis, are usually present in the coronary arteries,[27, 49] and in non-fatal myocardial infarction, multiple plaques with unstable characteristics in the coronary angiogram are present in 40 % of cases.[43] Rupture of the plaque surface occurs most often where the cap is thinnest and most heavily infiltrated by macrophages and, therefore, weakest, namely at the cap's shoulders[50] (Fig. 2-3). The weak shoulder regions are, however, also points where biomechanical and hemodynamic forces acting on plaques appear to be concentrated. At present, the exact mechanisms of plaque rupture are not known. Several theories have been proposed, including increased shear or circumferential stress, rupture of the vasa vasorum, vasospasm, and fatigue failure following exposure to repetitive, low-amplitude stress.[32]

VASOCONSTRICTION

Plaque rupture and vasospasm often coexist, and the former most likely gives rise to the latter.[17] Abnormal coronary vasoreactivity is common in acute coronary syndromes but 'spasm' is usually confined to the culprit lesion, suggesting that it is caused by vasoactive substances that are released locally.[51] Macrophages in ruptured plaques responsible for unstable angina contain potent vasoconstrictors such as endothelin-1,[52] and superimposed thrombosis may also contain or generate vasoconstrictors such as thrombin and platelet-derived serotonin and thromboxane A2.[25]

VISUALIZATION OF ATHEROSCLEROSIS

The vulnerability and thrombogenicity of atherosclerotic plaques, rather than their obstructive capability (severity of stenosis), together with the status of the collateral circulation have emerged as the most important determinants for the occurrence, type, and outcome of acute coronary events.[17] Although visual characteristics can be used,[43] coronary angiography is not a good method for identifying high-risk thrombosis-prone lesions. This is partly because the size of a plaque and its vulnerability correlate poorly, if at all,[34, 44, 45] and partly because vascular remodeling tends to preserve the lumen better with the larger but vulnerable plaques (compensatory enlargement) than with the smaller and stable plaques (shrinkage).[44] The great majority of heart attacks and ischemic strokes originate from atherosclerotic lesions that, prior to the acute events, were only mild-to-moderately stenotic, i.e., they were hemodynamically insignificant and probably asymptomatic. Although the risk of occlusion, and becoming a culprit for myocardial infarction or stroke, increases with the severity of stenosis, the great majority of coronary occlusions (71 %) and myocardial infarctions (86 %) in pooled studies originated from lesions that caused less than 70-80 % angiographic stenosis prior to the acute event.[17] The reason is that stenotic lesions are markers of plaque burden. Lower-risk non-stenotic lesions will always far outnumber the higher-risk stenotic lesions and, altogether, increase the risk of an acute event much more than the few stenotic lesions that carry a higher individual risk. The same holds for ischemic stroke. In a large trial,[46] only 19 % of new strokes were judged to have originated from initially symptomatic lesions that at baseline caused more than 70 % angiographic stenosis. The reason is that lower-risk non-stenotic carotid plaques (n = 2113) far outnumbered the stenotic plaques (n = 127) that carried a higher risk.

The visual appearance of the plaque is another way to evaluate plaque stability. It has been shown that yellow (lipid-rich) plaques evaluated by angioscopy have a high risk of becoming unstable.[47] Detection of heat released by activated inflammatory cells in atherosclerotic plaques may also predict plaque rupture and thrombosis.[48] Thermal heterogeneity correlates to both macrophage density in the plaque and outcome,[48] further emphasizing the importance of inflammation in unstable coronary syndromes. Several other invasive techniques have been tested.[44, 45] Non-invasive techniques, notably high-resolution magnetic resonance imaging (MRI), are promising. They theoretically allow plaque components to be differentiated on the basis of biophysical and biochemical parameters such as chemical composition and concentration, water content, physical state, molecular motion, or diffusion.

CLINICAL MANIFESTATIONS

As noted above, not every plaque rupture leads to the superimposition of a thrombus, and not every superimposed thrombus leads to occlusion or sub-occlusion. In some cases, however, plaque rupture does lead to an occlusive or subocclusive thrombus, presenting as an acute coronary syndrome. The development of a symptomatic thrombus is facilitated by three major factors: 1) the high thrombogenicity of the exposed plaque material, with *tissue factor* probably playing a major role, 2) local flow disturbances, and 3) an elevated systemic propensity to thrombosis. It is a highly dynamic process of alternating thrombus growth and lysis, which sometimes causes intermittent coronary blood flow reduction. The clinical symptoms and outcome depend on the severity and duration of impaired flow and myocardial ischemia.[53] While blood flow over the ruptured plaque continues, microemboli of plaque material and thrombus may be washed away, which can produce downstream microvascular ob-

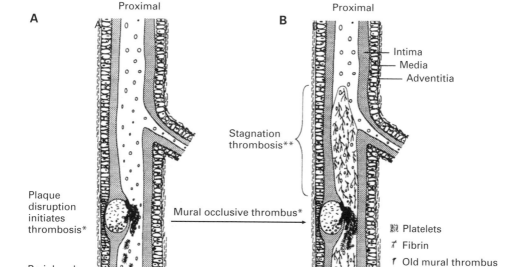

Coronary Thrombosis: Plaque, Flow, And Blood

Proximal

A

Plaque disruption initiates thrombosis*

Peripheral embolization

Mural occlusive thrombus*

Stagnation thrombosis**

Stagnation thrombosis**

Proximal

B

Intima
Media
Adventitia

Platelets
Fibrin
Old mural thrombus
Erythrocytes
Cholesterol crystals in atheromatous gruel

*White thrombus macroscopically   **Red thrombus macroscopically

Figure 2-4. Just after plaque rupture, a dynamic process builds up. A platelet-rich, white thrombus takes place, often with peripheral micro-embolization (A). After occlusion, a red, fibrin-rich thrombus builds up (B).

struction with compromised tissue perfusion[54] (Fig. 2-4). Such microembolization is associated with a poorer prognosis in unstable angina pectoris and myocardial infarction. In cases of non-fatal plaque rupture, a healing process ensues within the ruptured plaque (Fig. 2-5). Although the exact process has yet to be described, it is thought that it resembles the healing response that takes place after percutaneous transluminal coronary angioplasty. This consists of lysis or reorganization of the thrombus (or both), proliferation of smooth muscle cells followed by matrix deposition, and, ultimately, re-endothelization.[55] Clinically silent plaque rupture or intra-plaque hemorrhage and subse-

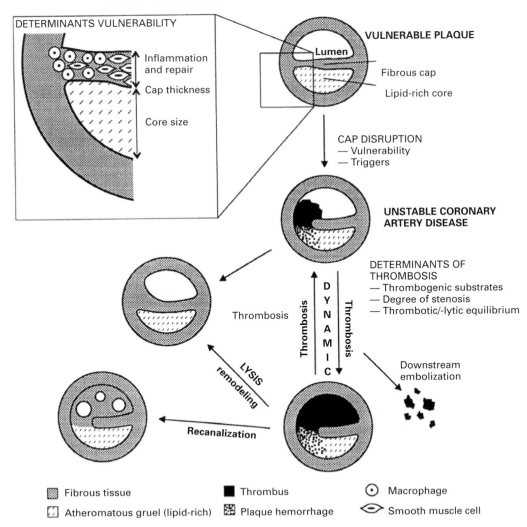

Figure 2-5. A vulnerable plaque is characterized by a thin, inflamed cap over a large lipid-rich core with a high risk of rupture. Plaque rupture can lead to partial or complete thrombotic obstruction. The thrombus either undergoes lysis or is organized and recanalized. Lysis often leads to an aggravation of the stenosis, and this increase in severity can be very rapid.

quent healing is probably the mechanism that underlies the episodic rather than linear development of coronary lesions detected in serial angiographic examinations, and may be a central step in the formation of high-grade stenoses.[56] Firstly, residual thrombi are consistently found in a fraction of lesions that cause stable angina.[57] Secondly, a special non-uniform pattern of denser (older) and loosely arranged (younger) collagen, which is thought to indicate healed plaque rupture, has been identified in many coronary plaques, particularly in those causing chronic high-grade stenosis.[57]

ACKNOWLEDGMENT

Many thanks to Jacob Fog Bentzon for helpful comments on the manuscript.

REFERENCES

1. Kannel WB. Some lessons in cardiovascular epidemiology from Framingham. *Am J Cardiol* 1976; 37:269-82.
2. Libby P, Sukhova G, Lee RT, Galis ZS. Cytokines regulate vascular functions related to stability of the atherosclerotic plaque. *J Cardiovasc Pharmacol* 1995; 25 Suppl 2:S9-12.
3. Ross R. Atherosclerosis an inflammatory disease. *N Engl J Med* 1999; 340:115-26.
4. Kinlay S, Libby P, Ganz P. Endothelial function and coronary artery disease. *Curr Opin Lipidol* 2001; 12:383-9.
5. Schachinger V, Britten MB, Zeiher AM. Prognostic impact of coronary vasodilator dysfunction on adverse long-term outcome of coronary heart disease. *Circulation 2000*; 101: 1899-1906.
6. Biegelsen ES, Loscalzo J. Endothelial function and atherosclerosis. *Coron Artery Dis* 1999; 10:241-56.
7. Gimbrone MA, Topper JN, Nagel T, et al. Endothelial dysfunction, hemodynamic forces, and atherogenesis. *Ann NY Acad Sci* 2000; 902:230-239; discussion 239-240.
8. Steinberg D, Lewis A. Conner Memorial Lecture: oxidative modification of LDL and atherogenesis. *Circulation* 1997; 95:1062-1071.
9. Horkko S, Binder CJ, Shaw PX, et al. Immunological responses to oxidized LDL. *Free Radic Biol Med* 2000; 28:1771-9.
10. Kol A, Libby P. The mechanisms by which infectious agents may contribute to atherosclerosis and its clinical manifestations. *Trends Cardiovasc Med* 1998; 8:191-99.
11. Witztum JL, Palinski W. Are immunological mechanisms relevant for the development of atherosclerosis? *Clin Immunol* 1999; 90:153-6.
12. Falk E, Fuster V. Atherogenesis and its determinants. Chapter 35 in Hurst's the Heart, 10th edition. Fuster V, Alexander RW, O'Rourke RA, Roberts R, King SB, Wellens HJJ, eds. McGraw-Hill, New York 2001.
13. Napoli C, D'Armiento FP, Mancini FP, et al. Fatty streak formation occurs in human fetal aortas and is greatly enhanced by maternal hypercholesterolemia. Intimal accumulation of low density lipoprotein and its oxidation precede monocyte recruitment into early atherosclerotic lesions. *J Clin Invest* 1997; 100:2680-90.
14. Stary HC, Chandler AB, Glagov S, et al. A definition of initial, fatty streak, and intermediate lesions of atherosclerosis. A report from the Committee on Vascular Lesions of the Council on Arteriosclerosis, American Heart Association. *Circulation* 1994; 89(5): 2462-78.
15. Zeiher AM, Schachlinger V, Hohnloser SH, et al. Coronary atherosclerotic wall thickening and vascular reactivity in humans. Elevated high-density lipoprotein levels ameliorate abnormal vasoconstriction in early atherosclerosis. *Circulation* 1994; 89:2525-32.
16. Shah PK, Yano J, Reyes O, et al. High-dose recombinant apolipoprotein A-I(milano) mobilizes tissue cholesterol and rapidly reduces plaque lipid and macrophage content in apolipoprotein E-deficient mice. Potential implications for acute plaque stabilization. *Circulation* 2001; 103:3047-50.
17. Falk E, Shah PK, Fuster V. Coronary plaque disruption. *Circulation* 1995; 92:657-71.
18. Martinet W, Kockx MM. Apoptosis in atherosclerosis: focus on oxidized lipids and inflammation. *Curr Opin Lipidol* 2001; 12:535-41.

19. Kockx MM. Apoptosis in the atherosclerotic plaque: quantitative and qualitative aspects. *Arterioscler Thromb Vasc Biol* 1998; 18:1519-22.

20. Moulton KS. Plaque angiogenesis and atherosclerosis. *Curr Atheroscler Rep* 2001; 3:225-33.

21. Glagov S, Weisenberg E, Zarins CK, Stankunavicius R, Kolettis GJ. Compensatory enlargement of human atherosclerotic coronary arteries. *N Engl J Med* 1987; 316: 1371-5.

22. Schoenhagen P, Ziada KM, Vince DG, Nissen SE, Tuzcu EM. Arterial remodeling and coronary artery disease: the concept of «dilated» versus «obstructive» coronary atherosclerosis. *J Am Coll Cardiol* 2001; 38: 297-306.

23. Nagai T, Luo H, Atar S, Lepor NE, Fishbein MC, Siegel RJ. Intravascular ultrasound imaging of ruptured atherosclerotic plaques in coronary arteries. *Am J Cardiol* 1999; 83: 135-7, A10.

24. Beckman JA, Ganz J, Creager MA, Ganz P, Kinlay S. Relationship of clinical presentation and calcification of culprit coronary artery stenoses. *Arterioscler Thromb Vasc Biol* 2001; 21:1618-22.

25. Fuster V, Fayad ZA, Badimon JJ. Acute coronary syndromes: biology. *Lancet* 1999; 353 (suppl II):5-9.

26. Falk E, Fernandez-Ortiz A. Role of thrombosis in atherosclerosis and its complications. *Am J Cardiol* 1995; 75:3B-11B.

27. Falk E. Plaque rupture with severe pre-existing stenosis precipitating coronary thrombosis. Characteristics of coronary atherosclerotic plaques underlying fatal occlusive thrombi. *Br Heart J* 1983; 50:127-34.

28. Muller JE. Circadian variation and triggering of acute coronary events. *Am Heart J* 1999; 137:S1-S8.

29. Yusuf S, Peto R, Lewis J, Collins R, Sleight P. Beta blockade during and after myocardial infarction: an overview of the randomized trials. *Prog Cardiovasc Dis* 1985; 27:335-71.

30. Tavel ME. Stress testing in cardiac evaluation: current concepts with emphasis on the ECG. *Chest* 2001; 119:907-25.

31. Toschi V, Gallo R, Lettino M, et al. Tissue factor modulates the thrombogenicity of human atherosclerotic plaque. *Circulation* 1997; 95:594-9.

32. Bank AJ, Versluis A, Dodge SM, Douglas WH. Atherosclerotic plaque rupture: a fatigue process? *Med Hypotheses* 2000; 55: 480-4.

33. Libby P. Molecular bases of the acute coronary syndromes. *Circulation* 1995; 91:2844-2850.

34. Mann JM, Davies MJ. Vulnerable plaque. Relation of characteristics to degree of stenosis in human coronary arteries. *Circulation* 1996; 94:928-31.

35. van der Wal AC, Becker AE, van der Loos CM, Das PK. Site of intimal rupture or erosion of thrombosed coronary atherosclerotic plaques is characterized by an inflammatory process irrespective of the dominant plaque morphology. *Circulation* 1994; 89:36-44.

36. Mach F, Schonbeck U, Bonnefoy JY, Pober JS, Libby P. Activation of monocyte/macrophage functions related to acute atheroma complication by ligation of CD40: induction of collagenase, stromelysin, and tissue factor. *Circulation* 1997; 96:396-9.

37. Parks WC. Who are the proteolytic culprits in vascular disease? *J Clin Invest* 1999; 104: 1167-8.

38. Shah PK, Galis ZS. Matrix metalloproteinase hypothesis of plaque rupture: players keep piling up but questions remain. *Circulation* 2001; 104:1878-80.

39. Shah PK, Falk E, Badimon JJ, et al. Human monocyte-derived macrophages induce collagen breakdown in fibrous caps of atherosclerotic plaques. Potential role of matrix-degrading metalloproteinases and implications for plaque rupture. *Circulation* 1995; 92: 1565-9.

40. Laine P, Kaartinen M, Penttila A, Panula P, Paavonen T, Kovanen PT. Association between myocardial infarction and the mast cells in the adventitia of the infarct-related coronary artery. *Circulation* 1999; 99:361-9.

41. Ridker PM, Cushman M, Stampfer MJ, Tracy RP, Hennekens CH. Inflammation, aspirin, and the risk of cardiovascular disease in apparently healthy men. *N Engl J Med* 1997; 336:973-9.

42. Folsom AR, Pankow JS, Tracy RP, et al. Association of C-reactive protein with markers of prevalent atherosclerotic disease. *Am J Cardiol* 2001; 88:112-7.

43. Goldstein JA, Demetriou D, Grines CL, Pica M, Shoukfeh M, O'Neill WW. Multiple complex coronary plaques in patients with acute myocardial infarction. *N Engl J Med* 2000; 343:915-22.

44. Fayad ZA, Fuster V. Clinical imaging of the high-risk or vulnerable atherosclerotic plaque. *Circ Res* 2001; 89:305-16.

45. Pasterkamp G, Falk E, Woutman H, Borst C. Techniques characterizing the coronary atherosclerotic plaque: influence on clinical decision making? *J Am Coll Cardiol* 2000; 36:13-21.

46. The European Carotid Surgery Trialists Collaborative Group. Risk of stroke in the distribution of an asymptomatic carotid artery. *Lancet* 1995; 345:209-12.

47. Thieme T, Wernecke KD, Meyer R, et al. Angioscopic evaluation of atherosclerotic plaques: validation by histomorphologic analysis and association with stable and unstable coronary syndromes. *J Am Coll Cardiol* 1996; 28:1-6.

48. Casscells W, Hathorn B, David M, et al. Thermal detection of cellular infiltrates in living atherosclerotic plaques: possible implications for plaque rupture and thrombosis. *Lancet* 1996; 347:1447-1451.

49. Davies MJ, Bland JM, Hangartner JR, Angelini A, Thomas AC. Factors influencing the presence or absence of acute coronary artery thrombi in sudden ischaemic death. *Eur Heart J* 1989; 10:203-8.

50. Moreno PR, Falk E, Palacios IF, Newell JB, Fuster V, Fallon JT. Macrophage infiltration in acute coronary syndromes: implications for plaque rupture. *Circulation* 1994; 90:775-8.

51. Bogaty P, Hackett D, Davies G, Maseri A. Vasoreactivity of the culprit lesion in unstable angina. *Circulation* 1994; 90:5-11.

52. Zeiher AM, Goebel H, Schachinger V, Ihling C. Tissue endothelin-1 immunoreactivity in the active coronary atherosclerotic plaque. A clue to the mechanism of increased vasoreactivity of the culprit lesion in unstable angina. *Circulation* 1995; 91:941-7.

53. Kristensen SD, Lassen JF, Ravn HB. Pathophysiology of coronary thrombosis. *Semin Interv Cardiol* 2000; 5:109-15.

54. Wu KC, Zerhouni EA, Judd RM, et al. Prognostic significance of microvascular obstruction by magnetic resonance imaging in patients with acute myocardial infarction. *Circulation* 1998; 97:765-72.

55. Falk E, Nobuyoshi M. Differences between atherosclerosis and restenosis. In: Atherosclerosis and coronary artery disease. Fuster V, Ross R, Topol EJ, editors. Philadelphia: Lippincott-Raven, 1996: 683-700.

56. Burke AP, Kolodgie FD, Farb A, et al. Healed plaque ruptures and sudden coronary death: evidence that subclinical rupture has a role in plaque progression. *Circulation* 2001; 103:934-40.

57. Mann J, Davies MJ. Mechanisms of progression in native coronary artery disease: role of healed plaque disruption. *Heart* 1999; 82:265-8.

3

General Concepts in Coronary Physiology

Morton J. Kern, MD

Fundamental Concepts. Coronary Flow Reserve. Relative Coronary Flow Velocity Reserve. Proximal-to-Distal Flow (P/D) Ratios and Diastolic-to-Systolic Flow Velocity Ratio (DSVR). Pressure-Derived Fractional Flow Reserve (FFR). Physiologic Techniques Differentiating Focal from Diffuse Atherosclerosis. Clinical Applications. Coronary Physiology in Acute Myocardial Infarction. Collateral Circulation. References.

Why do we need new intracoronary diagnostic techniques? The easiest and most straightforward answer is that the time-tested angiogram fails to provide critical information about the arterial wall and lumen morphology, and does not accurately describe the forces acting on blood flow to predict flow limitations in all but the most extreme ends of the spectrum of stenoses.

How do we know this need is real? One only has to stand next to an angiographer for 1 or 2 cases to hear the following lament, «I can't really tell if this lesion is severe. Let's take another view.» After 3 or 4 more views with different angulations, it would be no surprise to hear the next refrain of the angiographer's lament, «could you call in Dr. X so that I can ask him what he thinks the lesion severity is?» At this point, there should be little doubt that neither physician can accurately gauge what the true nature of the lesion in question is and that this is truly the rationale for critical application of new intracoronary diagnostic techniques.

The measurement of coronary blood flow and pressure provides unique information that complements the angiographic evaluation and in many cases facilitates decision-making regarding appropriateness of therapy.[1,2] From this perspective, we will discuss fundamental assumptions and describe several common clinical applications of coronary physiology that can be measured in the cardiac catheterization laboratory in patients.

FUNDAMENTAL CONCEPTS

Coronary blood flow can increase from a resting level to a maximum value depending on increases in myocardial oxygen demand, or in response to neurogenic or pharmacological hyperemic stimuli. Normally, the resistance to blood flow of large epicardial vessels is trivial. Most coronary flow is regulated by the myocardial pre-capillary arteriolar resistance vessels. In a normal artery supplying normal myocardium, coronary blood flow can increase >3-fold in adults. However, left ventricular hypertrophy, myocardial ischemia, diabetes, or other conditions can affect the microcirculation, blunting the maximal absolute increase in coronary flow or increase resting flow above the expected level for myocardial oxygen demand at rest. This reduces the relative increase in flow needed during increased oxygen demand.

Significant coronary atherosclerotic stenosis produces epicardial conduit resistance. In response to the loss of perfusion pressure and flow to the distal vascular bed, the resistance vessels dilate to maintain a satisfactory basal flow for myocardial oxygen demand. Viscous friction, flow separation forces, and flow turbulence at the site of the stenosis produce energy loss at the stenosis. Energy (heat) is extracted, which reduces pressure distal to the stenosis, producing a pressure gradient between proximal and distal artery regions. The pressure loss, or gradient, increases with increasing coronary flow in accordance with a curvilinear pressure-flow relationship of the specific coronary stenosis resistance.[3,4] There is an absolute post-stenotic myocardial perfusion pressure threshold below which myocardial ischemia may be easily induced.

In the catheterization laboratory, the hemodynamic significance of a given stenosis, as determined by the pressure-flow relationship, can be measured and incorporated into clinical practice. A hemodynamically significant coronary lesion is associated with one or more of the following parameters: post-stenotic absolute coronary flow reserve (CVR) < 2.0, relative coronary flow reserve (rCVR) < 0.8, proximal-to-distal flow velocity ratio (P/D) < 1.7, diastolic-to-systolic velocity ratio (DSVR) < 1.8. Using pressure sensor guidewires, the hyperemic translesional pressure ratio, also known as the fractional flow reserve (FFR), is < 0.75.

To determine the velocity of red blood cells flowing past an ultrasound emitter/receiver, the difference between the transmitted and returning frequency, called the frequency shift, is calculated as:

$$V = (F1 - F0) \cdot (C)/(2F0) \cdot (\cos \varnothing)$$

where V = velocity of blood flow, F0 = transmitting (transducer) frequency, F1 = returning frequency, C = constant for the speed of sound in blood, $\varnothing$ = angle of incidence. Volumetric blood flow can be determined multiplying the flow velocity (cm/s) by vessel area (cm^2) yielding a value in cm^3/s.

Intracoronary Doppler flow velocity can be measured using a 175-cm long, 0.014 to 0.018 inch (0.035 to 0.046 cm) diameter, flexible, steerable angioplasty type guidewire with a piezoelectric ultrasound transducer integrated into the tip (FloWire; JOMED, Inc., Sweden). Doppler guidewire velocity measurements have been validated and correlated with absolute coronary flow measurements *in vitro* and *in vivo*.[5,6]

CORONARY FLOW RESERVE

Absolute CVR is the ratio of maximal hyperemic-to-basal mean flow (or velocity) in the target vessel obtained *distal* to a stenosis. As stenosis severity increases, hyperemic flow becomes attenuated and CVR decreases. In vessels with intact endothelial function and flow-mediated vasodilation, coronary velocity reserve may be less than volumetric CVR. Absolute Doppler velocity flow represents volumetric coronary flow when the vessel cross-sectional area remains constant over the measurement period. Absolute CVR measures the capacity of the two-component system of coronary artery and supplied vascular bed to achieve maximal blood flow in response to a given hyperemic stimulation. Early studies report absolute CVR ranging from 3.5 to 5 in normal patients. Recently, in young patients intravascular ultrasound (IVUS) demonstrated in normal arteries that CVR commonly exceeds 3.0.[7] In patients with chest pain undergoing cardiac catheterization that exhibit angiographically normal vessels, the normal absolute CVR is 2.7 ± 0.6,[8] suggesting a degree of patient-patient variability and distal microvascular disease that is beyond the threshold of angiographic detection.

Coronary flow reserve is subject to variations in conditions that may alter resting flow and limit maximal hyperemic flow. Tachycardia increases basal flow; coronary flow reserve is reduced by 10% for every 15 beats of heart rate.[9] Increasing mean arterial pressure reduces maximal vasodilation, thus reducing hyperemia with less alteration in basal flow. Coronary flow reserve may be reduced in patients with essential hypertension and normal coronary arteries and in patients with aortic stenosis and normal coronary arteries.[10, 11] In some patients with moderate coronary artery disease, the stenosis configuration and surrounding vessel segments are subject to vasomotor stimuli. Thus, vasoconstrictor, neurologic or humoral influences, endothelial dysfunction, and extracardiac vasoconstrictor stimuli may produce dynamic or episodic ischemia-related symptoms with activities of daily life such as exercise, emotional stress, or adrenergic stimulation. For example, Weineke et al.[12] examined CVR in 242 unobstructed coronary arteries in 141 patients and found that individual CVR values obtained at different basal average peak velocities could be transformed and corrected for patient age, relating them to a mean basal average peak velocity (BAPV) of 15 cm/s and age of 55 years ($CVR_{corr} = 2.85 \cdot CVR_{measured} \cdot 10X$, where $X = 0.48 \log (BAPV) + 0.0025 \cdot age - 1.16$). Use of the corrected CVR standardizes for variations in basal average peak velocity and patient age and may discriminate between intrinsic and extracardiac factors impairing CVR.

RELATIVE CORONARY FLOW VELOCITY RESERVE

Because of a two-component system, (epicardial and microvascular) there is some uncertainty about accepting an abnormal CVR as the sole indicator of the significance of a lesion. To measure lesion severity independent of the microvascular influence, a relative CVR (rCVR), defined as the ratio of maximal flow in the coronary with stenosis (Q^S) to flow in a normal coronary without stenosis (Q^N), has been suggested.[3, 4] Relative CVR is independent of the aortic pressure and rate pressure product, and is well suited to assessing the physiological significance of coronary stenoses when an adjacent non-diseased coronary artery is available. For patient studies, rCVR is the ratio of CVR_{target}-to-CVR in an angiographically normal reference vessel, $rCVR = (Q^S/Q_{base})/(Q^N/Q_{base}) = (CVR_{target}/CVR_{reference})$.[13, 14] Basal flow in the two vessels is assumed to be similar and thus, rCVR mathematically resembles Gould's derivation. Relative CVR cannot be used in patients with three-vessel coronary disease who have no suitable reference vessel. Relative CVR relies on the assumption that the microvascular circulatory response is uniformly distributed among the myocardial beds, so rCVR is of no value in patients with myocardial infarction, left ventricular regional dysfunction, or heterogeneous microcirculatory responses. The normal range for rCVR in patients is 0.75-1.0.[15, 16]

PROXIMAL TO DISTAL FLOW (P/D) RATIOS AND DIASTOLIC TO SYSTOLIC FLOW VELOCITY RATIO (DSVR)

A significant epicardial stenosis produces characteristic alterations of phasic coronary blood flow patterns, hyperemic capacity, and regional flow responses compared to unobstructed arterial branches. For normal vessels with diameters >2.0 mm, arterial flow velocity remains within 15% from proximal to distal regions along the course of the artery. Because the blood flow *volume* and epicardial conduit cross-sectional *area* are proportionately reduced along the course of the vessel, there is generally no significant decline in distal velocity relative to proximal blood flow velocity. A proximal-to-distal velocity (P/D) ratio of 1 is a normal value. Significant stenosis with resting pressure gradients >30 mm Hg are associated with P/D ratios >1.7.[17]

Significant stenosis also blunts the dominant diastolic flow relative to the normally low systolic flow. As a stenosis increases in severity, the ratio of DSVR is reduced from >2.0 to around 1.0.[18] Unfortunately, the DSVR and P/D velocity ratios are weak indicators of the severity of the lesion, with a large variability and low specificity, and are no longer generally used.[19]

PRESSURE-DERIVED FRACTIONAL FLOW RESERVE (FFR)

Myocardial perfusion is closely linked to myocardial ischemia and is directly dependent on the coronary «driving» pressure associated with three major coronary vascular resistances (epicardial, arteriolar, and intramyocardial capillary resistance). The myocardial perfusion pressure (aortic pressure-left ventricular pressure or right atrial pressure) is reduced when an epicardial stenosis causes pressure loss distal to the stenosis in proportion to the flow rate. If the myocardial bed resistances are stimulated to maximal hyperemia and remain constant, then the post-stenotic hyperemic coronary artery pressure represents the maximal achievable perfusion available in that vessel and can be used to produce an estimate of normal coronary blood flow.

Using coronary pressure measured at constant and minimal myocardial resistances (i.e., maximal hyperemia), Pijls et al.[20, 21] derived an estimate of the percentage of normal (i.e., in the theoretical absence of the stenosis) coronary blood flow expected to go through a stenotic artery, called the fractional flow reserve (FFR). The FFR, calculated as the ratio of the post-stenotic or distal coronary pressure-to-aorta pressure (as the pressure in an unobstructed artery, i.e., the theoretical normal artery pressure) obtained at sustained minimal resistance (i.e., maximal hyperemia), reflects both antegrade and collateral myocardial perfusion rather than merely trans-stenotic pressure loss (i.e., a stenosis pressure gradient). Because it is calculated only at peak hyperemia, FFR is

further differentiated from CVR by being largely independent of basal flow, driving pressure, heart rate, systemic blood pressure, or status of the microcirculation.[22] The FFR, but not the resting pressure or hyperemic pressure gradient, is strongly related to inducible myocardial ischemia (FFR < 0.75) as established by rigorous comparisons to different clinical stress testing modalities in patients with stable angina.

Because FFR and rCVR are theoretically independent of hemodynamic and microcirculatory changes, the two variables should strongly correlate as compared to CVR. Indeed, Baumgart et al.[13] found that absolute CVR did not correlate with percent area stenosis or FFR. FFR and rCVR, showed a curvilinear correlation to percent area stenosis (r = 0.89 and r = 0.79; p < 0.0001) and there was a strong linear relationship between FFR and rCVR (0.91; p < 0.0001) but not absolute CVR, as expected, due to the influence of variable microvascular flow.

In patients with an abnormal microcirculation, it can be argued that a normal FFR indicates that conduit resistance is not a major contributing factor to perfusion impairment, and that focal conduit enlargement (e.g., stenting) would not restore normal perfusion. It is of interest that microvascular disease also originates discordance between FFR and CVR. Meuwissen et al.[23] compared FFR and CVR in 126 patients with intermediate stenosis. In 27% of patients there was disagreement between FFR and CFR. Patients with a normal FFR (i.e. >0.75), but abnormal CVR (<2.0), had a larger variability in minimum microvascular resistance (2.421 ± 0.77 vs 1.91 ± 0.70 mm Hg cm-^{1}.s-^{1}, p = 0.034) compared to patients with normal CVR, regardless of the FFR. This variance suggests that microvascular resistance modulates the relationship between FFR and CFR, and that both techniques should be considered for complete lesion assessment. The current physiologic criteria do not apply to patients with profound microvascular disease, acute or remote myocardial infarction, and unstable angina.

PHYSIOLOGIC TECHNIQUES DIFFERENTIATING FOCAL FROM DIFFUSE ATHEROSCLEROSIS

A diffusely diseased atherosclerotic coronary artery can be viewed as a series of branching units diverting and gradually distributing flow along the longitudinally narrowing conduit length. The perfusion pressure gradually diminishes along the artery. In this artery, CVR is reduced but not associated with a focal stenotic pressure loss. Thus, mechanical therapy directed at a presumed «culprit» plaque for the purpose of reversing this abnormal physiology would be ineffective in restoring normal coronary perfusion.

Using FFR during continuous pressure wire pullback from a distal to proximal location, the impact of a specific area of angiographic narrowing can be examined and the presence of diffuse atherosclerosis can be documented. Diffuse atherosclerosis, as opposed to focal narrowing, is characterized by a continuous and gradual pressure recovery without a localized abrupt increase in pressure related to an isolated region. Diffuse atherosclerosis would also explain the persistently abnormal distal FFR despite unobstructed proximal segments.[24] Table 3-1 summarizes characteristics of coronary flow reserves and FFR.

CLINICAL APPLICATIONS

Post-angioplasty CVR and FFR have been used to guide decisions regarding residual lumen impairment that is undetected by satisfactory angiographic results. Sequential flow velocity data have confirmed that the normalization of CVR occurs in only 50% of patients after PTCA alone and may be increased to 80% of patients after stenting. Serial measurements of CVR, rCVR, QCA, and IVUS in a 55-patient study after PTCA alone and again after stent placement[25] found that the cross-sectional area was significantly larger after stenting than with PTCA alone (7.6 mm^2 vs 4.5 mm^2; $p < 0.01$), and confirmed a relationship between lumen size and coronary flow. However, in 20% of patients, CVR remained <2.0 despite clearly patent target sites, which is consistent with co-existent microvascular disease. Nonetheless, the ability to restore a normal flow with an anatomically acceptable result might lead to improved long-term PCI outcomes.

From numerous studies over more than 5 years, coronary physiologic measurements are now associated with at least four major clinical outcomes (Table 3-2). For lesion as-

Table 3-1. Comparison of Absolute and Relative CFR and FFR

	Hemodynamic Independence	Independent of Microcirculation Abnormalities	Unequivocal Normal Values	Use in Multivessel CAD	Use for Collateral Measurements
CVR	–	–	Range >2.0	+	+
rCVR	+	+	Range >0.8	–	–
FFR	+	+	1.0	+	+

+ = useful;– = not useful. CAD = coronary artery disease.
Reprinted with permission, Kern MJ, *Circulation* 2000; 101:1344-1351.

Table 3-2. Catheter-based Anatomic and Physiologic Criteria Associated
with Clinical Outcomes

Application	IVUS	CVR	rCVR	FFR
Ischemia detection	$<3\text{-}4$ mm^2	<2.0	<0.8	<0.75
Deferred angioplasty	>4 mm^2	>2.0	—	>0.75
Endpoint of angioplasty	—	$>2.0\text{-}2.5$ with $<35\%$ DS	—	>0.90
Endpoint of stenting	>9 mm^2 $>80\%$ ref area, full apposition	—	—	>0.94

Modified from Kern MJ, Circulation 2000; 101:1344-1351.

sessment before intervention, strong correlations exist between myocardial stress testing and FFR or CVR. An FFR of <0.75 identifies physiologically significant stenoses associated with inducible myocardial ischemia, with a high sensitivity, specificity, positive predicted value, and overall accuracy. An abnormal CVR (<2.0) corresponded to reversible myocardial perfusion imaging defects with a similarly high sensitivity, specificity and predictive accuracy (Table 3-3).

Data supporting deferring coronary intervention for intermediate stenoses with normal physiology are remarkably consistent, with clinical event rates of <10% over a two-year follow-up period. Despite the excellent safety of the deferred approach, some patients may still have recurrent angina, requiring continued medical therapy. Like other clinical tests at a single point in time, in-laboratory translesional hemodynamics may not reflect the episodic ischemia-producing conditions of daily life. Physiologic thresholds have been validated by ischemic stress testing and clinical outcomes in order to support decisions to defer intervention while continuing medical therapy for endothelial dysfunction, hypertension, hyperlipidemia, and episodic coronary vasoconstriction.

Provisional stenting has been proposed whereby balloon angioplasty guided by an-

giographic anatomy and a physiologic end point is performed; stenting is performed only when end point criteria are not met. A multicenter prospective trial, the Doppler End Point Balloon Angioplasty Trial Europe (DEBATE), first demonstrated that the combination of optimal angiographic and coronary flow velocity measurements could identify a subset (22 %) of patients in whom a clinical event rate after balloon angioplasty alone was low (<16 %) at six months and comparable to results obtained after coronary stenting.[26] As a follow-up study, the DEBATE trial found the best outcome results in stented patients with optimal PTCA physiology. At least four other multicenter randomized trials have proved the concept of provisional stenting.[27-30] However, provisional stenting using coronary flow, pressure, or IVUS has not become common practice, probably for several reasons.[31] The results of routine stenting without adjunctive technology are excellent. A large percentage of provisional stenting procedures will still require stenting due to suboptimal anatomic physiologic results. Provisional stenting is more time-consuming than routine stenting. In some analyses, routine stenting appears less costly than provisional stenting,[82] and any cost differential is offset by the increased procedure time required to use adjunctive

Table 3-3. Comparison of Stress Testing (Ischemia) and Directly Measured Coronary Blood Flow Physiology

Author	Year	(n)	Ischemic Test	Physiologic Threshold	Sensitivity	Specificity	PV+	PV−	Accuracy
Poststenotic CVR									
Miller	1994	33	Adeno/Dipy MIBI	<2.0	82	100	100	77	89
Joye	1994	30	Exercise Thallium	<2.0	94	95	94	95	94
Deychak	1995	17	Exercise Thallium	<1.8	94	94	100	91	96
Heller	1995	100	Exercise Thallium	<1.8	89	92	96	89	92
Danzi	1998	30	Dipy Echo	<2.0	91	84	—	—	87
Schulman	1997	35	Exercise ECG	<2.0	95	71	—	—	86
Donahue	1996	50	Ex/Pharm Thallium	<2.0	98	76	88	88	—
Duffy	2001	43	Stress Echo	<2.0,	80	93	—	—	88
				rCVR <0.75	100	76	—	—	81
Chamuleau	2001	127	Dipy MIBI	CVR <2.0,	—	—	—	—	69
				rCVR <0.75	—	—	—	—	75
El Shafei	2001	53	Ex/Pharm Thall	CVR <0.20,	71	83	81	74	—
				rCVR <0.75	63	88	83	70	—
FFR									
Pijls	1995	45	4 test standard*	<0.75	88	100	100	88	93
de Bruyne	1995	60	Exercise ECG	<0.72	100	87	—	—	—
Bartunek	1999	37	Dobu/Exercise Echo	<0.68	95	90	—	—	—
Chamuleau	2001	127	Dipy MIBI	<0.75	—	—	—	—	75
Caymaz	2000	30	Ex Thallium	<0.75	—	—	91	100	—
Fearon	2000	10	Ex Thallium	<0.75	90	100	—	—	95

Adeno/Dipy MIBI = adenosine or dipyridamole sestamibi scan; CVR = coronary flow reserve; Dobu = dobutamine; Sens = sensitivity; Spec = specificity; PV+/PV− = predictive value positive/negative; Pharm = pharmacologic.
* 4 tests were ECG, Echo, pacing, nuclear stress tests.

technology (IVUS and coronary flow or pressure). Since significant reductions in major adverse clinical events after stenting are evident, provisional stenting seems unlikely to supplant routine stenting in clinical practice.

Major predictors of adverse cardiac events after stent implantation can be determined by intracoronary Doppler and quantitative coronary angiography. Haude et al.[32] examined both absolute and relative coronary reserve and angiographic results in 150 patients six months after stenting. Thirty-three of the 150 patients developed adverse cardiac events with a relative CVR < 0.88, defining an incidence of 6.8%. A combination of relative CVR > 0.88 and percent diameter stenosis < 11% predicted an adverse cardiac event rate of 1.5%. The measurement of relative CVR and percent diameter stenosis after stenting were highly significant for identifying those at risk for major adverse cardiac events six months after stenting.

Coronary physiology and IVUS measurements are more closely related than quantitative coronary angiography (QCA). In 73 patients, Abizaid et al.[33] reported that a minimum lumen cross-sectional area of <4.0 mm^2 or mean lumen diameter (MLDIVUS) of <2.0 mm has a diagnostic accuracy of 92% for identification of diseased vessels with a CVR of <2.0. QCA lesion length, but not lumen diameter, was an independent predictor of CVR. A similar study comparing IVUS, QCA, and FFR in 42 patients with 51 stenoses also demonstrated that QCA alone was not accurate in determining the significance of a physiologic lesion assessed by either IVUS or FFR.[34] There was, however, a strong correlation between minimal lumen area by IVUS <3.0 mm^2 and cross-sectional area stenosis > 60% with a measured FFR < 0.75 (IVUS sensitivity 83%, specificity 92%), respectively. Briguori et al.[35] also found that the percent area stenosis and lesional length had a significant inverse correlation with FFR (r = -0.58, p < 0.001 and r = -0.41, p < 0.004, respectively). Hanekamp et al.[36] found that a normal FFR after stent

deployment indicates good stent implantation. In 31 patients with 81 paired IVUS and FFR measurements, an FFR > 0.94 indicated a 91% concordance in the ability to predict suboptimum stent deployment (p < 0.00001). QCA alone showed a low concordance rate with either IVUS or FFR (48% and 46%) respectively. A similar U.S. multicenter trial (FUSION) study is currently under evaluation.

Van Liebergen et al.[37] demonstrated improved hyperemic coronary flow after optimized stent implantation guided by IVUS in 20 patients. When maximal hyperemia after optimal balloon angioplasty (guided by IVUS) is achieved, further flow increases after stenting are not expected. The absence of functional residual luminal obstruction after IVUS-guided balloon angioplasty may explain similar clinical outcomes reported for PTCA results in the provisional stent studies.

CORONARY PHYSIOLOGY IN ACUTE MYOCARDIAL INFARCTION

An impaired CVR appears related to the degree of residual stenoses and the amount of microcirculatory injury in the region adjacent to the infarct. Since microvascular stunning is partially reversible over time, a variable acute physiology limits the use of measurements in the first days of the index event. Some investigators reported that post-infarction CVR may be associated with preservation of the microcirculation while others found no relationship between CVR and myocardial viability by scintigraphy. CVR did not differentiate patients with an extensive versus small infarction, suggesting that coronary vasodilator capacity is not directly related to the extent of necrosis.

The capacitance of viable myocardium should be reflected in phasic CVR flow characteristics. Kawamoto et al.[38] measured systolic APV and diastolic flow velocity deceleration time (DDT) in 23 patients with acute anterior MI and found that if the systolic APV was >6.5 cm/s or the DDT >600 ms, there was more recovery in the infarcted region and improved regional wall motion as assessed by echocardiography. Similarly, Tsunoda et al.[39] evaluated continuous flow velocity measurements for 18 ± 4 hours after successful angioplasty in 19 patients with acute anterior MI. Two divergent flow-response groups were identified. In those patients in whom average peak velocity (APV) increased after only a transient decline, regional wall motion and overall left ventricular systolic function improved (ejection fraction increased 17 ± 9 %). However if the APV progressively decreased throughout the next day, left ventricular systolic function did not improve (ejection fraction increased only 4 ± 9%; p = 0.007). These findings suggest that maneuvers that might maintain or produce flow augmentation (e.g., intra-aortic balloon pumping or adenosine) might result in improved myocardial salvage. Improved microcirculation responses that may be related to new pharmacology promote the recovery of left ventricular function. Neumann et al.[40] measured CVR and regional left ventricular function immediately after stenting and again, 14 days later, in two groups of acute infarction patients: a control group treated with standard heparin and a group treated with heparin and glycoprotein IIb/IIIa inhibition with abciximab. Improved coronary vascular function by hyperemia was coupled with improved regional systolic wall motion in the abciximab group compared with the standard therapy group.

COLLATERAL CIRCULATION

One of the areas in which new information provided by the sensor guidewire techniques has been greatest is in the assessment of collateral function and physiology. Collateral circulation can be described by intracoronary pressure and flow relationships. Ipsilateral collateral flow and contralateral arterial responses have been described in numerous studies using both pressure and flow to provide new information regarding mechanisms, function, and clinical significance of collateral flow in patients and provide new insights into coronary artery disease.[41-43]

In summary, new intracoronary diagnostic techniques, principally involving physiology and IVUS, have now taken their place as important tools for documenting findings in support of research hypotheses, as well as documenting data useful for critical decision-making regarding clinical interventions.

REFERENCES

1. Kern MJ. Coronary physiology revisited: practical insights from the cardiac catheterization laboratory. *Circulation* 2000; 101: 1344-1351.
2. Topol EJ, Nissen SE. Our preoccupation with coronary luminology. The dissociation between clinical and angiographic findings in ischemic heart disease. *Circulation* 1995; 92:2333-2342.
3. Gould KL, Lipscomb K, Hamilton GW. Physiologic basis for assessing critical coronary stenosis: instantaneous flow response and regional distribution during coronary hyperemia as measures of coronary flow reserve. *Am J Cardiol* 1974; 33:87-94.
4. Gould KL, Kirkeeide RL, Buchi M. Coronary flow reserve as a physiologic measure of stenosis severity. *J Am Coll Cardiol* 1990; 15:459-474.
5. Doucette JW, Corl PD, Payne HM, Flynn AE, Goto M, Nassi M, Segal J. Validation of a Doppler guide wire for intravascular measurement of coronary artery flow velocity. *Circulation* 1992; 85:1899-1911.
6. Labovitz AJ, Anthonis DM, Cravens TL, Kern MJ. Validation of volumetric flow measurements by means of a Doppler-tipped coronary angioplasty guide wire. *Am Heart J* 1993; 126:1456-1461.
7. Baumgart D, Haude M, Liu F, Ge J, Goerge G, Erbel R. Current concepts of coronary flow reserve for clinical decision making during cardiac catheterization. *Am Heart J* 1998; 136:136-149.

8. Kern MJ, Bach RG, Mechem C, CaraccioloEA, Aguirre FV, Miller LW, Donohue TJ. Variations in normal coronary vasodilatory reserve stratified by artery, gender, heart transplantation and coronary artery disease. *J Am Coll Cardiol* 1996; 28:1154-1160.

9. McGinn AL, White CW, Wilson RF. Interstudy variability of coronary flow reserve: influence of heart rate, arterial pressure, and ventricular preload. *Circulation* 1990; 81: 1319-1330.

10. Marcus ML, Mueller TM, Gascho JA, Kerber RE. Effects of cardiac hypertrophy secondary to hypertension on the coronary circulation. *Am J Cardiol* 1979; 44:1023-1031.

11. Chauhan A, Millins PA, Petch MC, Schonfield PM. Is coronary flow velocity response really normal in syndrome X? *Circulation* 1994; 89:1998-2004.

12. Wieneke H, Haude M, Ge J, Altmann C, Kaiser S, Baumgart D, von Birgelen C, Welge D, Erbel R. Corrected coronary flow velocity reserve: a new concept for assessing coronary perfusion. *J Am Coll Cardiol* 2000; 35:1713- 1720.

13. Baumgart D, Haude M, Goerge G, Ge J, Vetter S, Dagres N, Heusch G, Erbel R. Improved assessment of coronary stenosis severity using the relative flow velocity reserve. *Circulation* 1998; 98:40-46.

14. Kern MJ, Puri S, Bach RG, Donohue TJ, Dupouy P, Caracciolo EA, Craig WR, Aguirre F, Aptecar E, Wolford TL, Mecham CJ, Dubois-Rande JL., Abnormal coronary flow velocity reserve after coronary artery stenting in patients: role of relative coronary reserve to assess potential mechanisms. *Circulation* 1999; 100:2491-2498.

15. Van Liebergen RAM, Piek JJ, Koch KT, Peters RJG, de Winter RJ, Schotborgh CE, Lie KI. Hyperemic coronary flow after optimized intravascular ultrasound-guided balloon angioplasty and stent implantation. *J Am Coll Cardiol* 1999; 34:1899-1906.

16. El-Shafei A, Chiravuri R, Stikovac MM, El-Badry MA, Donohue TJ, Bach RG, Aguirre FV, Caracciolo EA, Bitar S, Wolford TL, Miller DD, Kern MJ. Comparison of relative coronary Doppler flow velocity reserve to stress myocardial perfusion imaging in patients with coronary artery disease. *Cathet Cardiovasc Intervent* 2001; 53:193-201.

17. Donohue TJ, Kern MJ, Aguirre FV, Bach RG, Wolford T, Bell CA, Segal J. Assessing the hemodynamic significance of coronary artery stenoses: Analysis of translesional pressure-flow velocity relationships in patients. *J Am Coll Cardiol* 1993; 22:449-458.

18. Segal J, Kern MJ, Scott NA, King SB III, Doucette JW, Heuser RR, Ofili E, Siegel R. Alterations of phasic coronary artery flow velocity in man during percutaneous coronary angioplasty. *J Am Coll Cardiol* 1992; 20:276-286.

19. Gaster AL, Korsholm L, Thayseen P, Pedersen KE, Haghfelt TH. Reproducibility of Intravascular Ultrasound and Intracoronary Doppler Measurements. *Cathet Cardiovasc Intervent* 2001; 53:449-458.

20. Pijls NH, Van Gelder B, Van der Voort P, Peels K, Bracke FA, Bonnier HJ, el Gamal MI. Fractional flow reserve: a useful index to evaluate the influence of an epicardial coronary stenosis on myocardial blood flow. *Circulation* 1995; 92:3183-3193.

21. Pijls NH, De Bruyne B, Peels K, Van Der Voort PH, Bonnier HJ, Bartunek J, Koolen JJ. Measurement of fractional flow reserve to assess the functional severity of coronary-artery stenoses. *N Engl J Med* 1996; 334: 1703-1708.

22. De Bruyne B, Bartunek J, Sys SU, Pijls NH, Heyndrickx GR, Wijns W. Simultaneous coronary pressure and flow velocity measurements in humans: feasibility, reproducibility, and hemodynamic dependence of coronary flow velocity reserve, hyperemic flow versus pressure slope index, and fractional flow reserve. *Circulation* 1996; 94: 1842-1849.

23. Meuwissen J, Chamuleau AJ, Siebes M, Schotborgh CE, Koch KT, de Winter RJ, Bax M, De Jong A, Spaan JAE, Piek JJ. Role of variability in microvascular resistance on fractional flow reserve and coronary blood flow velocity reserve in intermediate coronary lesion. *Circulation* 2001; 103:184-187.

24. Kern MJ. Focus for the new millennium: Diffuse coronary artery disease and physiologic measurements of severity. *Am Coll Cardiol Curr J Rev* March/April 2000:13-19.

25. Kern MJ, Dupouy P, Drury JH, Aguirre FV, Aptecar E, Bach RG, Caracciolo EA, Donohue TJ, Dubois-Rande J, Geschwind HJ,

Mechem CJ, Kane G, Teiger E, Wolford TL. Role of coronary artery lumen enlargement in improving coronary blood flow after balloon angioplasty and stenting: a combined intravascular ultrasound Doppler flow and imaging study. *J Am Coll Cardiol* 1997; 29: 1520-1527.

26. Serruys PW, Di Mario C, Piek J, Schroeder E, Vrints C, Probst P, De Bruyne B, Hanet C, Fleck E, Haude M, Verna E, Voudris V, Geschwind H, Emanuelsson H, Muhlberger V, Danzi G, Peels HO, Ford AJ, Boersma E, for the DEBATE Study Group. Prognostic value of intracoronary flow velocity and diameter stenosis in assessing the short and long-term outcomes of coronary balloon angioplasty: the DEBATE study (Doppler Endpoints Balloon Angioplasty Trial Europe). *Circulation* 1997; 96:3369-3377.

27. Lafont A, Dubois-Rande JL, Steg PG, Dupouy P, Carrie D, Coste P, Furber A, Beygui F, Feldman LJ, Rahal S, Tron C, Hamon M, Grollier G, Commeau P, Richard P, Colin P, Bauters C, Karrillon G, Ledru F, Citron B, Marie FN, Kern M, for the F.R.O.S.T. Study Group. The French Randomized Optimal Stenting Trial: A prospective evaluation of provisional stenting guided by coronary velocity reserve and quantitative coronary angiography. *J Am Coll Cardiol* 2000; 36:404-9.

28. DiMario C, Moses JW, Anderson TJ, Bonan R, Muramatsu T, Jain AC, de Lezo JS, Cho SY, Kern M, Meredith IT, Cohen D, Moussa I, Colombo A, on behalf of the DESTINI Study Group (Doppler Endpoint STenting INternational Investigation). Randomized comparison of elective stent implantation and coronary balloon angioplasty guided by online quantitative angiography and intracoronary Doppler. *Circulation* 2000; 102:2938-2944.

29. Serruys PW, de Bruyne B, Carlier S, Sousa JE, Piek J, Muramatsu T, Vrints C, Probst P, Seabra-Gomes R, Simpson I, Voudris V, Gurne O, Pijls N, Belardi J, Van Es GA, Boersma E, Morel MA, Van Hout B, on behalf of the Doppler Endpoints Balloon Angioplasty Trial Europe (DEBATE) II Study Group. Randomized comparison of primary stenting and provisional balloon angioplasty guided by flow velocity measurement. *Circulation* 2000; 102:2930- 2937.

30. Dupouy P, Pelle G, Garot P, Kern MJ, Kane G, Woscoboinick J, Aptecar E, Belarbi A, Pernes JM, Rande JLD, Teiger E. Physiologically guided angioplasty in support to a provisional stenting strategy: immediate and six-month outcome. *Cathet Cardiovasc Intervent* 2000; 49:369-375.

31. Anderson HV, Carabello BA. Provisional versus routine stenting - routine stenting is here to stay. *Circulation* 2000; 102:2910-2914.

32. Haude M, Baumgart D, Verna E, Piek JJ, Vrints C, Probst P, Erbel R. Intracoronary Doppler —and quantitative coronary angiography— derived predictors of major adverse cardiac events after stent implantation. *Circulation* 2001; 103:1212-1217.

33. Abizaid A, Mintz GS, Pichard AD, Kent KM, Satler LF, Walsh CL, Popma JJ, Leon MB. Clinical, intravascular ultrasound, and quantitative angiographic determinants of the coronary flow reserve before and after percutaneous transluminal coronary angioplasty. *Am J Cardiol* 1998; 82:423-428.

34. Takagi A, Tsurumi Y, Ishii Y, Suzuki K, Kawana M, Kasanuki H. Clinical potential of intravascular ultrasound for physiological assessment of coronary stenosis: relationship between quantitative ultrasound tomography and pressure-derived fractional flow reserve. *Circulation* 1999; 100:250-255.

35. Briguori C, Anzuini A, Airoldi F, Gimelli G, Nishida T, Adamian M, Corvaja N, Di Mario C, Colombo A. Intravascular ultrasound criteria for the assessment of the functional significance of intermediate coronary artery stenoses and comparison with fractional flow reserve. *Am J Cardiol* 2001; 87:136-141.

36. Hanekamp CEE, Koolen JJ, Pijls NHJ, Michels HR, Bonnier HJRM. Comparison of quantitative coronary angiography, intravascular ultrasound, and coronary pressure measurement to assess optimum stent deployment. *Circulation* 1999; 99:1015-1021.

37. Van Liebergen RAM, Piek JJ, Koch KT, Peters RJG, de Winter RJ, Schotborgh CE, Lie KI. Hyperemic coronary flow after optimized intravascular ultrasound-guided balloon angioplasty and stent implantation. *J Am Coll Cardiol* 1999; 34:1899-906.

38. Kawamoto T, Yoshida K, Akasaka T, Hozumi T, Takagi T, Kaji S, Ueda Y. Can

coronary blood flow velocity pattern after primary percutaneous transluminal coronary angiography predict recovery of regional left ventricular function in patients with acute myocardial infarction? *Circulation* 1999; 100:339-345.

39. Tsunoda T, Nakamura M, Wakatsuki T, Nishida T, Asahara T, Anzai H, Touma H, Mitsuo K, Soumitsi Y, Sakatani H, Nakamura S, Degawa T, Yamaguchi T. The pattern of alteration in flow velocity in the recanalized artery is related to left ventricular recovery in patients with acute infarction and successful direct balloon angioplasty. *J Am Coll Cardiol* 1998; 32:338-344.

40. Neumann FJ, Blasini R, Schmitt C, Alt E, Dirschinger J, Gawaz M, Kastrati A, Schomig A. Effect of glycoprotein IIb/IIIa receptor blockade on recovery of coronary flow and left ventricular function after the placement of coronary artery stents in acute myocardial infarction. *Circulation* 1998; 98:2695-2701.

41. Seiler C, Fleisch M, Billinger M, Meier B. Simultaneous intracoronary velocity —and pressure— derived assessment of adenosine —induced collateral hemodynamics in patients with one— to two-vessel coronary artery disease. *J Am Coll Cardiol* 1999; 34:1985-1994.

42. Pijls NHJ, Bech GJW, el Gamal MIH, Bonnier HJ, De Bruyne B, Van Gelder B, Michels HR, Koolen JJ. Quantification of recruitable coronary collateral blood flow in conscious humans and its potential to predict future ischemic events. *J Am Coll Cardiol* 1995; 25:1522-1528.

43. Piek JJ, van Liebergen RAM, Koch KT, Peters RJG, David GK. Clinical, angiographic and hemodynamic predictors of recruitable collateral flow assessed during balloon angioplasty coronary occlusion. *J Am Coll Cardiol* 1997; 29:275-282.

4

Limitations of Coronary Angiography: Rationale for New Intracoronary Diagnostic Techniques

Fernando Alfonso, MD
Javier Botas, MD

Perspective. Angiography vs Postmortem Findings. Limitations of Angiography. Morphological and Physiological Considerations: Angiography vs the New Intracoronary Techniques. References.

PERSPECTIVE

Until very recently, selective coronary angiography was the only tool available for the study of coronary anatomy in patients. Discrete luminal stenoses are readily visualized by angiography, a technique well suited for depicting the silhouette of the coronary lumen.[1-4] However, the limitations of conventional angiography are currently well established. Even when a detailed angiographic examination is made by experienced personnel, we frequently encounter lesions that escape precise assessment, including the nature of the stenosis (underlying pathophysiological substrate), relevant associated anatomic findings (thrombus, calcification, eccentricity) and, more importantly, the severity and functional significance of the lesion. Therefore, in the last decade the perception of coronary angiography as the «gold standard» for the diagnosis of the extent and severity of coronary artery disease has been critically challenged.[1-4] Previously, «luminology» was considered a valid surrogate for gauging all the information required for diagnostic purposes.[1] Angiography provides excellent resolution of the lumen but it simply does not depict the vessel wall (Fig. 4-1). The luminogram provides little insight into plaque disposition and the underlying pathology[1-4] (Figs. 4-2 and 4-3). Although angiography is widely available and provides a valid road map of the entire coronary tree, as well as a rough estimate of stenosis severity in discrete luminal narrowing, this technique often fails to provide the critical anatomic insights that are currently required for clinical decision-making during percutaneous coronary interventions. This has brought into question both its utility during routine clinical practice and its value as a reliable research tool.[1-4]

In the last decade, several new intracoronary diagnostic techniques have been developed and accepted as valuable adjuncts to angiography in providing unique and complementary insights that have changed conventional paradigms in diagnosis and therapy.[1-10] It is hoped that these technical refinements will help to minimize discrepancies between the images and reality.[1-10]

In this chapter, we will summarize the value and limitations of conventional angiography. With this aim, we will review: 1) classical correlations between angiography and histological findings, 2) common prob-

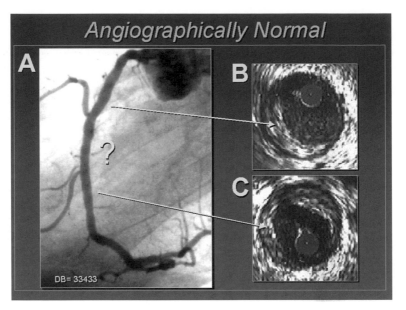

Figure 4-1. (A) Coronary angiogram of the right coronary artery showing a normal looking coronary lumen. Angiography, however, fails to detect a significant atherosclerotic plaque burden on the vessel wall that is readily detected by intravascular ultrasound. (B) Eccentric plaque (C) Concentric plaque.

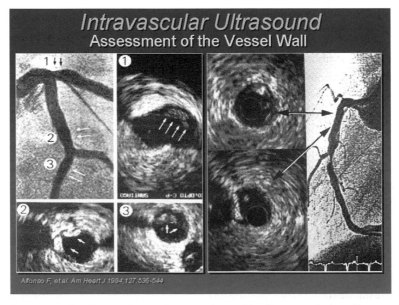

Figure 4-2. Atherosclerotic plaques (arrows) on angiographically normal sites. Large atherosclerotic plaques are also detected at sites with just mild lumen irregularities on angiography (ostium of the left anterior descending coronary artery).

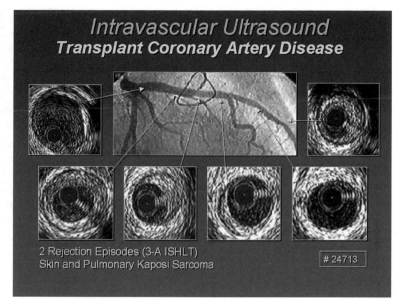

Figure 4-3. Cardiac transplantation recipient with angiographically normal coronary arteries. In this patient every type of atherosclerotic plaque (intimal thickening, eccentric plaque, concentric plaque, calcified plaque) could be detected using intravascular ultrasound.

lems and limitations in the performance and interpretation of coronary angiograms using either visual assessment or quantitative methods, and also certain difficult situations that represent angiographic challenges, 3) angiography versus true anatomic and physiological insights obtained by the new diagnostic intracoronary techniques.

ANGIOGRAPHY VS POSTMORTEM FINDINGS

Until the introduction of selective coronary angiography, the only available information on coronary anatomy came from the study of postmortem specimens. The advent of angiography made it possible, for the first time, to visualize coronary artery stenoses in living patients and this information was soon used not only for diagnostic purposes but also to establish the need for coronary revascularization procedures, at that time coronary bypass operations.[1-3] Nevertheless, many investigators were soon interested in cor-

relating angiographic findings with the classical data from detailed autopsy studies and, later on, from observations made during coronary surgery.[1-3, 11-16]

Reports from autopsy series obviously have the problem of selection bias in that they only include the oldest and sickest patients from the broad spectrum of patients with coronary artery disease.[11-16] Therefore, care should be taken when postmortem data are extrapolated directly for comparison with findings from living patients. In addition, some technical considerations may also explain the limitations of characterizing coronary artery disease from postmortem observations. In many early studies, atherosclerosis was judged qualitatively on gross inspection. In other preliminary studies, quantitative data about atherosclerosis was obtained from longitudinal analysis (not cross-sectional measurements) or was limited to selected coronary segments. Examination of fresh, unfixed specimens avoids artifacts produced by fixation and shrinkage. However, such studies do not reproduce the physiological conditions of the coronary vessel during life, which so greatly influence lumen size and wall configuration. Vessel should be fixed after physiological pressure-distention to ensure proper comparisons. Nevertheless, it should be kept in mind that this technique is complex and can also induce artifacts. Careful pressurization of the artery is required since it has been suggested that excessive intravascular pressure may artificially distend and deform a weakened sclerotic wall.[11]

Comparative studies have shown important discrepancies between the extent and severity of coronary artery disease as depicted by angiography and the results of postmortem histology.[11-16] Most anatomopathologic observations suggest that angiography grossly underestimates the extent and severity of coronary artery disease.[11-16] The angiographically «normal» reference segment is universally involved in the atheromatous process and most lesions exhibit positive remodeling, which explains why the severity of lesions is underestimated by angiography.[1-3] This is in complete contrast with comparisons between *in vitro* histological measurements of the atherosclerotic plaque burden (on arteries distended to physiological pressure) and intravascular ultrasound (IVUS) findings, where an excellent correlation has been found.[11-16]

In a classical study, Vlodaver et al.[12] correlated antemortem coronary angiograms with postmortem specimens (134 coronary segments) and suggested that major discrepancies between the two techniques were due mainly to five reasons: 1) incorrect radiological technique; 2) type of projections used; 3) presence of a slit-like lumen adjacent to the atheroma; 4) true degree of obstruction, and 5) misinterpretation of true obstructions present in life based on findings from the postmortem specimen. The problem of lumen shape and need for multiple projections was clearly appreciated at that time. In addition, they also suggested that «... *the roentgenologist's anticipation of the normal caliber of a given coronary segment may be*

an underestimation....» In fact, in that study many false negative readings were made from segments that showed only a uniform, but relatively small vessel in arteriography, while diffuse disease was evident in histological studies.

Arnett et al.[13] compared the amount of narrowing in 61 coronary arteries studied angiographically during life by three experienced angiographers (reduction in diameter), with that observed histologically (cross-sectional area) at necropsy. They suggested that a reduction in lumen diameter >50 % on angiography represents a reduction >75 % in the luminal cross-sectional area. Alternatively, a reduction in lumen diameter >75 % on angiography was associated with a reduction in the luminal cross-sectional area >95 % on histologic examination. This study also stressed that the presence of diffuse atherosclerosis seems to account for most of the angiographic underestimation of the degree of lumen narrowing. Finally, they further emphasized that unless angiography is obtained in multiple views, luminal narrowing of segments with a non-round residual section will be greatly underestimated.

The Montreal[14] group reported in another classical study appreciable, potentially relevant, discrepancies between cineangiographic and postmortem findings in more than 30 % of patients undergoing coronary revascularization. They suggested that the particular transverse orientation of the initial left coronary artery frequently caused angiographic superposition of multiple branches that could not be properly separated despite multiple projections in the transverse plane. The use of additional projections in the sagittal plane was therefore recommended.

The interobserver variability of coronary angiogram interpretation was a problem that was recognized early and prospectively assessed in a clinicopathological correlation using histological findings as the standard of accuracy.[17, 18] In the study by Galbraith et al.,[18] a barium gelatin cast was used to assess the degree of obstruction. In this study, a reduction in lumen diameter >50% was also considered equivalent to a reduction in the cross-sectional area of >75%. A total of 624 luminal sections were available for comparison. In most instances (>80% of cases), the interpretation of noteworthy lesions by angiography correlated well with histological findings. However, interobserver variability between three experienced observers was significant, including false negative interpretation (ranging from 20% to 45%) and even false positive interpretation (ranging from 20% to 53%). It is interesting that the same error was made by 2 of the 3 interpreters in more than half of the misinterpreted luminal areas. It was suggested at that time that a more accurate interpretation could be obtained by reaching a «consensus opinion» among several observers reading the coronary angiogram at the same time.

On the other hand, there has been very limited information on angiographic-histological correlation of coronary artery disease in young patients. Symptomatic coronary artery disease typically manifests after the age of 40 years but some postmortem studies have unequivocally demonstrated that atherosclerotic changes can be found earlier in life, even in asymptomatic individuals with no evidence of atherosclerotic heart disease.[19-23] Gross inspection of the coronary arteries from American soldiers demonstrated definite atherosclerosis in >50% of the hearts examined.[19-22] In a recent study[23] involving 262 heart transplant recipients (mean donor age 33 years), 52% of patients had at least one atherosclerotic site on IVUS whereas coronary arteriography was completely normal in 92% of these patients and only mild angiographic irregularities were visible in 8% of cases. No angiogram was abnormal in any patient <30 years old, yet IVUS was abnormal in 28% of them.

Finally, much interest has focused on correlating angiographic and histological findings in the left main coronary trunk. Isner et al., in a now classical study,[24] analyzed the accuracy of angiography in determining left main coronary artery narrowing as compared with postmortem findings from 28 patients with symptomatic coronary artery disease in which angiography had been performed within 40 days of death. Major angiographic errors were appreciated (mainly gross underestimation of the severity of the lesion) which, once again, resulted primarily from an undetected atherosclerotic plaque on the left main coronary artery and an insufficient number of angiographic projections.

Last, but not least, it is important to keep in mind that the famous «Glagow phenomenon» (positive remodeling) was initially described by this pathologist in histologic sections of the left main coronary artery from 136 hearts obtained at autopsy.[25] In his pioneering pathologic description of coronary lumen preservation despite the presence of a large amount of plaque, Glagow concluded that this finding «...*should be taken into account in evaluating coronary artery disease with the use of angiography....*»

LIMITATIONS OF ANGIOGRAPHY

Conventional Angiography

Forty-five years ago Sones[26] performed the first selective coronary angiography and described a technique that enabled the direct visualization of coronary artery disease *in vivo*, heralding a paradigm shift in the diagnosis and treatment of coronary artery disease. Since then, cardiologists have relied on coronary angiography to guide clinical practice and research. The seminal contributions of coronary angiography during the last decades generated an enormous impulse for cardiovascular medicine, leading to unprecedented advances and developments.[1] Although angiography has endured all these years as the predominantly used method for defining coronary anatomy, many studies have challenged its accuracy and reproducibility.

Reproducibility

Soon after the introduction of coronary angiography into routine clinical practice, some investigators began to question its reproducibility. Initial studies suggested that a visual «eyeball» interpretation of coronary angiograms was convenient and rapid, but showed a significant interobserver and intraobserver variability within the range to interfere with clinical decisions.[17,18] The variability is highest for lesions producing stenosis equivalent to 30 % to 80 % of diameter.[27] The clinical implications of marked interobserver variability in coronary angiography were disturbing, so methods to overcome this problem were soon proposed. Firstly, «group opinion,» based on independent readings, was suggested as a way of reducing interobserver variability. Alternatively, «consensus opinion,» based on several observers reading the coronary angiogram at the same time, was also proposed.[17] Secondly, the use of calipers reduced variability compared with visual assessment but tended to underestimate lesions >75 % and overestimate lesions <75 %.[28] Moreover, caliper measurements are not as reproducible as computer-assisted quantification.[29]

Extent and Severity of Disease

The traditional visual method of assessing the severity of stenosis has been «percent diameter stenosis.» This method entails the comparison of diameters in the target lesion and a «normal» reference segment. Accordingly, angiography has two major problems: 1) the presence of diffuse disease and 2) remodeling.[1-3] Histological and IVUS studies have demonstrated that coronary artery disease is universally diffuse and that in most cases a truly normal segment cannot be identified (Figs. 4-1 to 4-3). This explains the predictable underestimation of disease severity when the angiographic percent stenosis of diameter is used to characterize the lesion. In extreme circumstances, false negative angiograms may be present. Diffuse, concentric, and symmetrical disease affecting the coronary segment of interest usually gives the angiographic appearance of a completely normal coronary artery.[1-3] Secondly, as described above, the remodeling phenomenon affects most coronary lesions and induces an enlargement of the external elastic lamina (with outward displacement of the bulk of the atherosclerotic mass), resulting in preservation of the lumen.[1-3,25] This phenomenon tends to oppose luminal encroachment by the plaque —and might be considered a compensatory mechanism— concealing the presence of disease in the early stages of atherosclerosis and preserving the lumen to some extent even when plaque growth is significant. Eventually, this mechanism fails, resulting in «undercompensation» (roughly when the plaque area exceeds 40 % of the total vessel section). Any further increase in plaque volume is necessarily linked to progressive luminal narrowing.[25] Even when remodeled lesions do not restrict coronary flow, this finding may also be relevant clinically because these lesions could have, as the underlying substrate, vulnerable plaques.[2,3] Furthermore, small plaques can be associated with «overcompensation» at the initial phase of the disease and serial angiographic studies could be misinterpreted as atherosclerosis regression. Finally, in some cases a «negative remodeling» phenomenon may be the main cause of luminal narrowing.[5] In these cases, the external elastic lamina actually shrinks in size, contributing to a large extent to luminal stenosis.[5]

The diffuse nature of atherosclerosis and the remodeling phenomenon are two key factors that explain why the percentage of stenosis determined by IVUS is often substantially greater than angiographic determinations. These limitations also explain why coronary angiography should not be considered a reliable tool for assessing atherosclerosis progression or regression.[30] Nevertheless, if this is the case, absolute values (minimal lumen diameter) are more accurate and reproducible (see below) than relative measurements such as percent luminal narrowing. Multiple controlled lipid-lowering trials have revealed major discrepancies between marginal changes in lumen caliber at follow-up and a striking reduction in the event-rate. A potential explanation for this staggering dissociation could be that major changes in plaque volume or underlying characteristics leading to plaque stabilization (accounting for differences in clinical outcome) are systematically missed by angiographic analysis. By virtue of its ability to directly depict the vessel wall by «visualizing atherosclerosis,» IVUS appears more appropriate in this setting. In fact, most large-scale regression/progression studies currently underway are now using IVUS, [2, 3]

Technical considerations

Technical issues are major factors in image quality. The vessel lumen should be perfectly opacified by the contrast agent. Inadequate filling of the lumen with contrast medium may lead to angiographic overestimation of the degree of narrowing. In some patients with aortic valve disease (mainly those with severe aortic regurgitation), underfilling of the coronary arteries may be a problem (Fig. 4-4).[15, 24] In addition, the use of ever smaller catheters should always be controlled with checks of image quality. Even in the best-case scenario, the resolution of cineangiography is limited. As a rule of thumb, features that are smaller than 0.2 mm remain angiographically invisible. Moreover, the widespread use of the digital angiographic format, while very versatile and attractive, may lead to a significant loss of spatial resolution. In addition, image compression is a very appealing strategy for handling archiving problems and speeding up electronic information exchanges. Nevertheless, image compression >2:1 should be avoided, as recently concluded in a consensus document,[31, 32] in order to guarantee accurate resolution and preservation of diagnostic value. Obviously, the use of direct digitalization of the video signal grossly compromises image resolution. Finally, most recent

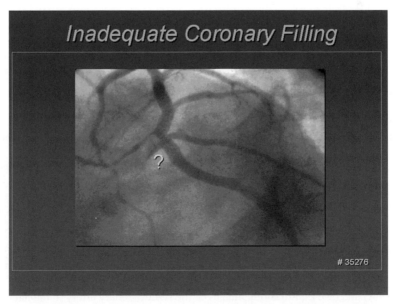

Figure 4-4. Inadequate filling of the left main coronary artery (?) in a patient with severe aortic regurgitation (left anterior oblique projection with caudal angulation). Despite forceful manual injections, the coronary tree did not properly opacify with contrast agent due to the high flow.

technical advances reflect a widespread concern about the need to limit radiation doses to patients and health care personnel. However, there is always a price to pay in terms of image quality, which decreases with the increment in the quantum noise artifact (an image flaw that reduces sharpness and contrast between the contrast-filled lumen and background). This flaw can only be overcome by increasing radiation doses. The entire angiographic X-ray system requires continuous attention by experienced personnel to maintain an optimal resolution.

Coronary motion is yet another factor accounting for image degradation (Fig. 4-5).[33] Motion blur may become clinically significant when rapid coronary motion occurs (typically from the right coronary artery) and recording settings are fixed, with a relatively large pulse duration, at 12.5 images/s. This again could be perceived as a current limitation of modern equipment when a trade-off is made between image quality and archiving

possibilities. Image blurring, poor resolution, and higher radiation doses also become a significant problem when the image intensifier is not located immediately adjacent to the patient. Finally, other radiological factors, such as veiling glare or pincushion distortion, should be taken into consideration.[34]

Nevertheless, before complaining of the caveats and limitations of angiography, we need to make sure that we are using it properly, getting the best possible information from our X-ray equipment. In many cases, information missed by angiography (and eventually revealed by alternative diagnostic techniques), could indeed have been detected by angiography if the technique had been wisely performed with adequate X-ray settings, by an experienced angiographer looking for excellence.

Challenging/Complex Situations

«Tortuous segments» with multiple and unpredictable turns and bends frequently

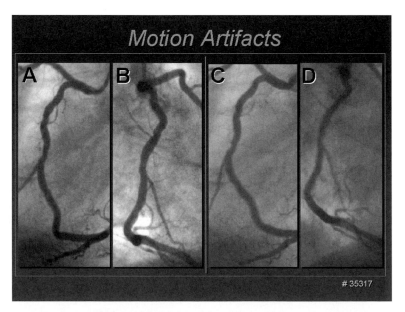

Figure 4-5. (A) and (B): End-diastolic images of the right coronary artery in the lateral and right anterior oblique projections, respectively. (C) and (D), similar images showing poor delineation of luminal contours leading to inadequate resolution. Motion artifact secondary to high heart rate and the limited temporal resolution of the system.

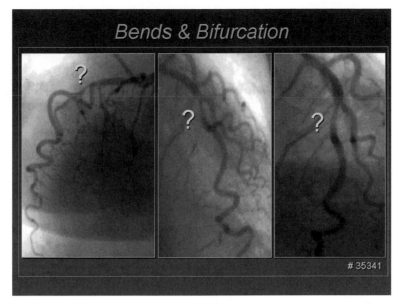

Figure 4-6.   Severe tortuosity of the left coronary artery in a patient with a moderate lesion (significant ?) on the left anterior descending coronary artery. The lesion was only recognized in a 10° right anterior oblique projection with 25° of cranial angulation. Bending and overlapping branches prevented a full delineation of the severity of the lesion.

constitute a complex anatomy (Fig. 4-6). Many lesions are located on these troublesome sites. In this setting, angiography can only identify lesions when the projection is perpendicular to the long-axis of the vessel. Only when this is achieved can significant vessel foreshortening be prevented. In addition, as previously discussed, multiple projections are always required to obtain at least two orthogonal views that are perpendicular to the long axis of the vessel and to avoid overlapping structures (Fig. 4-7).[1-3] Meticulous angiographers should check multiple unconventional angles in challenging anatomical situations without forgetting about the toxicity of contrast agents and X-ray exposure.

«*Bifurcations*» are another anatomic challenge because confluence shadows from overlapping vessels may completely obscure a lesion despite the use of multiple projections. This is of particular relevance precisely because flow dividers are well known triggers for the development of coronary atheroma. Both the parent and daughter branches may conceal atherosclerosis.[1-4] The same applies to «*ostial*» lesions (Fig. 4-8). Steep angulations should always be tested. The ostium of the right coronary artery is especially prone to «catheter-induced spasm» which may be difficult to distinguish from a true coronary lesion.

A special anatomic situation is the «*left main*». Accurate identification of the degree of luminal narrowing in the left main coronary artery is of paramount importance because it constitutes a *prima facie* indication for revascularization. However, this segment is particularly difficult to analyze with angiography and, as previously discussed, the correlations with postmortem findings have been particularly poor at this site.[24, 35, 36] The funnel-shaped and angled origin of the left main coronary artery as it arises from the aorta often makes it more difficult to adequately fill its proximal segment. The os-

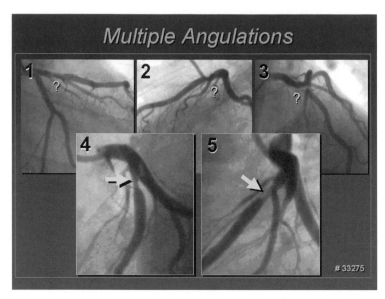

Figure 4-7.   Left coronary angiograms in different views (1 to 3) that failed to identified a severe lesion on the proximal left anterior descending coronary artery. Only very steep angulated views (4 = left anterior oblique and 5 = lateral view) were able to unravel the lesion. The lesion was near the ostium of the left coronary artery and some overlapping branches were also present further compromising its angiographic evaluation.

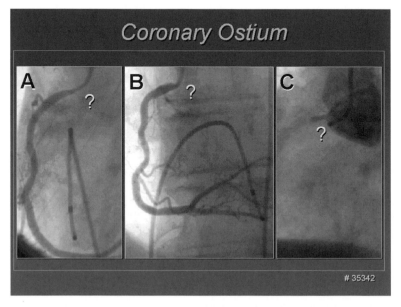

Figure 4-8.   Catheter-induced spasm on the ostium of the right coronary artery. Despite the use of intracoronary nitroglycerin severe damping of the aortic pressure was induced every time the catheter engaged the ostium (A and B). A final view (C) obtained with the catheter disengaged ten minutes later revealed moderate disease (severity ?) of the ostium of the right coronary artery, just when the contrast agent was entering the artery.

tium of the left main coronary artery may be difficult to evaluate since the catheter may be deeply engaged. In fact, ostial disease of the left main may be missed when the catheter tip seats beyond the lesion site. Although a forceful injection of contrast may be required to obtain an adequate reflux of contrast into the aorta and proper visualization of the ostium, this maneuver could be hazardous, especially if some pressure damping is recognized. Aortic cusp opacification or streaming of contrast may also obscure the ostium. In addition, disease at the distal edge of the left main and at the bifurcation between the left anterior descending coronary artery and left circumflex coronary artery may escape angiographic recognition. Confluence shadows of these arteries may obscure a lesion located at this junction. Further complicating the general problem of diffuse involvement and positive remodeling, angiographic assessment of the left main coronary artery is especially challenging due to its short length,

making it especially difficult to identify a «normal» reference segment.

«Eccentricity.» The validity of angiography to assess the «circumferential distribution» of atherosclerotic plaques in relation to the coronary lumen (eccentricity) has been critically challenged. This emphasizes the limitations of using the luminogram to predict atherosclerotic plaque location (Fig. 4-9). It is important to keep this in mind when an eccentric angiographic appearance is used to define a lesion as unstable or culprit, or when angiography is used to indicate or guide debulking techniques. IVUS, as a tomographic technique, allows direct cross-sectional visualization of plaques surrounding a vessel lumen and is therefore the method of choice for assessing plaque distribution and eccentricity. The pathologic definition of eccentricity is an atherosclerotic plaque that fails to involve the entire coronary circumference, leaving an arc of disease-free arterial wall. Histological stu-

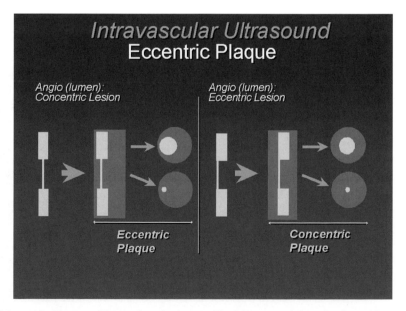

Figure 4-9. Schematic diagram illustrating the issue of lesion eccentricity. Angiography cannot detect the atherosclerotic plaque on the vessel wall so a typical appearance of concentric narrowing on the shadowgram may in fact be the result of a highly eccentric lesion (left). Alternatively, an eccentric lumen at the lesion site in relation to the adjacent-angiographically normal-reference segment may be caused by the concentric disposition of the atherosclerotic plaque (right).

dies by Waller et al.[37, 38] of 500 severe coronary lesions (cross-sectional area >75 %), revealed that 73 % had eccentric plaques whereas 27 % were concentric lesions. In eccentric lesions, the arc of disease-free wall ranged from 2 % to 32 % (mean 17 %). These histological studies suggested that eccentric plaques, in particular those narrowing the lumen to a slit, are most likely to lead to underestimation of lesion severity during angiographic assessment. In a study involving 1446 lesions, Mintz et al.[39] compared angiographic and IVUS criteria for lesion eccentricity. On angiography, 55 % of target lesions were eccentric. On IVUS, 15 % of lesions were eccentric, defined as those with an arc of normal arterial wall (equivalent to histological criteria). The concordance with angiography was only 48 %. On IVUS, an eccentricity index >3 was documented in 46 % of lesions and, using this criterion, the concordance with angiography was only 54 %. Determinants of angiographic eccentricity included lesion length and plaque thickness, but not the IVUS eccentricity index. Eccentric lesions on IVUS had a larger lumen, smaller plaque area, and smaller arcs of calcification, suggesting that they may represent less advanced atherosclerotic disease. This study demonstrated the profound discordance between angiography and IVUS in assessing plaque distribution, which underlines the limitations of angiography in this respect. Furthermore, the use of angiography to guide the orientation of atherectomy devices toward the area of maximum plaque thickness may be absolutely misleading.

«Calcium.» Several studies have demonstrated that angiography is relatively specific but not very sensitive for the detection of coronary calcification (Fig. 4-10). This may be relevant because coronary calcification represents advanced coronary artery disease and also has implications during coronary interventions. Tuzcu et al.[40] demonstrated that, compared with IVUS, the sensitivity of an-

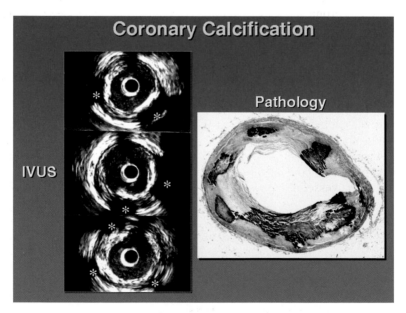

Figure 4-10.   Angiography is unable to detect mild to moderate calcification of the coronary arteries. Conversely, intravascular ultrasound is very sensitive in detecting coronary calcification, its extent and distribution (deep versus superficial). In addition, unusual patterns of coronary calcification, as evident in the image (mimicking stent struts), may be readily recognized. Pathologic specimen: courtesy of Paloma Aragoncillo MD.

giography for the detection of calcification was 40 %, with a specificity of 82 %. When calcification was visible on angiography, the arc of calcification was likely to be large and superficial on IVUS. The only predictor of calcification by IVUS was angiographic calcification elsewhere in the coronary tree. In addition, angiographic calcification at remote sites was a predictor of angiographically undetected calcification at the target lesion site. Three additional studies, all from the Washington Hospital Center, have expanded our current knowledge of this problem.[41-43] In the first report,[41] IVUS was able to detect calcification in 73 % of target coronary lesions, whereas angiography only detected calcification in 38 % of these lesions. Overall, concordance was relatively low. Again, the ability of angiography to identify target lesion calcification depended on its location, the presence of calcification in the reference segment, the arc of calcification at the lesion, and the arc of superficial calcification. In a subsequent study,[42] IVUS was used to determine coronary calcification in 1442 consecutive patients. Overall, 72 % of lesions were calcified (mean arc of calcification = 110°). The arc of calcification was larger in older patients, in patients with stable angina, and in lesions with a larger plaque burden at the target site or in the reference segment. However, calcification was not related to the degree of luminal compromise. Finally, the same group demonstrated with IVUS[43] that there was a consistent relation between decreasing vessel lumen size and calcification of the target lesion, the calcification length, and the arc of calcification. However, there was no relation between decreasing angiographic vessel size and angiographic calcification. This finding underscores that coronary calcification is particularly common in small vessels with severe lesions, but these findings are not clearly appreciated by angiography.

«Acute lesions,» that is, those causing acute coronary syndromes, are complex by definition. Classically, the angiographic «footprint» of a ruptured plaque has been well described and different classifications have been proposed.[44-46] A filling defect near the culprit lesion, in an adequate clinical setting, constitutes the hallmark of intracoronary thrombus (Figs. 4-11, 4-12, 4-13). However, in most cases, angiography cannot identify the anatomic substrate of these acute lesions.[2-4, 44-46] In addition, when the lumen is complex, some arbitrarily selected projections may misrepresent the extent of narrowing. Orthogonal multiple views may improve recognition of the coronary anatomy in these situations.

«Results of coronary intervention.» After intervention, a hazy, artifactually enlarged silhouette frequently overestimates the actual gain in minimal lumen diameter and cross-sectional area. Plaque fracture caused by the balloon exaggerates the extent of luminal irregularity and eccentricity, leading to unclear luminal contours (haziness) with a broadened silhouette that typically causes overestimation of the true extent of lumen gain.[2-4, 47] After balloon angioplasty, an intimal tear or fracture with variable degrees of medial penetration is recognized.[2-4, 47] These cracks, which extend from the lumen for variable lengths into the plaque, improve vessel patency by creating additional channels for coronary blood flow.[47] However, these channels are difficult to identify by angiography and may account for the hazy appearance of lesions after dilation. The false impression obtained from angiography may explain why some angiographic parameters, used as surrogates for clinical end-points, often fail to demonstrate clinical value. On angiographic grounds alone, it is sometimes difficult to differentiate between the true lumen and the dissected lumen. In addition, a better angiographic image can be obtained from an intervention yielding a complex lumen than from an intervention resulting in a circular lumen, despite a similar final increase in lumen area. Conversely, resistance to flow can be higher in a lumen with complex tears than in a round, smooth lumen, despite a similar absolute lumen area.[1, 47]

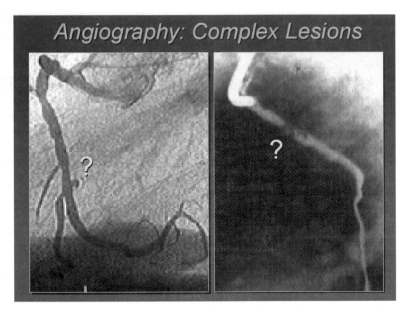

Figure 4-11. Right: Coronary angiogram of an ulcerated lesion on the right coronary artery. The lesion was not associated to significant lumen narrowing. Left: Complex angiographic lesion with an associated intraluminal filling defect on a degenerated old saphenous vein graft.

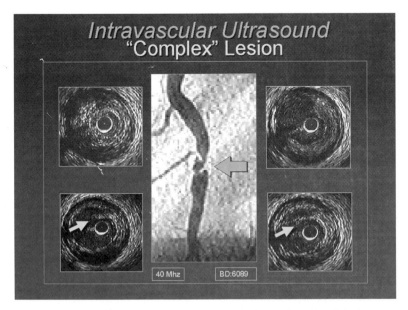

Figure 4-12. Complex angiographic lesion on the middle segment of the right coronary artery in a patient with unstable angina. Intravascular ultrasound demonstrated the pathologic substrate, namely, a ruptured soft plaque with positive remodeling. The site of plaque rupture was accurately identified by intravascular ultrasound.

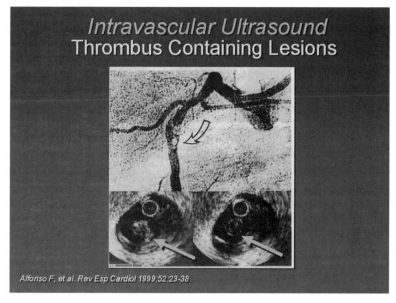

Figure 4-13. Angiographic image of intraluminal filling defect on the proximal right coronary artery after successful thrombolysis. On intravascular ultrasound, a pediculated thrombus was recognized. The thrombus originated from a soft plaque that caused just mild lumen narrowing.

In addition, the mechanism of lumen gain after balloon angioplasty is difficult to elucidate using angiography alone. IVUS studies, however, have often demonstrated plaque fracture and dissection, as well as stretching of the total vessel. Plaque compression appears to play a minor role, whereas axial redistribution of the plaque burden can also be demonstrated. After directional atherectomy, the most striking discrepancy consists of a significant amount of residual plaque burden despite an optimal angiographic result.[2-4, 47] This may be relevant because in many studies, such as the GUIDE II,[48] residual plaque burden was the most powerful predictor of clinical outcome. Obviously, residual plaque burden cannot be detected by angiography. Finally, probably more importantly than the results of randomized trials, the cardinal feature motivating the exponential growth of coronary stenting is its ability to «readily ensure an optimal coronary luminogram.» The initial angiographic gratification of coronary stenting (a smooth, round, large lumen) is

more real —as assessed by IVUS— than the frequently misleading angiographic result obtained after balloon angioplasty. Therefore, it can produce better long-term angiographic results. On the other hand, many stents are nearly invisible on angiography and IVUS examination may be required to precisely define the position of the stent struts with respect to angiographic landmarks or even in relation to luminal stenoses.

Quantitative Coronary Angiographic Analysis

Quantitative coronary angiography (QCA) has been used in the last decade to ensure accurate and reproducible measurements of luminal diameters and stenosis severity. In fact, this technique has become the gold standard for clinical studies and research purposes.[49, 59] The advent of QCA introduced a new jargon of terms that soon became widely accepted in research, including minimal lumen diameter, acute gain, late loss, and the loss index. This challenged the relevance of the traditional visual method for assessing the severity of stenosis, namely percent diameter stenosis. QCA constitutes an excellent and widely available tool for coronary lumen measurement, herein we will review some of its limitations.

Computerized analysis of vessel borders is an objective and highly reproducible technique that yields (in contrast with visual assessment) a very low inter- and intraobserver variability.[29] However, reproducibility should not be confused with accuracy. In fact, the performance of QCA may be influenced by a wide array of factors.[49-59] Even in experienced core laboratories, significant differences may be detected in relation to minor technical issues, and comparisons between different algorithms may yield major differences. Early studies suggested a low variability in measurements of minimal lumen diameter using the same frame (standard deviation 0.08 mm) but increased significantly (standard deviation 0.14) with measurements from different frames. Such measurements appear to be independent of vessel size and stenosis severity.[58] The performance (accuracy and precision) of QCA-derived measurements against true values obtained from phantom stenoses has been validated recently.[53] Minimum lumen diameter is simple to obtain and more reproducible than other potential end-points because it does not depend on measurements of the «normal» arterial dimension. Therefore, its major advantage is that it does not take vessel size into account. The diameter of stenosis is more appealing clinically and still widely appreciated, but less reproducible. Initial studies suggested[58] that changes of 0.4 mm for minimal lumen diameter and 15 % for percentage stenosis are required to define progression or regression in coronary artery disease. Coronary angiographic changes could then be used as surrogate end-points for clinical trials. Interestingly, in a comprehensive review of all available progression-regression studies,[30] the reported changes in positive studies were small (<0.3 mm or 10 % change). In fact, in many studies the reported changes fell within the standard deviation of repeated measurements. The primary aim of measurements from serial coronary arteriograms is to detect changes in the extent and severity of coronary atherosclerosis reliably and accurately. However, angiography simply «*does not measure atherosclerosis.*» In this regard, the assessment of plaque area (and its three-dimensional counterpart, plaque volume) was also initially attempted using QCA. This required the use of very restrictive assumptions and was defined as the area between the reference vessel boundary (extrapolated proximally to distally) and the lumen boundary at the lesion site. However, as has been extensively discussed in this book, such measurements are, by definition, incorrect and since the advent of IVUS have been largely abandoned.

On the other hand, it is important to keep in mind that in the clinical setting most of the limitations of conventional angiography also apply to QCA.[49-59] As a matter of fact, some angiographers still believe that visual assessment of stenosis based on moving images may better integrate anatomic details than a still frame taken in end-diastole. This may explain why QCA is not systematically performed on-line during coronary interventions in many laboratories throughout the world. In a critical study, Gurley et al.[59] analyzed the potential value of QCA for routine clinical use. Of all the lesions unanimously identified by four experienced angiographers, nearly 50 % could not be analyzed with a fully automatic arterial border detection system. The reasons were the presence of stenosis at bifurcations (72 %), diffuse stenosis (44 %), excessive vessel tortuosity (22 %), and poor image quality 28 %. This suggests that QCA is impractical for routine use for diagnostic purposes. However, in that study the same algorithm was very successful for the analysis (in pre-selected frames) of discrete lesions referred for coronary angioplasty.

Currently, two different QCA techniques are used, namely edge-detection QCA and videodensitometry.[49-59] In edge-detection QCA, the boundaries of the selected coronary segment are automatically detected by a threshold method, an algorithm using the weighted sum of the first and second derivative functions of the brightness profile. Smoothing procedures and minimal cost algorithms are applied to detect lumen contours. The reference segment is either selected by the operator or automatically interpolated by the system. The user-defined method has a higher variability. The catheter, used as a scaling device, allows absolute measurements. Eventually, luminal cross-sectional areas are «calculated» from orthogonal projections (assuming an elliptic model) or from the worst view (as a circle).[49-59] *Therefore, it is important to remember that QCA does not directly measure luminal area but rather provides «an estimate» based on geometric assumptions and minimal lumen diameter.* All QCA algorithms require a pathline as an approximation of the course of the vessel segment. In the minimum-cost algorithm, the image is analyzed along scanlines perpendicular to the selected pathline. For each point to be detected, first and second derivative values of the brightness profile are calculated. Points with a low-cost value (inverse value of the weighted sum of the first and second derivatives) have a higher probability of being included in the detected contour. Then, a path of minimal cost is identified within the matrix of values. This methodology is fast and robust.[29, 60] However, when the scanline is not perpendicular but nearly parallel to the true vessel boundary, most edge information is entirely discarded. This is a major limitation in the analysis of complex lesions with sharp, twisting edges. Although manual editing may partially overcome this problem, whenever gross errors are detected, this sacrifices precision and reproducibility. Nevertheless,

the recent development of the «gradient field transform,» based on the *shortest-path* algorithm[61] rather than the classical *smoothing* algorithm, renders eccentric and complex lesions more amenable to reliable edge-detection QCA analysis. The gradient field transform is not limited in its search directions and incorporates directional information on the brightness of each point in the image assessed from all directions. Therefore, it is especially suited for lesions with abrupt changes in luminal shape, where minimum-cost algorithms severely overestimate the diameter of the obstruction.[61]

Alternatively, videodensitometry calculates the depth of the column of dye and appears to be superior to the edge-detection method in eccentric lesions.[58] However, this technique also requires the assumption that a linear relation exists between the image optical density and thickness of contrast material. Therefore, ideal radiographic conditions, absence of calcifications, a homogeneous background, and a homogeneous mixture of blood and dye are required.[58] The cross-sectional area function is obtained from brightness values calibrated for the amount of X-ray absorption after subtracting the background contribution. Accordingly, this technique measures vessel dimensions more independently of lesion contour and luminal shape, and is relatively independent of the projection selected for analysis. In fact, when IVUS is used as the standard for lumen area measurements, videodensitometry always yields results closer to IVUS measurements than edge-detection QCA.[54, 55] This difference may be striking in patients with complex lesions and following coronary interventions.

Finally, we should address the problem of «*serial studies*». Serial angiographic studies need to pay special attention to the details of image acquisition to ensure valid comparisons. These include attainment of maximal vasodilation, the use of similar radiographic equipment, the same position of the table and intensifier, and precise reproduction of the selected projections. In addition, these studies should avoid producing motion vessel artifacts (end-diastolic frames selected from runs obtained while the patient holds his or her breath). The region of interest (and the catheter tip) should be relatively centered in the image to avoid pincushion distortion. Furthermore, angiographic sizing requires calibration to correct for radiographic magnification. However, the density of the catheter wall may also influence QCA measurements. The varying composition of the catheter in different brands and sizes results in different X-ray attenuation. Calculated catheter diameter varies in relation to the actual catheter diameter as determined by measurements with a micrometer. Therefore, similar catheters (baseline, post-intervention and follow-up) should be used to guarantee appropriate comparisons. In addition, contrast-filled catheters cannot be compared with similar, but empty, catheters.

MORPHOLOGICAL AND PHYSIOLOGICAL CONSIDERATIONS: ANGIOGRAPHY VS THE NEW INTRACORONARY TECHNIQUES

Morphological Considerations

Most of the limitations of coronary angiography were well established before the advent of IVUS. However, only the systematic use of IVUS during routine diagnostic and interventional procedures was able to put into perspective the striking morphological disparities frequently revealed by the two techniques in many patients.[1-4] Accordingly, angiographic limitations ceased to be a potential theoretical concern, becoming «real problems» in patients in which a correct diagnosis was required for the decision-making process involved in clinical management. The unique ability of IVUS to provide a direct tomographic visualization of the atherosclerotic plaque *in vivo*[1-4] completely challenged our traditional approach to the

study of coronary artery disease, disease of the vessel wall. The two key contributions of IVUS to assessing coronary morphology were *a*) its ability to image the vessel wall and *b*) its unique tomographic perspective. Tomographic visualization of IVUS allows full visualization of the entire circumference of the vessel wall, not just two surfaces.[2-3] This explains why IVUS provides valuable information in most cases where angiographic information may be misleading. The exhaustive and comprehensive information provided by IVUS about both atherosclerotic involvement of the vessel wall and plaque impingement on the coronary lumen has been a major breakthrough in our understanding of coronary atherosclerosis and has had major clinical implications, as outlined above. Measurements of IVUS and edge-detection QCA correlate closely in undiseased vessels with circular lumens. However, when lumen shape becomes progressively more irregular, the results of angiography and IVUS diverge significantly.[1,49-56] In diseased coronary arteries, only a moderate correlation has been found between the two techniques (r = 0.5 to 0.8), with standard errors in the range of 0.5 mm. This discrepancy is best detected after interventions where, in fact, correlations between these two imaging modalities can be very poor.[49-56]

Physiological Aspects

The second challenge that angiography is facing today is physiological assessment. Coronary «cosmetology»[1] should never be the driving force for performing coronary interventions. With this in mind, the following questions are relevant: What is an angiographically severe lesion? What does it represent —from a physiological or functional point of view— for the patient? Many studies have demonstrated a marked disparity between the apparent severity of coronary lesions on angiography and their physiological consequences. IVUS has been invaluable in providing morphological insights that cannot be obtained with angiography, but this technique can also yield some indirect physiological information.[62-66] In angiographically ambiguous or indeterminate coronary lesions, IVUS may be helpful not only in the decision to intervene or defer intervention, but also in selecting the interventional device of choice. Intermediate stenoses (angiographic severity ranging from 40 % to 60 %) are particularly problematic, especially in patients with a symptomatic status that is difficult to assess.[62-66] In some studies, IVUS was useful in changing the operator's appreciation of target vessel severity, leading to a change in the decision to perform or defer the intervention.[67]

Nevertheless, the use of conventional angiography or even QCA to assess the physiological implications of a given coronary stenosis has only been seriously challenged by the introduction of new techniques for direct intracoronary physiological assessment, namely Doppler studies and the pressure wire. As will be discussed in the corresponding chapters, these techniques are quite different but both of them rely largely on the achievement of maximal vasodilation of the microvascular bed.

In animal models with coronary constrictors, Gould demonstrated that coronary flow reserve deteriorates when the reduction of luminal diameter exceeds a determined value.[69] Stenotic flow reserve values can also be obtained from several QCA systems but, in general, rely on multiple angiographic assumptions and are therefore frequently unreliable and have been abandoned since the introduction of techniques that provide direct physiological information. The method of Kirkeeide et al.[70] allows stenotic flow reserve to be calculated as an index of the functional significance of a narrowing based on lesion morphology and geometric dimensions. Coronary flow reserve derived from digital angiography, intracoronary Doppler, or positron emission tomography[71-74] has revealed major discrepancies between the angiographic severity of coronary lesions and

their physiological consequences. Interestingly, coronary flow reserve remains normal until the percent diameter stenosis approaches 75 %.[1] From this point on, a progressive fall in coronary flow reserve is encountered with further increases in percentage diameter stenosis. However, minor differences in luminal diameter, within the range of the limits of angiographic resolution, may be responsible for an abnormal flow reserve and, consequently, for differentiating between moderate and severe lesions. Currently, coronary flow reserve is readily obtained with intracoronary Doppler.[72]

In addition, the pressure wire —with its ability to measure the fractional flow reserve— has emerged as a major tool for physiological evaluation. Therefore, comparison of angiographic findings with this new index, currently considered the «gold standard» for the functional evaluation of the severity of epicardial coronary stenosis, has generated great interest. Piljs et al.[9] demonstrated that the hyperemic absolute distal coronary pressure, rather than the resting pressure gradient, was closely related to the potential of a given coronary stenosis to induce ischemia and reflects both antegrade and collateral blood flow. Therefore it is a lesion-specific parameter that is very attractive to interventional cardiologists.

The possibility of readily obtaining «angiographic gratification» is a strong inducement to proceed with a coronary intervention on any «angiographically significant» lesion following only the «oculostenotic reflex,» with complete disregard for the evidence of inducible ischemia or the results of physiologically based techniques.[1] Nevertheless, we should resist this temptation because the above findings remind us of the hazards of formulating clinical decisions solely on the basis of angiographic estimates of lesion severity.

REFERENCES

1. Topol TJ, Nissen SE. Our preoccupation with coronary lumenology: the dissociation

between clinical and angiographic findings in ischemic heart disease. *Circulation* 1995; 92:2333-2342.

2. Nissen SE, Yock P. Intravascular ultrasound: novel pathophysiological insights and current clinical applications. *Circulation* 2001; 103:604-616.

3. Mintz GS, Nissen SE, Anderson WD, et al. American College of Cardiology clinical expert consensus document on standards for acquisition, measurement and reporting of intravascular ultrasound studies (IVUS). *J Am Coll Cardiol* 2001; 37:1478-1492.

4. Di Mario C, Görge G, Peters R, et al. Clinical application and image interpretation in intracoronary ultrasound. *Europ Heart J* 1998; 19:207-219.

5. Mintz GS, Kent KM, Pichard AD, Satler LF, Popma JJ, Leon MB. Contribution of inadequate arterial remodeling to the development of focal coronary artery stenoses. An intravascular ultrasound study. *Circulation* 1997; 95:1791- 1798.

6. Botas J, Clark DA, Pinto F, Chenzbraun A, Fischell TA. Balloon angioplasty results in increasing segmental coronary distensibility: a likely mechanism of percutaneous transluminal coronary angioplasty. *J Am Coll Cardiol* 1994; 23:1043-1052.

7. Alfonso F, Goicolea J, Hernandez R, Goncalves M, Segovia J, Bañuelos C, Zarco P, Macaya C. Angioscopic findings during coronary angioplasty of coronary occlusions. *J Am Coll Cardiol* 1995; 26:135-141.

8. Abizaid A, Mintz GS, Pichard A, Kent KM, Satler LF, Walsh CL, Popma JJ, Leon MB. Clinical, intravascular ultrasound and quantitative angiographic determinants of the coronary flow reserve before and after percutaneous transluminal coronary angioplasty. *Am J Cardiol* 1998; 82:423-428.

9. Pijls NH, De Bruyne B, Peels K, van der Voort PH, Bonnier HJ, Bartunek J, Koolen JJ. Measurement of fractional flow reserve to assess the functional severity of coronary-artery stenoses. *N Engl J Med* 1996; 334: 1703-1708.

10. Kern MJ. Coronary physiology revisited. Practical insights from the cardiac catheterization laboratory. *Circulation* 2000; 101:1344-1351.

11. Gray CR, Hoffman HA, Hammond WS, Miller KL, Oseasohn RO. Correlation of arteriographic and pathologic findings in the coronary arteries in man. *Circulation* 1962; 26:494-499.

12. Vlodaver Z, Frech R, Van Tassel RA, Edwards JE. Correlation of antemortem coronary arteriogram and the postmortem specimen. *Circulation* 1973; 47:162-169.

13. Arnett EN, Isner JN, Redwood DR, Kent KM, Baker WP, Ackerstein H, Roberts WC. Coronary artery narrowing in coronary heart disease: comparison of cineangiographic and necropsy findings. *Ann Intern Med* 1979; 91:350-356.

14. Grondin CM, Dyrda I, Pasternac A, Campeau L, Bourassa MG, Lesperance J. Discrepancies between cineangiographic and postmortem findings in patients with coronary artery disease and recent coronary revascularization. *Circulation* 1974; 49: 703-708.

15. Roberts WC, Jones AA. Quantitation of coronary artery narrowing at necropsy in sudden coronary death. Analysis of 31 patients and comparison with 25 control subjects. *Am J Cardiol* 1979; 44:39-46.

16. Dietz WA, Tobis JM, Isner JM. Failure of angiography to accurately depict the extent of coronary artery narrowing in three fatal cases of percutaneous transluminal coronary angioplasty. *J Am Coll Cardiol* 1992; 19: 1261-1270.

17. Zir LM, Miller SW, Dinsmore RE, Gilbert JP, Harthorne JW. Interobserver variability in coronary angiography. *Circulation* 1976; 53:627-632.

18. Galbraith JE, Murphy ML, de Soyza N. Coronary angiogram interpretation. Interobserver variability. *JAMA* 1978; 240:2053-2056.

19. Enos WF, Holmes RH, Beyer J. Coronary artery disease among United States soldiers killed in action in Korea: Preliminary report. *JAMA* 1953; 152:1090-1093.

20. McNamara JJ, Molot MA, Stremple JF, et al. Coronary artery disease in combat casualties in Vietnam. *JAMA* 1971; 216:1185-1187.

21. Velican D, Velican C. Atherosclerotic involvement of the coronary arteries of adolescents and young adults. *Atherosclerosis* 1980; 36:449-460.

22. Strong JP. Landmark perspective. Coronary atherosclerosis in soldiers a clue to the natural history of atherosclerosis in the young. *JAMA* 1986; 256:2863-2866.

23. Tuzcu EM, Kapadia SR, Tutar E, Ziada KM, Hoobs RE, McCarthy PM, Young JB, Nissen SE. High prevalence of coronary atherosclerosis in asymptomatic teenagers and young adults. Evidence from intravascular ultrasound. *Circulation* 2001; 103: 2705-2710.

24. Isner JM, Kishel J, Kent KM, Ronan JA, Ross AM, Roberts WC. Accuracy of angiographic determination of left main coronary arterial narrowing. Angiographic-Histologic correlative analysis in 28 patients. *Circulation* 1981; 63:1056-1065.

25. Glagov S, Weisenberg E, Zarins CK, Stankunavicious R, Koletti GK. Compensatory enlargement of human atherosclerotic coronary arteries. *N Engl J Med* 1987; 316:1371-1375.

26. Sones FM, Shirey EK. Cine coronary arteriography. *Mod Concepts in Cardiovasc Dis* 1962; 31:735-738.

27. Detre KM, Kelsey SF, Passamani ER, et al. Reliability of assessing change with sequential coronary angiography. *Am Heart J* 1982: 104:816-823.

28. Kalbfleisch SJ, McGillem MJ, Pinto IM, et al. Comparison of automated quantitative coronary angiography with caliper measurements of percent diameter stenosis. *Am J Cardiol* 1990; 65:1181:1184.

29. Mancini GBJ. Quantitative coronary arteriographic methods in the interventional catheterization laboratory: an update and perspective. *J Am Coll Cardiol* 1991; 17:23B-33B.

30. Hong MK, Mintz GS, Popma JJ, Kent KM, Pichard AD, Satler LF, Leon MB. Limitations of angiography for analysing coronary atherosclerosis progression or regression. *Ann Intern Med* 1994; 121;348-354.

31. Brennecke R, Burgel U, Simon R, et al. American College of Cardiology / European Society of Cardiology international study of angiographic data compression phase III. Measurements of image quality differences at varying levels of data compression. *Eur Heart J* 2000; 21:687-696.

32. Tuinenburg JC, Koning G, Hekking E, et al. American College of Cardiology / European Society of Cardiology international study of angiographic data compression phase II. The effect of varying JPEG data compression levels on the quantitative assessment of the degree of stenosis severity in digital coronary angiography. *Europ Heart J* 2000; 21:679-686.

33. Nissen SE. Radiographic principles in cardiac catheterization. In Roubin GS, Califf RM, O'Neill W, Phillips H, Stack R. Eds. Interventional Cardiac Catheterization. Principles and Practice. New York, NY. *Churchill Livingstone Inc.* 1993; 409-425.

34. Takahashi T, Honda Y, Rosso RJ, Fitzgerald PJ. Intravascular ultrasound and quantitative coronary angiography. *Cathet Cardiovasc Interv* 2002; 55:118-128.

35. Abizaid AS, Mintz GS, Abizaid A, Mehran R, Lansky AJ, Pichard AD, Satler LF, Wu H, Kent KM, Leon MB. One-year follow-up after intravascular ultrasound assessment of moderate left main coronary artery disease in patients with ambiguous angiograms. *J Am Coll Cardiol* 1999; 34:707-715.

36. Hermiller JB, Buller CE, Tenaglia AN, et al. Unrecognized left main coronary artery disease in patients undergoing interventional procedures. *Am J Cardiol* 1993; 71:153-176.

37. Waller BF. The eccentricity of coronary atherosclerotic plaque. Morphological considerations and clinical relevance. *Clin Cardiol* 1989; 12;14-20.

38. Waller BF. Coronary luminal shape and the arc of disease free wall: morphologic observations and clinical relevance. *J Am Coll Cardiol* 1985; 6:1100-1101.

39. Mintz GS, Popma JJ, Pichard A, Kent KM, Satler LF, Chuang YC, DeFalco RA, Leon MB. Limitations of angiography in the assessment of plaque distribution in coronary artery disease. A systematic study of target lesion eccentricity in 1446 lesions. *Circulation* 1996; 93:924-931.

40. Tuzcu EM, Berkalp B, De Franco AC, et al. The dilemma of diagnosing coronary calcification: Angiographic versus intravascular ultrasound. *J Am Coll Cardiol* 1996; 15:832-838.

41. Mintz GS, Popma JJ, Pichard AD, et al. Patterns of calcification in coronary artery disease. A statistical analysis of intravascular

ultrasound and angiographic lesions. *Circulation* 1995; 91:1959-1965.

42. Mintz GS, Pichard AD, Popma JJ, et al. Determinants and correlates of target lesion calcium in coronary artery disease: a clinical angiographic and intravascular ultrasound study. *J Am Coll Cardiol* 1997; 29: 268-274.

43. Mintz GS, Pichard AD, Kent KM, et al. Interrelation of coronary angiographic reference lumen size and intravascular ultrasound target lesion calcium. *Am J Cardiol* 1998; 81:387-391.

44. Ambrose JA, Winters SL, Arora RR, Eng A, Riccio A, Gorlin R, Fuster V. Angiographic evolution of coronary artery morphology in unstable angina. *J Am Coll Cardiol* 1986; 7:472-478.

45. Alfonso F, Fernandez-Ortiz A, Goicolea J, Hernandez R, Segovia J, Phillips P, Bañuelos C, Macaya C. Angioscopic evaluation of angiographically complex lesions. *Am Heart J* 1997; 134:703-711.

46. von Birgelen C, Klinkhart W, Mintz GS, et al. Plaque distribution and vascular remodeling of ruptured and nonruptured plaques in the same vessel: an intravascular ultrasound study in vivo. *J Am Coll Cardiol* 2001; 37:1864- 1870.

47. Waller BF. «Crackers, Breakers, Stretchers, Drillers, Scrapers, Shavers, Burners, Welders and Melters» The future treatment of atherosclerotic coronary artery disease? A clinical-morphologic assessment. *J Am Coll Cardiol* 1989; 13;969-987.

48. Fitzgerald PJ, Yock PG. Mechanisms and outcomes of angioplasty and atherectomy assessed by intravascular ultrasound imaging. *J Clin Ultrasound* 1993; 21:579-588.

49. Alfonso F. Videodensitometric versus edge-detection quantitative angiography. Insights from intravascular ultrasound imaging. *Europ Heart J* 2000; 21:604-607.

50. Nakamura S, Mahon DJ, Maheswaran B, Gutfinger DE, Colombo A, Tobis JM. An explanation for discrepancy between angiographic and intravascular ultrasound measurements after percutaneous transluminal coronary angioplasty. *J Am Coll Cardiol* 1995; 25:633-639.

51. Alfonso F, Macaya C, Goicolea J, Iñiguez A, Hernandez R, Zamorano J, MJ Pérez-Vizcayno, Zarco P. Intravascular ultrasound imaging of angiographically normal coronary segments in patients with coronary artery disease. *Am Heart J* 1994;127:536-544.

52. von Birgelen C, Umans VA, Di Mario C, Keane D, Gil R, Prati F, de Feyter P, Serruys PW. Mechanisms of high-speed rotational atherectomy and adjunctive balloon angioplasty revisited by quantitative coronary angiography: edge-detection versus videodensitometry. *Am Heart J* 1995; 130:405-412.

53. Keane D, Haase J, Slager CJ, van Swijndregt EM, Lehmann KG, Ozaki Y, Di Mario C, Kirkeeide R, Serruys PW. Comparative validation of quantitative coronary angiography systems. Results and implications from a multicenter study using a standardized approach. *Circulation* 1995; 91:2147-2183.

54. Ozaki Y, Violaris AG, Kobayashi T, Keane D, Camenzind E, Di Mario C, de Feyter P, Roelandt JRTC, Serruys PW. Comparison of coronary luminal quantification obtained from intracoronary ultrasound and both geometric and videodensitometric quantitative angiography before and after balloon angioplasty and directional atherectomy. *Circulation* 1997; 96:491-499.

55. Peters RJG, Kok WEM, Pasterkamp G, von Birgelen C, Prins M, Serruys PPW, on behalf of the PICTURE study group. Videodensitometric quantitative angiography after coronary balloon angioplasty, compared to edge-detection quantitative angiography and intracoronary ultrasound imaging. *Europ Heart J* 2000; 21:654-661.

56. von Birgelen C, Kutryk MJB, Gil R, Ozaki Y, Di Mario C, Roelandt JRTC, de Feyter PJ, Serruys PW. Quantification of the minimal luminal cross-sectional area after coronary stenting by two- and three-dimensional intravascular ultrasound versus edge-detection and videodensitometry. *Am J Cardiol* 1996; 78:520-525.

57. Bermejo J, Botas J, García E, Elizaga J, Osende J, Soriano J, Abeytua M, Delcan JL. Mechanisms of residual lumen stenosis after high pressure stent implantation: a quantitative coronary angiography and intravascular ultrasound study. *Circulation* 1998; 98:112-118.

58. Waters D, Lesperance J, Craven TE, Hudon G, Gillam LD. Advantages and limitations

of serial coronary arteriography for the assessment of progression and regression of coronary atherosclerosis. Implications for clinical trials. *Circulation* 1993; 87(Suppl II): II38-II47.

59. Gurley JC, Nissen SE, Booth DC, DeMaria AN. Influence of operator and patient dependent variables on the suitability of automatic quantitative coronary arteriography for routine clinical use. *J Am Coll Cardiol* 1992; 19;1237-1243.

60. Reiber JHC, Serruys PW, Kooyman CJ et al. Assessment of short-medium-and long-term variations in arterial dimensions from computer assisted quantification of coronary cineangiograms. *Circulation* 1985;71;280-288.

61. van der Zwet PM, Reiber JHC. A new approach for the quantitation of complex lesion morphology: The gradient field transform, basic principles and validation results. *J Am Coll Cardiol* 1994; 24:216-224.

62. Takagi A, Tsurumi Y, Ishii Y, Suzuki K, Kawana M, Kasanuki H. Clinical potential of intravascular ultrasound for physiological assessment of coronary stenosis. Relationship between quantitative ultrasound tomography and pressure derived fractional flow reserve. *Circulation* 1999;100: 250-255.

63. Baumgart D, Haude M, Goerge G, et al. Improved assessment of coronary stenosis severity using the relative flow velocity reserve. *Circulation* 1998; 98:40-46.

64. Nishioka T, Amanullah AM, Luo H, Berglund MD, Kim CJ, Nagai T, Hakamata N, Katsushika S, Uehata A, Takase B, Isojima K, Berman DS, Siegel RJ. Clinical validation of intravascular ultrasound imaging for assessment of coronary stenosis severity. Comparison with stress myocardial perfusion imaging. *J Am Coll Cardiol* 1999; 33:1870- 1878.

65. Abizaid AS, Mintz GS, Mehran R, Abizaid A, Lansky AJ, Pichard AD, Satler LF, Wu H, Pappas C, Kent KM, Leon MB. Long-term follow-up after percutaneous transluminal coronary angioplasty was not performed based on intravascular ultrasound

findings. Importance of lumen dimensions. *Circulation* 1999; 100;256-261.

66. Briguori C, Anzuini A, Airoldi F, Gimelli G, Nishida T, Adamian M, Di Mario C, Colombo A. Intravascular ultrasound criteria for the assessment of the functional significance of intermediate coronary artery stenoses and correlation with fractional flow reserve. *Am J Cardiol* 2001; 87:136-141.

67. Lee DY, Eigler N, Luo H, et al. Effect of intracoronary ultrasound imaging on clinical decision making. *Am Heart J* 1995; 129:1084-1093.

68. Mintz GS, Pichard AD, Kovach JA, et al. Impact of preintervention intravascular ultrasound imaging on transcatheter treatment strategies in coronary artery disease. *Am J Cardiol* 1994; 73:423-430.

69. Gould KL. Quantification of coronary artery stenosis in vivo. *Circ Res* 1985; 57:341-353.

70. Kirkeeide RL, Gould KL, Parsel L. Assessment of coronary stenosis by myocardial perfusion imaging during pharmacologic coronary vasodilation VII. Validation of coronary flow reserve as a single integrated functional measure of stenosis severity reflecting all its geometric dimensions. *J Am Coll Cardiol* 1986; 7:103-113.

71. White CW, Wright CB, Doty DB, et al. Does visual interpretation of the coronary arteriogram predict the physiological importance of a coronary stenosis? *N Engl J Med* 1984;310:819-824.

72. Kern MJ, Donohue TJ, Aguirre FV, et al. Assessment of angiographically intermediate coronary artery stenosis using the Doppler flow wire. *Am J Cardiol* 1993; 71:26D-33D.

73. Vogel RA, LeFree MT, Bates ER, et al. Application of digital techniques to selective coronary arteriography: use of myocardial appearance time to measure coronary flow reserve. *Am Heart J* 1983; 107:153-164.

74. Nissen SE, Elion JL, Booth DC. Value and limitations of computer analysis of digital subtraction angiography in the assessment of coronary flow reserve. *Circulation* 1986: 73:562-571.

SECTION II

Intracoronary Ultrasound

5

Historic Perspective. Imaging Catheters. Practical Issues and Technological Developments

Javier Botas, MD
Fernando Alfonso, MD

Basic principles for obtaining images and equipment available. Spatial orientation, image acquisition and the most frequent errors and artifacts. Tissue characterization. References.

Contrast angiography has, until now, been the gold standard for the assessment of the existence and severity of coronary atheromatosis. Nonetheless, this technique only provides a two-dimensional representation of the silhouette of the vessel's lumen and cannot directly visualize the object of study, the atheroma plaque. By the very nature of the examination, angiography has numerous limitations, which are particularly evident when compared with histology,[1-4] and have been reviewed in detail in chapter 4. These limitations have spurred interest in developing *techniques,* such as ultrasound, that enable tomographic assessment of the vessel and provide a direct view of the item under analysis or intervention, namely the atheroma plaque, also allowing a certain degree of tissue characterization. In addition to the direct visualization of the vessel wall, there are other direct advantages of using ultrasound in comparison with angiography. Ultrasound systems use an electronically generated scale so that measurements can be made directly using planimetry. There is no need for calibration as in angiography, where it is necessary to correct for radiographic enlargement, a frequent source of error. In addition, the inherent tomographic

nature of ultrasound is particularly useful for resolving situations that are especially difficult to assess using angiography, such as the presence of diffuse disease, ostial or bifurcation lesions, eccentric plaques, or arterial segments that have been shortened or darkened by branch crossover.[1-7]

Ultrasound is routinely used in other areas of cardiovascular medicine to make non-invasive transcutaneous assessments of the vessel architecture, but this can only be done in limited areas of the peripheral circulatory system.[1-10] It is also possible, using transesophageal echocardiography, to assess the most proximal segment of the coronary arteries. Once more, this is feasible only in a small number of patients and the image quality usually is not suitable for diagnostic use.[11-13] Furthermore, epicardial echography has been used in operating theaters for the study of coronary arteries, obtaining images of sufficient quality and further confirming that angiography underestimates the degree of coronary disease.[14] The use of ultrasound to study coronary anatomy from inside the vessel is more recent. This is fundamentally due to the technical requirements involved, including a miniature transducer and a flexible, non-traumatic transport system, elements that have only recently become available. Ultrasound catheters began to be used inside coronary arteries in the late 1980s. In 1987, Mallery et al.,[15] and in 1988, Yock et al.[16] and Pandian et al.[17] described the use of single-element systems for the assessment of the vessel wall to obtain cross-sectional images of the artery. The transducer located inside the transport catheter emits an ultrasound beam that explores the vessel, with a sweep that is perpendicular to the catheter, by rotating either the transducer or an acoustic mirror around it. In 1989, Hodgson et al.[18] described the use of a multi-element system with an integrated circuit for examining the coronary arteries. The images initially obtained with these prototypes were of poor quality, but in the last ten years the images obtained have markedly improved, and are currently comparable to that of low-powered histology. In addition, over the years the size of the transducers and catheters has decreased from 6 Fr to <3 Fr (<1 mm in diameter), thanks to miniaturization of their components. Catheters commercially available at present range from 2.6 to 3.5 Fr (0.87 to 1.17 mm), can be introduced through a 6-Fr guide catheter, and are capable of assessing even the distal segments of epicardial arteries.

BASIC IMAGING PRINCIPLES AND EQUIPMENT AVAILABLE

The sound waves used to obtain coronary images are in the spectrum of millions of cycles per second (MHz) and are therefore within the range of ultrasound (>20,000 cycles per second, inaudible to the human ear). Ultrasound waves are generated by passing an electric current through a piezoelectric element, usually ceramic, which emits sound waves as it expands and contracts in response to excitation by an electric signal. Therefore, this electric signal is transformed or transduced into a mechanical movement that creates sound waves. A small part of the transmitted waves are reflected back to the transducer, basically at the interfaces of tissues with differing acoustic impedances (Table 5-1). The magnitude of the ultrasound reflected depends on the difference in mechanical impedance of the two adjacent tissues. The greater the ability to reflect ultrasound, the greater the echogenicity and, therefore, the brighter its image representation. Reflected ultrasound reaches the transducer, which converts the signal into electrical energy and, finally, after an external process of filtering and amplification, into images. The ultrasound beam emitted by the transducer initially remains fairly parallel, gradually diverging as it goes away from the source. It is in the first part of the tightly bunched, parallel beam, known as the *near field,* that image quality and resolution are greater, when compared with the *far field.* The length of the near field depends directly on the size of the transducer, specifically, the size of its active part or aperture, and is inversely proportional to the ultrasound wavelength. The transducers used for intracoronary imaging are, logically, small and operate at high frequencies, but coronary arteries are also small, so insufficient penetration is usually not a problem. On the other hand, the high frequencies of these transducers give them an excellent spatial resolution, or a great ability to discriminate between objects close together in the image obtained. The axial spatial resolution, in the direction of the ultrasound beam, is of an order of 80-150 microns for 30-40 MHz transducers. The lateral resolution, i.e.,

Table 5-1. Attenuation Coefficients for Different Tissues at 1 MHz (25)

Tissue	Attenuation Coefficients (dB/cm)
Blood	0.2
Fat	0.6
Muscle	1.5
Bone	10

the resolution perpendicular to the ultrasound beam and to the catheter, is about 200-250 microns.[19, 20] The other factor that decisively influences image quality is the dynamic range, that is, the distribution of the gray scale of the reflected signal. The dynamic range, generally expressed in decibels, indicates the difference between the strongest and weakest signals in the gray scale. A low dynamic range provides images with few shades of gray, thus making it difficult to distinguish between different structures. A high dynamic range is, therefore, a desirable characteristic, with current systems reaching 17 to 55 decibels.

There are currently two systems of intracoronary ultrasound transducers available: mechanical and solid-state (Fig. 5-1). In the mechanical systems, a single transducer spins on its own axis at 1800 rpm (30 revolutions per second) by means of a flexible drive cable connected to an external motor drive unit. The transducer scans the vessel with an ultrasound beam perpendicular to the catheter, providing 256 scanlines for each image.[19] The transducer is located inside a protective sheath to prevent it from coming into contact with the artery and the sheath must be filled with saline solution to permit the transmission of the ultrasound waves. In fact, one of the artifacts most often responsible for poor quality imaging is inadequate purging of air from the transducer sheath.

In the solid-state or electronic systems, instead of a single transducer that spins 360°, there are an array of small transducers (up to 64 in modern systems) arranged around the circumference of the catheter, which emit, and receive, co-ordinated ultrasound signals to scan specific areas of the image. These systems do not need saline flushing and, in addition, they currently allow blood-flow to be colored to facilitate the visualization of the blood-vessel wall boundary. The images obtained are recorded on videotape or stored directly as digital data that can be later transfer onto a CD-ROM.

SPATIAL ORIENTATION, IMAGE ACQUISITION AND MOST FREQUENT ERRORS AND ARTIFACTS

It is often difficult to remain spatially oriented while looking at intravascular ultrasound images. Axial orientation, along the vessel's long axis, can be achieved by observing the take-offs of various arterial branches and correlating them with the ones viewed using angiography. It is also possible to use perivascular structures as a reference, as discussed in the following chapter on image interpretation. In order to keep oriented rotationally, attention must be paid to the perivascular structures and arterial branches. It must be remembered that intracoronary imaging with ultrasound does not have any absolute reference for up/down or left/right.

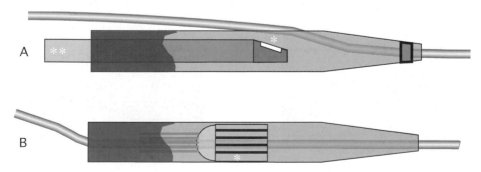

Figure 5-1. Schematic drawing of mechanical (A) and solid state systems (B). * transducer(s). ** drive shaft (see text).

It is necessary to observe the relationship of the artery under study to the take-offs of different side branches to orient the image rotationally and understand where the plaque being studied is located (see Chapter 12). Some systems allow the image to be rotated electronically to facilitate interpretation, although most operators do not routinely use this feature. For instance, if we are interrogating the anterior descending artery and the circumflex artery emerges at the 9 o'clock position, the other, more distal, branches emerging in the same direction will correspond to diagonal branches and the septal branches will appear perpendicularly to the diagonal arteries (Fig. 5-2).

Typically, an ultrasound examination is performed after administering 5,000-10,000 U of intravenous heparin. In addition, unless contraindicated, intracoronary nitroglycerin is routinely given to prevent the most frequent complication, coronary spasm (see Chapter 6). The ultrasound catheter is advanced until the transducer is located at least 10 mm distal to the area of interest and then it is pulled back, ideally to the ostium of the artery under study. Our routine practice, also used by most other groups, is to pull the transducer back automatically at a speed of 0.5 mm/s with the assistance of an external device. Automated pull-back has the advantage of allowing the operator to concentrate on interpreting the image instead of manipulating the catheter. It obtains images that can be used for longitudinal reconstruction and helps to avoid overlooking areas of potential

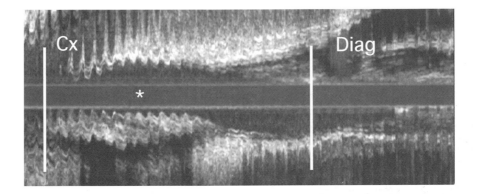

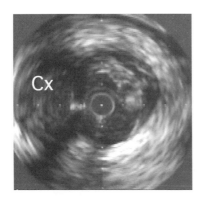 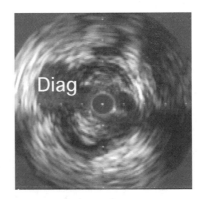

Figure 5-2.   Longitudinal view and cross sections of the distal left main, at the circumflex (Cx) artery, and left anterior descending artery, at the take-off of the first diagonal (Diag). Note that both the circumflex and the diagonal arteries emerge from the parent vessel at 9 o'clock. *IVUS catheter artifact.

interest as a result of scanning them too quickly. It is, however, a good idea, particularly if there are difficult-to-interpret areas, to return to these areas of interest under manual control for a more detailed examination. Furthermore, if necessary, contrast or saline solution can be injected through the guide catheter to better delimit any structures that are not clearly visible, such as dissections. It is important to recall that if the area of interest is located at the ostium of the left or right coronary artery, then the guide catheter must be pulled back into the aorta to truly scan the ostium with the ultrasound catheter.

If the pull-back is performed automatically, a longitudinal reconstruction can be made of the study segment, with volumetric measurements of the lumen and vessel, in addition to the cross-sectional slices.[11] Longitudinal reconstruction requires the transducer to be pulled back at a constant speed, while digitally storing each vessel cross-section acquired at equal, regular intervals. Over and above the evident interest of this type of image analysis, there are a number of limitations that should be pointed out. First of all, because of the systolic and diastolic movement of the catheter within the vessel, regardless of the pull-back movement, the intervals at which images are acquired may not be truly equal, thus limiting the volumetric analysis. This out-of-sync movement of the catheter and vessel gives rise to a characteristic *saw-tooth image* artifact (Fig. 5-3). To overcome this problem, there are systems in which image capture takes place with elec-

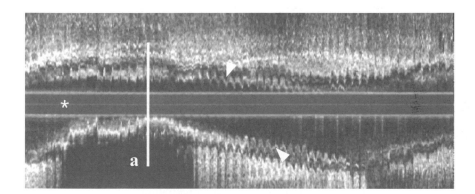

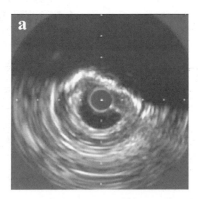

Figure 5-3. Longitudinal reconstruction showing the characteristic *saw-tooth* artifact (white arrow heads), produced by the *out-of-sync* movement of the IVUS catheter (*), and the systolic and diastolic movement of the vessel. Note the acoustic shadowing due to superficial calcification at site *a*.

trocardiographic synchronization to eliminate part of these artifacts.[12, 23] Another important limitation is that in commercially available systems, the vessel is always represented as a straight segment, without any of its natural curvature. Its on-screen presentation, although it can later be altered, can only be viewed from a single longitudinal plane, thus hindering interpretation. Despite these limitations, longitudinal reconstruction is of particular interest in studies where calculation of the volume of the plaque or intimal hyperplasia is an important goal, as in studies of regression/progression of atheromatosis, or in trials of drugs that inhibit intimal proliferation after stent implantation.

There are a number of artifacts and problems during image acquisition that may affect image quality and should be taken into account when it comes to interpreting ultrasound examinations. Most of these artifacts will be discussed in depth in the next chapter on image interpretation and are only mentioned here for the sake of reference.

From the transducer to the periphery of the vessel, the first visible artifact is known as the *ring down*, a series of bright halos surrounding the catheter that are produced by acoustic oscillations of the transducer. This artifact means that the area immediately adjacent to the catheter may not be studied well and, in fact, the acoustic size of the transducer may be somewhat greater than its anatomic size. In solid-state catheters, this artifact can be eliminated in part by using image subtraction techniques, but once more with the risk of losing potentially valid data adjacent to the catheter.

The blood around the catheter produces a characteristic speckling, which is particularly striking in areas of slow blood flow, as may occur when the catheter is placed in a severe lesion where blood flow is reduced. This speckling occurs due to the reflection of ultrasound waves from the blood's firm elements, particularly red blood cell aggregates. The transmission frequency of the transducers also influences the intensity of the signal: the higher the operating frequency (MHz) of the transducer, the greater the speckling produced by blood. In fact, this phenomenon is what has limited the use of transducer frequencies above 45 MHz, although it is possible that automatic systems for reducing blood-speckling may overcome this problem in the future. Although blood-induced speckling is not in itself an artifact, it may hinder the differentiation of the lumen and the plaque, particularly if the plaque is sparsely echogenic or there is a thrombus. The key to differentiating speckling from the arterial wall is that there is always a small continuous movement of blood, which is not seen in the thrombus. If there are difficulties in interpreting the image, saline solution or contrast can always be injected through the guide catheter to clarify the lumen-vessel wall interface.

In large vessels or in curved arterial segments, the ultrasound catheter may be placed eccentrically in the vessel lumen and its axis may not be parallel to the long axis of the vessel (Fig. 5-4). As a result, the image may be deformed and the measurements may not be accurate, so special care must be taken not to take measurements in clearly deformed images.

In mechanical systems, an additional artifact may arise, namely non-uniform rotational distortion. If the transducer cannot turn freely at a uniform speed, for example because the catheter is in a tortuous part of the artery or is compressed by a too-tight hemostatic valve, the image is distorted by the appearance of a characteristically blurred sector (see chapter 6).

In studies using longitudinal reconstruction, it is of particular interest that catheters can be displaced axially by a few millimeters within the vessel during systole and diastole. Consequently, sampling of the images to be analyzed may not coincide with the distance intervals intended, unless they are synchronized with the heartbeat.

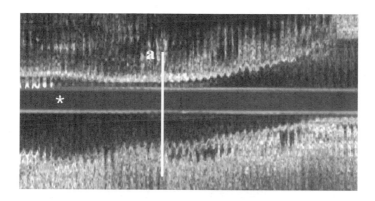

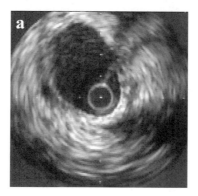

Figure 5-4. Longitudinal reconstruction showing the eccentric position of the IVUS catheter (*) within the vessel, which yields an elliptical deformation of the cross-section at site *a*.

TISSUE CHARACTERIZATION

Detailed analysis of the radiofrequency signal can provide useful information for tissue characterization.[24] The ultrasound signal reflected from the tissues is turned into electrical signals in the radiofrequency range prior to processing. In order to represent conventional ultrasound images, only the radiofrequency signal wrapper is used. The detailed analysis of the frequency components in this signal may offer information for a degree of tissue characterization, thus allowing the components of the plaque to be assessed more objectively. Despite the interest in the detailed analysis of the reflected radiofrequency signal, its usefulness in practice is as yet unconfirmed so it must be considered a research tool for the time being.

REFERENCES

1. Vlodaver Z, Frech R, Van Tassel RA, Edwards JE. Correlation of the antemortem coronary arteriogram and the postmortem specimen. *Circulation* 1973; 47:162-9.
2. Grondin CM, Dyrda I, Pasternac A, Campeau L, Bourassa MG, Lesperance J. Discrepancies between cineangiographic and postmortem findings in patients with coronary artery disease and recent myocardial revascularization. *Circulation* 1974; 49:703-8.
3. Arnett EN, Isner JM, Redwood DR, Kent KM, Baker WP, Ackerstein H, et al. Coronary artery narrowing in coronary heart dis-

ease: comparison of cineangiographic and necropsy findings. *Ann Intern Med* 1979; 91:350-6.

4. Isner JM, Kishel J, Kent KM, Ronan JA, Jr., Ross AM, Roberts WC. Accuracy of angiographic determination of left main coronary arterial narrowing. Angiographic-histologic correlative analysis in 28 patients. *Circulation* 1981; 63:1056-64.

5. Porter TR, Sears T, Xie F, Michels A, Mata J, Welsh D, et al. Intravascular ultrasound study of angiographically mildly diseased coronary arteries. *J Am Coll Cardiol* 1993; 22:1858-65.

6. Alfonso F, Macaya C, Goicolea J, Iniguez A, Hernandez R, Zamorano J, et al. Intravascular ultrasound imaging of angiographically normal coronary segments in patients with coronary artery disease. *Am Heart J* 1994; 127:536-44.

7. Mintz GS, Painter JA, Pichard AD, Kent KM, Satler LF, Popma JJ, et al. Atherosclerosis in angiographically «normal» coronary artery reference segments: an intravascular ultrasound study with clinical correlations. *J Am Coll Cardiol* 1995; 25:1479-85.

8. Acker JD, Cole CA, Mauney KA, Joly DM, Machin JE. Duplex carotid ultrasound. *Neuroradiology* 1986; 28:608-17.

9. Pignoli P, Tremoli E, Poli A, Oreste P, Paoletti R. Intimal plus medial thickness of the arterial wall: a direct measurement with ultrasound imaging. *Circulation* 1986; 74:1399-406.

10. Blankenhorn DH, Chin HP, Conover DJ, Nessim SA. Ultrasound observation on pulsation in human carotid artery lesions. *Ultrasound Med Biol* 1988; 14:583-7.

11. Ryan T, Armstrong WF, Feigenbaum H. Prospective evaluation of the left main coronary artery using digital two dimensional echocardiography. *J Am Coll Cardiol* 1986; 7:807-12.

12. Taams MA, Gussenhoven EJ, Cornel JH, The SH, Roelandt JR, Lancee CT, et al. Detection of left coronary artery stenosis by transesophageal echocardiography. *Eur Heart J* 1988; 9:1162-6.

13. Yoshida K, Yoshikawa J, Hozumi T, Yamaura Y, Akasaka T, Fukaya T, et al. Detection of left main coronary artery stenosis by transesophageal color Doppler and two-dimensional echocardiography. *Circulation* 1990; 81:1271-6.

14. McPherson DD, Hiratzka LF, Lamberth WC, Brandt B, Hunt M, Kieso RA, et al. Delineation of the extent of coronary atherosclerosis by high-frequency epicardial echocardiography. *N Engl J Med* 1987; 316:304-9.

15. Mallery JA, Gregory K, Morcos NC, et al. Evaluation of an ultrasound balloon dilatation imaging catheter (abstr.). *Circulation* 1987; 76:371.

16. Yock PG, Linker DT, Thapliyal HV, et al. Real-time, two-dimensional catheter ultrasound: a new technique for high resolution intravascular imaging (abstr.). *J Am Coll Cardiol* 1988; 11:130.

17. Pandian NG, Kreis A, Brockway B, Isner JM, Sacharoff A, Boleza E, et al. Ultrasound angioscopy: real-time, two-dimensional, intraluminal ultrasound imaging of blood vessels. *Am J Cardiol* 1988; 62:493-4.

18. Hodgson JM, Graham SP, Savakus AD, Dame SG, Stephens DN, Dhillon PS, et al. Clinical percutaneous imaging of coronary anatomy using an over-the-wire ultrasound catheter system. *Int J Card Imaging* 1989; 4:187-93.

19. Mintz GS, Nissen SE, Anderson WD, Bailey SR, Erbel R, Fitzgerald PJ, et al. American College of Cardiology Clinical Expert Consensus Document on Standards for Acquisition, Measurement and Reporting of Intravascular Ultrasound Studies (IVUS). A report of the American College of Cardiology Task Force on Clinical Expert Consensus Documents. *J Am Coll Cardiol* 2001; 37:1478-92.

20. Nissen SE, Yock P. Intravascular ultrasound: novel pathophysiological insights and current clinical applications. *Circulation* 2001; 103:604-16.

21. Gil R, von Birgelen C, Prati F, Di Mario C, Ligthart J, Serruys PW. Usefulness of three-dimensional reconstruction for interpretation and quantitative analysis of intracoronary ultrasound during stent deployment. *Am J Cardiol* 1996; 77:761-4.

22. Dhawale PJ, Griffin N, Wilson DL, Hogdson JM. Calibrated 3-D reconstruction of intracoronary ultrasound images with cardiac gating and catheter motion compensation. In:

Computers in Cardiology. Washington D.C.: Institute of Electrical and Electronics Engineers Computer Society; 1992:31-34.

23. Bruining N, von Biergelen C, Di Mario C, et al. Reconstruction of ICUS images based on an ECG-Gated pull back device. En: *Computers in Cardiology*. Los Alamitos: Institute of Electrical and Electronics Engineers Computer Society; 2000:633-636.

24. Linker DT, Kleven A, Gronningsaether A, Yock PG, Angelsen BA. Tissue characterization with intra-arterial ultrasound: special promise and problems. *Int J Card Imaging* 1991; 6:255-63.

25. Evans DH, McDicken WN, Skidmore R, Woodcock JP. In: Doppler Ultrasound: Physics, Instrumentation and Clinical Applications. (New York: Wiley, 1989).

6

Image Interpretation. Basic Diagnostic Concepts. Normal Morphology and Patterns of Disease

Jaime Elízaga, MD
Javier Botas, MD
Javier Soriano, MD

Characteristics of the Arterial Layers and Vessel Lumen. Perivascular References. Characterization of Arteriosclerotic Disease. Quantification of Images. Artifacts and Limitations of IVUS. Safety of Examinations with IVUS. References.

When a normal coronary artery is examined using intravascular ultrasound, a characteristic three-layer image of the vessel wall is usually observed. This image is the result of the differing acoustic properties of the arterial layers, leading to the perception of an interface between two tissues whenever there is an abrupt and significant change in their acoustic impedances. Various *in vitro* and *in vivo* studies have characterized the findings obtained with ultrasound techniques in coronary arteries and have established a correlation between the images obtained using this diagnostic technique and histological studies.[1-4] Of the three layers visible, the innermost echogenic layer is bound internally by the interface between the blood present inside the vessel lumen and the edge of the intima, and externally by the internal elastic membrane, which is highly echogenic due to its high elastic content. The outermost layer is bound internally by the interface between the external elastic membrane and adventitia, and the external portion cannot be defined because the adventitia is indistinguishable from the periadventitial tissue. Between these two layers is another layer, the media, made up mostly by smooth muscle cells in muscular arteries such as coronary or femoral arteries. Its low content in elastic tissue and collagen gives it a low level of echogenicity (Figs. 6-1 and 6-2). In the elastic arteries, the media is more echogenic because of its greater elastic fiber content, which makes it difficult to distinguish from the intima and adventitia using IVUS. In summary, the three layers observed in ultrasound images of muscular arteries could be considered to correspond to the intima, media, and adventitia.

CHARACTERISTICS OF THE ARTERIAL LAYERS AND THE VESSEL LUMEN

At an early age, the intima is thin, comprising a single layer of endothelial cells covering a fine subendothelial layer of connective tissue. Consequently, in 30-40 % of normal coronary arteries, particularly in young people, the axial resolution of the ultrasound catheter does not allow the fine intimal layer to be distinguished and the triple-layer appearance of the arterial wall is lost. With age, the intima gradually thickens, reaching about 220 μ at the age of 30 years

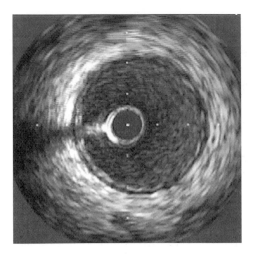

Figure 6-1. Image of a normal coronary artery in a 58-year-old man. In the vessel lumen can be seen an ultrasound catheter artifact, with a high-density image at 9 o'clock produced by the guide causing an acoustic shadowing that hinders visualization of part of the arterial wall. The characteristic three-layer image can be seen on a large part of the wall. The innermost layer corresponds to the intima and the high-density outermost layer to the adventitia, which merges into the periadventitial tissue. A low-density muscle layer is located between them.

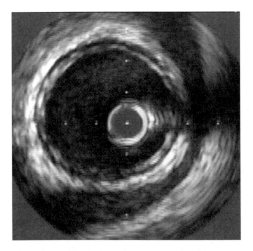

Figure 6-2. Image of a right coronary artery in which an anterior vein can be seen surrounding the coronary artery between 1 and 7 o'clock. These veins are not parallel to the artery, as in other locations, but cross over it.

and 250 μ at the age of 40. Fitzgerald[5] studied 16 intact hearts in autopsies of patients without any history of coronary disease, carrying out intracoronary ultrasound and histological analysis of 72 coronary segments. These segments were divided into two groups depending on whether or not they presented a three-layer image. Segments with a triple-layer image had a thicker intima (243 ± 105 μ versus 112 ± 55 μ) and belonged to older patients (42.8 ± 9.8 versus 27.1 ± 8.5 years), the cutoff value between the two groups was 178 μ thickness. Therefore, the presence of a three-layer image suggests thickening of the intima to at least 178 μ and is seen more frequently in older patients.

Unlike the intima, the media thins as arteriosclerosis progresses, with a median thickness ranging from 0.8 mm in uninjured coronary segments to 0.3 mm in those with the most severe arteriosclerosis.[6] An inverse relationship is observed between the severity of the lesion and thickness of the media layer. As will be seen later in this chapter, this affects the quantification of the thickness of the plaque using intracoronary ultrasound.

The vessel lumen is between the vessel wall and ultrasound transducer. Normally, it is possible to observe some low-density speckling of changing patterns and with a certain continuous movement produced by blood flow in the vessel lumen. The intensity of this blood-generated image increases as the ultrasound frequency increases and blood flow decreases, as in the case of the retention of blood in severe lesions. This makes it difficult to differentiate the edge of the intima, particularly in the case of «soft» plaques. Nonetheless, even in cases of severe stagnation, the blood presents an internal, flickering movement that allows it to be distinguished. The injection of contrast material through the guide catheter may assist in differentiating the edge of the intima, hyperplasia, or dissection, if doubts persist.

PERIVASCULAR REFERENCES

Ultrasound examination allows visualization not only of the vessel but also its adjacent structures. These include the cardiac veins, pericardium, and myocardium. Familiarity with the perivascular structures, their situation, and distribution helps to improve axial and rotational orientation (see *study techniques*) in the vessel. The main perivascular structures displayed using intracoronary ultrasound are:

In the proximal portion of the left coronary trunk, a very low-density space can be seen surrounding the artery, corresponding to the transthoracic sinus. It is due to a pericardial fold that comes from the ascending aorta and heads towards the anterior descending coronary. If the catheter is advanced distally into the proximal anterior descending coronary, the Brocq-Mouchet triangle is visible, i.e., the pericardial space bound by the proximal anterior descending coronary, proximal circumflex, and fork in the anterior interventricular vein and large cardiac vein. Once inside the middle third of the anterior descending coronary, it is usually possible to see the pericardium (with the pericardial space, which normally contains fluid), myocardium, and anterior interventricular cardiac vein, which in 90 % of cases runs to the left of the anterior descending coronary. The cardiac veins are characterized by thin walls, a more undulating wall movement, and a denser blood content due to its lower velocity. Inside the circumflex artery, a large venous structure is visible that corresponds to the large cardiac vein and runs above the artery in 95 % of cases. The branches departing this vein correspond to marginal branches and those approaching it are atrial branches. In the right coronary artery, the most striking feature is the venous structures surrounding the artery (Fig. 6-2), which correspond to the anterior cardiac veins that do not run parallel to the artery but cross over it, coinciding with outflow from the acute marginal branches that irrigate the right ventricle. In the distal portion of the right coronary artery, before and after the crux, the small cardiac vein runs parallel to the right coronary and the posterolateral branches, whereas the medial cardiac vein runs parallel to the posterior interventricular artery.

CHARACTERIZATION OF ARTERIOSCLEROTIC DISEASE

Initial Phases. Remodeling

Intravascular ultrasound examination is the best diagnostic method for studying coronary disease in vivo, as has been shown in numerous trials comparing the tomographic images obtained using ultrasound with histological findings.[7, 8] When the study of coronary arteries began with ultrasound techniques, the first thing that was noticed was the diffuse nature of arteriosclerosis. In fact, segments considered angiographically «normal» and used as reference values in comparison with diseased segments were found to contain a considerable amount of plaque occupying the arterial wall, with a mean of 51 % of the vessel area being occupied by plaque.[9] In the initial stages of arteriosclerosis, intimal thickening is detectable by intracoronary ultrasound scan but not by angiography. Assessment of this factor is important in certain subgroups of patients, such as transplant recipients, or in trials studying the progression/regression of arteriosclerosis. As the arteriosclerotic plaque develops in a coronary artery, there is normally an adaptive change, or remodeling, which affects the size of the vessel. Normally, as the amount of plaque on the arterial wall increases, the size of the vessel increases to maintain the size of the vessel lumen constant. However, in advanced lesions this compensation becomes impossible and the lumen size decreases, normally coinciding with an accumulation of plaque in excess of 40 % of the area of the vessel.[10-13] This is known as positive remodeling and was first described by Glagov[11] in 1987 in a study of autopsy samples. However, subsequent studies with intravascular ultrasound scan[14, 15] have shown that remodeling may also be negative (smaller vessel sizes in areas with the greatest accumulation of plaque or smaller lumen with respect to the reference), contributing to a reduction in the lumen, or even neutral (with no variation in vessel size with respect to «healthy» segments).

Composition of Arteriosclerotic Plaques

Types of Plaque

In the more advanced stages of arteriosclerosis, the lesions are morphologically more complex and can be grouped into three different types depending on the echogenicity of the predominant tissues in the arteriosclerotic plaque.

Low echogenicity: In order to assess the echogenicity of the plaque in practice, it is compared with adventitial and periadventitial tissue (which are highly echogenic). Thus, this type of lesion shows less echogenicity than adventitial and periadventitial tissue (Figs. 6-3A and 6-4). From a histological standpoint, the predominant tissues in low-echogenicity lesions are the fibromuscular cellular component and fatty deposits. On occasions, dark areas (very low density) may be observed in the plaque, which correspond to extensive lipid deposits with areas of necrotic degeneration, often covered by a fine layer of fiber that is not always detected by IVUS. When the fatty deposits are small and numerous, they may pass unnoticed due to the limited resolution and dynamic range of ultrasound waves. This type of lesion is also known as a «soft» plaque because it is theoretically less rigid than «hard» plaques and has a different response to balloon dila-

tion, stenting, or atherectomy. This terminology, however, is ambiguous as it fails to reflect accurately the plaque's mechanical properties. Many plaques defined as «soft» have offered great resistance to balloon dilation.[16] The term «soft» is currently associated with the acoustic signal deriving from the low level of echogenicity.

High echogenicity: The degree of echogenicity is equal to or greater than that of the adventitial tissue. These lesions contain predominantly dense, fibrous tissue that produces bright, heterogeneous echoes, that are occasionally speckled. These plaques are also called «hard» or fibrous plaques (Fig. 6-3B). This is the kind of plaque most frequently observed in intravascular ultrasound scans.

High echogenicity with acoustic shadowing: The presence of acoustic shadowing with a high degree of echogenicity (i.e., more than the adventitia) is specifically indicative of calcium. Calcium prevents ultrasound penetration, obscuring the vessel underneath (acoustic shadowing) so that only the internal edge is detected. IVUS cannot determine the thickness of the calcification. The calcification may cause reverberations as a result of the oscillation of the ultrasound waves between the transducer and margin of calcification, originating concentric images at a reproducible distance (Fig. 6-3C). Occasionally, densely fibrotic lesions may produce bright echoes with considerable progressive attenuation of the echo signal and acoustic shadowing, simulating areas of calcification. The attenuation of the signal will depend on the density and thickness of fibrosis and the power of the ultrasound transducer. Nonetheless, in calcifications the loss of the signal is abrupt, not progressive, and reverberation is present, thus allowing it to be differentiated from attenuation with an acoustic shadow due to extensive fibrosis.

Intracoronary ultrasound has been shown to be more sensitive than angiography in the detection of calcification. When the angio-

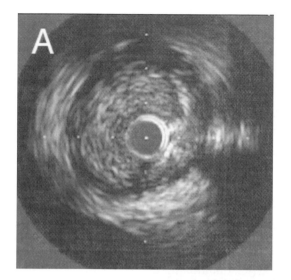

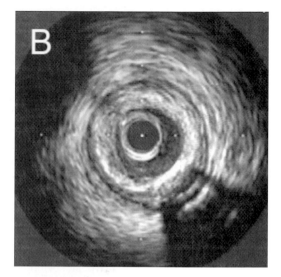

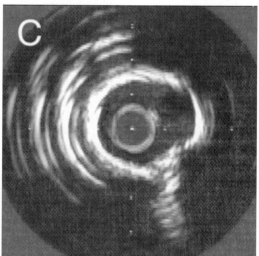

Figure 6-3. Classification of arteriosclerotic plaques by echogenicity. Low-echogenicity or «soft» plaque, with a small area of calcification and fibrosis between 2 and 4 o'clock (A). Mainly fibrous plaque, with acoustic shadowing between 4 and 6 o'clock (B). Plaque with severe superficial calcification affecting almost the entire circumference, causing acoustic shadowing and reverberation (C).

graphic findings of patients who have undergone surgery are analyzed, the presence of calcifications is detected in 10-35 % of cases, as opposed to 70-80 % of patients studied with ultrasound scanning.[17, 18]

The division of plaques into the three categories mentioned is useful from a theoretical standpoint, but in practice most lesions are mixed and show fibrotic, «soft» and/or calcified areas.

Thrombi

One of the main limitations of IVUS scanning is the identification of thrombi.

Whenever a thrombus reflects ultrasound waves, it produces a bright, heterogeneous image with a sparkling speckle. Microchannels are occasionally visible within the thrombus and/or lobulated images protruding into "the lumen. These characteristics suggest a fresh thrombus, particularly if it presents an undulating movement during systole and diastole, but some of these features are only rarely identified. An organized thrombus of longer evolution has characteristics very similar to those of a «soft» plaque, thus hindering its differentiation. On occasions, linear or layered images are seen inside the plaque, corresponding to the acoustic interface between the thrombus and plaque, and suggesting the presence of an organized thrombus. The future development of new tissue characterization techniques using ultrasound may improve thrombus characterization.

Ruptures and Dissections

Ultrasound scans have allowed certain aspects of plaque pathology, such as spontaneous dissection, fractures, or fissures, to be assessed with greater precision than with angiography. These images occur above all in patients with acute coronary syndromes. Plaque fracture or rupture is the term used when the tear is perpendicular to the arterial layers, whereas the lesion is parallel to the arterial layers in dissection. The diagnosis of fracture or dissection is based on the observation of blood inside the new lumen, frequently requiring the injection of contrast media to define the borders more clearly. In dissections, it is important to determine certain characteristics that yield significant information about their severity and prognosis: 1) *maximum depth*, classified as partial or superficial (dissection does not reach the media, some plaque remains between the lumen and media), or as complete or deep (the media is involved); 2) *axial length*, which can be calculated when automatic or motorized pull-back mechanisms are used to withdraw the ultrasound catheter. The area of dissection can be calculated in degrees (up to 360°) or quadrants.

Eccentricity

Intracoronary ultrasound scans provide information not only about the characteristics of the plaque but also its disposition on the circumference and along the axis of the vessel (Fig. 6-4). The eccentricity of the plaque is one of the factors that can affect the short-term and long-term results of angioplasty, conditioning the treatment to be used. Angiography has a limited value in assessing the eccentricity of a plaque. In a trial by Mintz et al.,[19] 1446 lesions in 1349 patients were analyzed and the assessment of eccentricity by both techniques was compared. Angiography found 55 % of the lesions to be eccentric, while intracoronary ultrasound imaging showed that 45.6 % of the lesions had an eccentricity index greater than 3.0 (maximum plaque thickness divided by

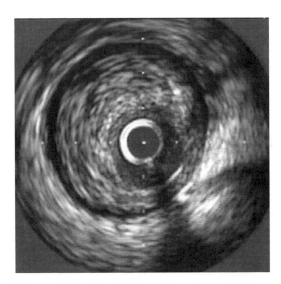

Figure 6-4. Distribution of the plaque on the arterial wall. Eccentric low-echogenicity plaque («soft» plaque) with an eccentricity index of 0.77.

minimum thickness). The concordance was only 53.8 %.

QUANTITATIVE ANALYSIS OF IVUS IMAGES

Study Techniques with IVUS

When an ultrasound catheter is inserted into a coronary artery for the first time, it is rather difficult to find one's bearings. The orientation of the catheter can be specified in two ways, axially, or longitudinally, and by reference to the circumference, or rotationally. Longitudinal orientation refers to the position of the catheter in relation to the length of the coronary artery (proximal-distal), whereas rotational orientation refers to the location of the structures (pericardium, myocardium, branches, veins, etc.) with respect to the cross-section or circumference of the artery displayed by the ultrasound scan.

For the purposes of longitudinal orientation, angiography is used to identify the image of the transducer (a radiopaque mark that must be distinguished from the sheath in which it moves) and its relationship to the branches viewed using angiography with contrast injection during the ultrasound study. Once the transducer is in place distal to the area of interest, automatic pull-back to the guide catheter is carried out at a constant speed. The angiographic position of the transducer is confirmed before beginning pull-back. After completing the first pull-back, the transducer is inserted manually to analyze any doubtful areas or areas of special interest, or to inject contrast medium to help position the transducer correctly with respect to the angiographic reference and better delineate the structures. Nonetheless, although the angiographic reference is very important, it is not sufficiently precise to identify specific areas (for the purpose of comparing measurements made before and after interventions at the same site). For this reason, it is important to use the features of the artery

under study as a reference for the lesion or area of the vessel to be assessed. The features most often used are:

— *Plaque composition, distribution, and shape:* Calcifications are frequent (70-80 %) in arteriosclerotic plaques and always have a characteristic distribution and shape, which differs for each case, but is easily identified each time the ultrasound scan is repeated. Any morphological characteristic of the plaque or its disposition on the arterial wall, such as fractures, areas of eccentricity or large-scale remodeling, etc., may serve as a reference.

— *Arterial branches:* The outflow from a branch proximal to the area under study may provide a clear reference. In the anterior descending coronary, the septal branches usually have a more pronounced and abrupt outflow angle (around 90°), whereas this angle is smaller and gradual in the diagonal branches. During pull-back from a distal to a proximal point, the diagonal branches are first visible as vessels parallel to the anterior descending coronary that gradually come closer until they connect. The circumflex artery contains atrial and marginal branches. The first, less numerous, are destined for the large cardiac vein, which can be seen as a vessel with a large lumen and thin walls. It often cannot be seen in its entirety because of the limited depth of the ultrasound waves. The larger-caliber marginal branches emerge from the circumflex opposite the atrial branches.

— *Perivascular references:* The perivascular structures previously described in this chapter are very useful for finding one's bearings inside a coronary artery.

If more precision in terms of axial orientation is needed, particularly for serial comparative studies, the best solution is to make at least one rigorous automatic pull-back in each sequence to be studied. If the velocity is constant, each image, or frame, becomes a time marker. For instance, if the pull-back is carried out at 0.5 mm/s and 30 images/s, the distance between two images will be 0.0167 mm, which means that if a reference is taken at the first frame in which the coronary structure (for example the start of a branch) is seen, the subsequent frame count will give a close approximation to the distance that can be repeated on a later occasion.

As was mentioned above, rotational orientation refers to the location of structures (pericardium, myocardium, branches, veins, etc.) in relation to the section or circumference of artery displayed by the ultrasound scan. The way this is displayed on the screen depends on where the device assigns an arbitrary start to the transducer's rotation, so the location of a diagonal branch may, for instance, be different each time the intracoronary ultrasound catheter is inserted (in the first pull-back of the transducer it might be located at twelve o'clock and later at 6 o'clock). Once the transducer has been activated, however, the image may be rotated electronically to place the structures on-screen in the desired position.

Image Measurements

Unlike angiography, quantification using ultrasound does not require routine calibration. Calibration is carried out automatically by the ultrascan device and is calculated using the speed of transmission of ultrasound waves through the blood and adjacent tissue. The ultrasound image has certain calibration points superimposed on it, normally in the form of a hairline cross, with an onscreen indication of the distance in millimeters between points, which allows speedy calculation of the distances as the image is being displayed.

Once a study has been made with IVUS and a specific part of the artery is to be quantified or analyzed, which image should be selected? The luminal section in a coronary artery varies throughout each cardiac cycle,

reaching its peak area in the systolic phase and minimal area in the diastolic phase, except in intramyocardial segments where systolic pressure is produced extrinsic to the artery.[20] The luminal section varies by about 8 % in normal coronary arteries during heartbeat cycles, and less in the presence of a coronary plaque, depending on the plaque thickness, composition, and eccentricity.[21] While angiographic images are quantified at the end of the diastole, when the movement of the heart and contrast medium, as well as the superimposition of branches, is minimal, in intracoronary ultrasound scans images are quantified at the end of systole. At this point in the cycle, arterial dimensions are greater and more accurate, and catheter movement is minimal, thus aiding in the interpretation of the images. In addition, residual lesions after angioplasty (dissections, fissures, fractures, etc.) have less impact on quantification due to vessel distension.

Determination of the Reference Segment

In order to assess the severity of a coronary lesion, it must be compared with a «healthy» reference segment, «healthy» being a relative term because coronary disease will often be present (Fig. 6-5). A reference segment is the segment with the largest luminal section in the proximity of the lesion. This may not be the site with the least amount of plaque. The diameter and cross-sectional area (CSA) of the reference segment are the parameters considered. Among the reference segments, the following segments can be distinguished:

— Proximal reference: The site with the largest luminal section proximal to a stenosis but in the same segment (usually within 10 mm of the stenosis with no major intervening branches).
— Distal reference: The site with the largest luminal section distal to a stenosis but in the same segment (usually with-

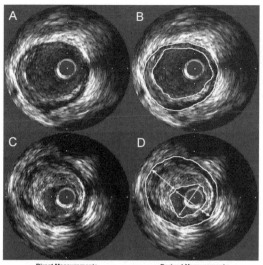

Direct Measurements

Reference lumen area= 10 mm²
Reference EEM area= 17 mm²
Lesion lumen area= 4.13 mm²
Lesion EEM area= 17.2 mm²
Maximum atheroma thickness= 2.04 mm
Minimum atheroma thickness= 0.91 mm
Maximum lumen diameter= 2.52 mm
Minimum lumen diameter= 2.03 mm

Derived Measurements

Lesion atheroma area= 13.07 mm²
Atheroma burden= 0.76
Lesion area stenosis= 0.59
Remodeling index= 1.01
Lesion lumen eccentricity index= 0.19
Atheroma eccentricity index= 0.55

Figure 6-5. Example of the measurement of a coronary lesion. The lower part of the image shows all the measurements made directly on the image and those calculated using these data, as described in the text. Panels A and B show the reference segment, which presents coronary disease. In panel B, the cross-section of the lumen and external elastic membrane has been marked. Panels C and D show the area of the lesion, with an indication of the lumen cross-section and the external elastic membrane in panel D, together with the maximum and minimum diameters of the plaque (solid arrows) and lumen.

Measurement of the Vessel Lumen

In order to measure the vessel lumen, it is necessary to define the interface between the

blood inside the lumen and the leading edge of the intimal layer. Usually there are no problems in defining this interface, except in healthy arterial segments of young people in which the intima is very thin (in this case the intima-muscle edge is used), and in cases of very soft plaques or neo-intimal hyperplasia of the stent. In the case of measurements in segments that have suffered dissection after an intervention, it should be clarified as to whether only the true lumen is considered or whether the measurement also includes the false lumen. Once the edge of the lumen has been defined, its perimeter and the maximum and minimum diameters are drawn (Fig. 6-5). In all cases, measurements are made relative to the center of mass of the lumen, not relative to the center of the IVUS catheter. The following parameters are obtained:

— *Lumen CSA:* The area bounded by the luminal border.
— *Minimum lumen diameter:* The shortest diameter through the center of the lumen.
— *Maximum lumen diameter:* The longest diameter through the center of the lumen.
— *Lumen eccentricity:* (Maximum Lumen Diameter —Minimum Lumen Diameter) divided by Maximum Lumen Diameter.
— *Lumen area stenosis:* (Reference Lumen CSA —Minimum Lumen CSA) divided by Reference Lumen CSA. The reference used (proximal, distal, average) must be indicated.

in 10 mm of the stenosis, with no intervening branches).
— Average reference: The average value of the luminal sections at the proximal and distal reference sites.

Vessel Measurements

The true size of the vessel comprises the three arterial layers but, as was mentioned at the beginning of this chapter, the adventitia is indistinguishable from the periadventitial tissue. Therefore, the outside edge of the vessel is drawn at the external portion of the media (external elastic membrane or EEM)

(Fig. 6-5). In any case, given the scant thickness of the adventitia (300-500 μ), the error with respect to true vessel size is negligible. Instead of the vessel CSA, the recommended term would be external elastic membrane CSA (EEM CSA).

There are circumstances that limit or impede the definition of the external elastic membrane. In areas of calcification, when the calcification arc and its acoustic shadow cover less than 90° (1 quadrant), the lumen edge can be extrapolated from the identifiable EEM borders, although measurement accuracy and reproducibility are reduced. If acoustic shadowing involves more than 90° of the circumference, the measurement should not be made (Fig. 6-3C). The same rule applies to cases of certain stent designs that limit the visibility of the vessel or, as will be discussed later, when the vessel image is deformed by artifacts or distortion.

If maximum and minimum EEM diameters are reported, measurements should intersect the geometric center of the vessel.

Plaque Measurements

IVUS cannot determine the true histological plaque because the internal elastic membrane is not well delimited for several reasons. Firstly, although the internal elastic membrane is composed of echogenic elastic tissue, fibrous changes in the inner third of the media reduce the difference in acoustic impedance between adjacent layers. Secondly, the transition of ultrasound signals from an area of high echogenicity (intima/plaque) to one of low echogenicity (media) produces a «blooming» effect, in which the signal is disseminated and the media appears thinner. For this reason, and considering that the external elastic membrane is generally visible as a sharp edge, quantification of the plaque includes the media and is referred to as plaque plus media. This measurement has been shown to

correlate well with histological measurements (Fig. 6-5).[22] Consequently, when reference is made to the plaque, it is understood to be the plaque + media (distance between the internal edge of the intima and external elastic membrane).

The main plaque parameters assessed are:

— *Plaque area*: Area of the vessel section minus the lumen section.
— *Maximum plaque thickness*: The part of the plaque corresponding to the greatest distance between the internal intimal edge and external elastic membrane.
— *Minimum plaque thickness*: The part of the plaque corresponding to the shortest distance between the internal intimal edge and external elastic membrane.
— *Plaque eccentricity*: (Maximum Plaque Thickness —Minimum Plaque Thickness) divided by Maximum Plaque Thickness. Occasionally, plaque eccentricity is assessed by dividing Maximum Plaque Thickness by Minimum Plaque Thickness.
— *Plaque burden*: Plaque Area divided by Vessel Area. This represents the proportion of the vessel (in CSA) occupied by the atheroma plaque, without taking into account the impact it has on the lumen. In contrast, lumen area stenosis assesses the impact of the plaque on the lumen in relation to the reference, and is equivalent to the angiography assessment. This parameter is also known as the atheroma burden.

Calcium Measurements

Calcium deposits are described qualitatively according to their location and disposition:

— Superficial calcification: The internal edge of the calcification is located within the 50 % of the plaque closest to the vessel lumen.

— Deep calcification: The internal edge of the calcification is located in the 50 % of the plaque furthest from the vessel lumen.

The parameters most often used to quantify calcification are:

— *Arc of calcification, in degrees*: This is measured using an electronic protactor centered on the vessel lumen. It reflects the involvement of the wall section. A semi-quantitative assessment of quadrant involvement can also be used (1 to 4).
— *Calcification length*: If an automatic pull-back system has been used, the longitudinal involvement of the vessel can be assessed.

Remodeling Measurement

In order to describe the magnitude and direction of remodeling, the following index is used: Lesion EEM CSA divided by Reference EEM CSA (without any major intervening side branches). If the index is >1, remodeling is positive; and if it is <1, remodeling is negative. However, the index only provides a relative assessment of remodeling because the reference segment itself may present remodeling. Direct evidence of remodeling can only be derived from serial studies.

ARTIFACTS AND LIMITATIONS OF IVUS

Limitations

Although IVUS accurately determines the thickness, areas, and echogenicity of vessel wall structures, it cannot consistently provide histological measurements. This is because different tissues may have the same acoustic properties. It is uncertain whether radiofrequency analysis will be reliable enough to assess tissue properties.

The physical size of ultrasound catheters, despite the reduction to about 1 mm achieved in recent years, is still an important limitation for the assessment of severe lesions. This means that the lumen and plaque cannot be quantified appropriately at the site of the lesion.

Artifacts

A. Non-Uniform Rotation Distorsion (NURD)

This artifact is unique to mechanical catheter[23] systems and results from mechanical binding of the drive cable that rotates the transducer. This can happen for various reasons, including : sharp bends in the coronary artery, excessive tightening of a hemostatic valve, twisting of the guide catheter, or, in a very small vessel, kinking of the catheter sheath, etc. In extreme situations, the drive cable may even break. The IVUS image would indicate vessel distortion due to oscillations in rotational speed (Fig. 6-6). When NURD is visually apparent, the degree of distortion may be significant (artifact >90°) and measurements are unreliable.

B. Motion Artifacts

These occur when the position of the catheter inside the coronary artery is unstable due to the movement of the artery during systole and diastole. Occasionally, the vessel moves before a complete circumferential image of the arterial section has been obtained, causing cyclic deformation of the image. When this occurs, it impedes the accurate assessment of phenomena that depend on the cardiac cycle (compliance, arterial pulsation) and affects the longitudinal reconstruction of the coronary artery.

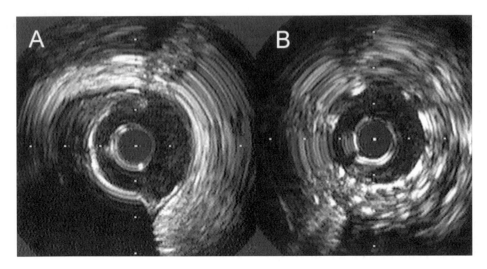

Figure 6-6. Examples of artifacts due to non-uniform transducer rotation. In panel A, a vessel deformation can be seen, with the characteristic linear images in between 1 and 6 o'clock. Panel B corresponds to the study of a stent. Due to the non-uniform rotation of the transducer, the struts (high-density points on the edge of the intima) can be seen far apart from 8 to 1 o'clock, where as they are close together on the rest of the circumference.

C. Proximity Artifacts

Proximity artifacts occur in the region close to the ultrasound catheter. Ring-down is the most common of them and consists of halos of variable thickness surrounding the catheter, sometimes resembling the layers of an onion (Fig. 6-7). These rings are caused by the acoustic oscillation transducer producing large-amplitude ultrasound signals that obscure the region immediately adjacent to the transducer, resulting in an acoustic catheter size larger than its physical size. The artifact can be attenuated in mechanical transducers by reducing the proximal gain (manipulating the device's time gain compensation, or TGC), and in solid-state transducers by using digital subtraction and a reference mask. In both cases, excessive reduction of the ring-down effect may reduce detail in the area close to the catheter, which could have important consequences in certain situations (severe soft lesions, small vessels, etc.).

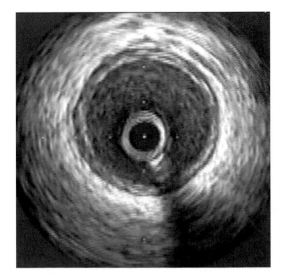

Figure 6-7. Proximity artifact. The ultrascan catheter can be seen inside the lumen, surrounded by a thick white layer corresponding to the ring-down artifact. This occurs with different degrees of intensity in almost all catheters, increasing the acoustic size of the transducer.

D. Position-related Alignment Artifacts

In order to achieve an optimal image with ultrasound, the transducer must be placed in the center of the vessel lumen, parallel to the arterial axis. If the catheter lies obliquely in the lumen, an elliptical image of the vessel is obtained, resulting in overestimation of arterial dimensions and a loss of image quality. The latter phenomenon occurs because the amplitude of the ultrasound signal reflected from an interface depends in part on the angle of incidence; maximum amplitude being obtained when the angle is 90° (the catheter lies co-axial in the vessel lumen). Alignment problems are less important in coronary arteries than in other vessels of the body because they are more frequent in large vessels.

SAFETY OF IVUS EXAMINATIONS

A potential constraint on the use of intracoronary ultrasound is the possibility of complications associated with this diagnostic technique. The incidence of complications reported in the literature is low, the most frequent being coronary spasm.[24-27] In the largest study published, with 2207 patients recruited at 28 centers in the U.S.,[25] the overall incidence of complications with a definite or possible link to the ultrasound scan was 3.9 %: 2.9 % due to spasm (reversible with nitroglycerin), 0.7 % due to other procedure-related causes (dissection, acute occlusion, embolism, or thrombus), and 0.3 % major complications (non-fatal AMI or need for urgent coronary surgery). The complication rate was significantly higher in patients with acute coronary syndromes and in those undergoing interventions. The European Registry[24] has compiled retrospective data from 12 centers and 718 studies. The overall incidence of complications was 1.1 % (8 cases), with transient coronary spasm again being the most frequent complication (4 cor-onary spasms, 2 possible dissections, and 2 guide wire entrapments). All these complications were resolved without further complications. At our hospital,[26] we collated data retrospectively on the complications that occurred in the first 18 months of regular use of IVUS. Over this period, 239 vessels were studied in 209 procedures (74 % involving interventions). No major complication occurred, but 3 patients (1.4 %) had minor complications: 1 acute occlusion resolved with PTCA, 1 ventricular fibrillation without consequences, and one coronary spasm resolved with nitroglycerin. Unlike the American and European studies mentioned above, all of our patients were treated with intravenous heparin and intracoronary nitroglycerin.

REFERENCES

1. Di Mario C, The SHK, Madretsma S, et al. Detection and characterization of vascular lesions by intravascular ultrasound: an in vitro study correlated with histology. *J Am Soc Echocardiogr* 1992; 5:135-46.
2. Nishimura RA, Edwards WD, Warnes CA, et al. Intravascular ultrasound imaging: in vitro validation and pathologic correlation. *J Am Coll Cardiol* 1990; 16:145-54.
3. Siegel RJ, Chae JS, Maurer G, Berlin M, Fishbein MC. Histopathologic correlation of the three-layered intravascular ultrasound appearance of normal adult human muscular arteries. *Am Heart J* 1993; 126:872-8.
4. Tobis JM, Mallery J, Mahon D, et al. Intravascular ultrasound imaging of human coronary arteries in vivo. Analysis of tissue characterizations with comparison to in vitro histological specimens. *Circulation* 1991; 83:913-26.
5. Fitzgerald PJ, St Goar FG, Connolly AJ, et al. Intravascular ultrasound imaging of coronary arteries. Is three layers the norm? *Circulation* 1992; 86:154-8.
6. Gussenhoven EJ, Frietman PA, The SH, et al. Assessment of medial thinning in atherosclerosis by intravascular ultrasound. *Am J Cardiol* 1991; 68:1625-32.

7. Gussenhoven EJ, Essed CE, Lancee CT, et al. Arterial wall characteristics determined by intravascular ultrasound imaging: an in vitro study. *J Am Coll Cardiol* 1989; 14:947-52.

8. Potkin BN, Bartorelli AL, Gessert JM, et al. Coronary artery imaging with intravascular high-frequency ultrasound. *Circulation* 1990; 81:1575-85.

9. Mintz GS, Painter JA, Pichard AD, et al. Atherosclerosis in angiographically «normal» coronary artery reference segments: an intravascular ultrasound study with clinical correlations. *J Am Coll Cardiol* 1995; 25:1479-85.

10. Ge J, Erbel R, Zamorano J, et al. Coronary artery remodeling in atherosclerotic disease: an intravascular ultrasonic study in vivo. *Coron Artery Dis* 1993; 4:981-6.

11. Glagov S, Weisenberg E, Zarins CK, Stankunavicius R, Kolettis GJ. Compensatory enlargement of human atherosclerotic coronary arteries. *N Engl J Med* 1987; 316:1371-5.

12. Hermiller JB, Tenaglia AN, Kisslo KB, et al. In vivo validation of compensatory enlargement of atherosclerotic coronary arteries. *Am J Cardiol* 1993; 71:665-8.

13. Losordo DW, Rosenfield K, Kaufman J, Pieczek A, Isner JM. Focal compensatory enlargement of human arteries in response to progressive atherosclerosis. In vivo documentation using intravascular ultrasound. *Circulation* 1994; 89:2570-7.

14. Mintz GS, Kent KM, Pichard AD, Satler LF, Popma JJ, Leon MB. Contribution of inadequate arterial remodeling to the development of focal coronary artery stenoses. An intravascular ultrasound study. *Circulation* 1997; 95:1791-8.

15. Pasterkamp G, Wensing PJ, Post MJ, Hillen B, Mali WP, Borst C. Paradoxical arterial wall shrinkage may contribute to luminal narrowing of human atherosclerotic femoral arteries. *Circulation* 1995; 91:1444-9.

16. Hiro T, Leung CY, Guzman S, et al. Are «soft echoes» really soft?: ultrasound assessment of mechanical properties in human atherosclerotic tissue. *Circulation* 1995; 92:I-649.

17. Mintz GS, Douek P, Pichard AD, et al. Target lesion calcification in coronary artery disease: an intravascular ultrasound study. *J Am Coll Cardiol* 1992; 20:1149-55.

18. Tuzcu EM, Berkalp B, De Franco AC, et al. The dilemma of diagnosing coronary calcification: angiography versus intravascular ultrasound. *J Am Coll Cardiol* 1996; 27:832-8.

19. Mintz GS, Popma JJ, Pichard AD, et al. Limitations of angiography in the assessment of plaque distribution in coronary artery disease: a systematic study of target lesion eccentricity in 1446 lesions. *Circulation* 1996; 93:924-31.

20. Ge J, Erbel R, Rupprecht HJ, et al. Comparison of intravascular ultrasound and angiography in the assessment of myocardial bridging. *Circulation* 1994; 89:1725-32.

21. Weissman NJ, Palacios IF, Weyman AE. Dynamic expansion of the coronary arteries: implications for intravascular ultrasound measurements. *Am Heart J* 1995; 130:46-51.

22. Wong M, Edelstein J, Wollman J, Bond MG. Ultrasonic-pathological comparison of the human arterial wall. Verification of intima-media thickness. *Arterioscler Thromb* 1993; 13:482-6.

23. ten Hoff H, Korbijn A, Smith TH, Klinkhamer JF, Bom N. Imaging artifacts in mechanically driven ultrasound catheters. *Int J Card Imaging* 1989; 4:195-9.

24. Batkoff BW, Linker DT. Safety of intracoronary ultrasound: data from a Multicenter European Registry. *Cathet Cardiovasc Diagn* 1996; 38:238-41.

25. Hausmann D, Erbel R, Alibelli-Chemarin MJ, et al. The safety of intracoronary ultrasound. A multicenter survey of 2207 examinations. *Circulation* 1995; 91:623-30.

26. Lopez-Palop R, Botas J, Elizaga J, et al. Feasibility and safety of intracoronary ultrasound. Experience of a single center. *Rev Esp Cardiol* 1999; 52:415-21.

27. Pinto FJ, St Goar FG, Gao SZ, et al. Immediate and one-year safety of intracoronary ultrasonic imaging. Evaluation with serial quantitative angiography. *Circulation* 1993; 88:1709-14.

7

Vascular Remodeling. Intravascular Ultrasound Patterns of Different Clinical Presentations

RAIMUND ERBEL, MD
CLEMENS VON BIRGELEN, MD
JUNBO GE, MD
DIETRICH BAUMGART, MD
MICHAEL HAUDE, MD

Introduction. Development of coronary artery disease. Remodeling. Preclinical disease. Acute coronary syndromes. Stary VIa lesions. Stary VIb lesions. Stary VIc lesions. Plaque healing. Angioplasty in acute coronary syndromes. Clinical implications. References.

INTRODUCTION

In coronary artery disease (CAD), preclinical disease has to be differentiated from clinical situations of stable and chronic CAD as well as from acute coronary syndromes (ACS), which include unstable angina, acute myocardial infarction, and sudden death. Using histological/anatomical studies, it can be shown that these three ACSs have many common morphological characteristics. Recently, characteristic coronary angiographic features were described for coronary lesions leading to ACS.[1-3] However, compared to histology and coronary angioscopy, the sensitivity and specificity of this technique is low.[5-7] Intravascular ultrasound (IVUS) has overcome some of these limitations and provides new insights into the natural history of CAD.

DEVELOPMENT OF CORONARY ARTERY DISEASE

Stary et al.[8] described different stages (Fig. 7-1) in the development of CAD, which were regarded as a recommendation for the use of imaging techniques. This classification has been appropriated for IVUS imaging of coronary arteries (Table 7-1).

Already in childhood and young adulthood, the beginning of the arteriosclerotic process can be demonstrated, including stages Stary I-III.[9] Intimal thickening can only be visualized by IVUS when it exceeds the resolution (Fig. 7-2) of ultrasound and the axial resolution of ultrasound is currently in the range of 100 μm.[10] This intimal thickness is regularly reached in men at an age of about 30 years.[11] At this time the single layer appearance of the vessel wall disappears and a three-layer appearance is appreciated, indicating that intimal thickness is at least 100 μm. The inner layer corresponds to the endoluminal vessel border, and the echolucent area to the media.[12-18] The outer layer corresponds to the external elastic lamina (EEL), or the border of adventitia and surrounding tissue.[10] This three-layer appearance is typical for arteries of the muscular type, but can also be seen in arteries of the elastic type like the aorta and iliac arteries.[12] The three-layer appearance is usually circular, but may be eccentric when tangential imaging is pres-

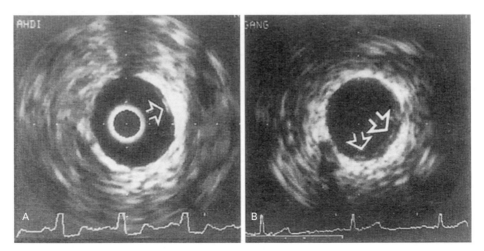

Figure 7-1. Stary I-II lesions. A type II lesion characterized by intimal thickening shows a «three-layer» appearance. On the opposite side, the vessel shows a single-layer appearance. Imaging with a centrally positioned catheter. Calibration marker indicates 1 mm.[19]

ent.[12, 17] The intima-media diameter represents vessel wall thickness.[10]

Whereas Stary I corresponds to arteries that show a single-layer, three layers are typical of Stary II and their appearance is part of the normal process of aging.[19, 20] With the increase in vessel wall thickness, the intermediate stage (Fig. 7-3), Stary III, devel-

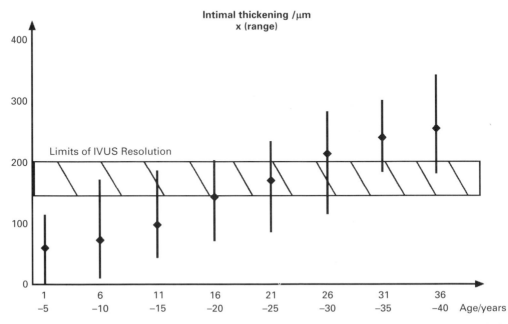

Figure 7-2. Demonstration of how intimal thickness increases with age in relation to the resolution of intravascular ultrasound. At the age of 30-40 years, the resolution is higher than intimal thickening, so the vessel wall has a three-layer appearance. Adapted from Velican D et al. Atherosclerosis 1981; 38:39-50 reference 11.

Table 7-1. Classification of Atherosclerotic Lesions Based on Histological Findings (modified from references [18-20]), in Relation to IVUS Features

Types	Histological appearance	IVUS features
Type I (initial lesion)	Accumulation of lipoprotein in intima; lipid in macrophages. No tissue damage.	Monolayer appearance; border zone of the vessel with bright reflectivity, representing adventitia. Aging originates a three-layered appearance, with interfaces at the lumen–intima and media-adventitia at 30-40 years.
Type II (fatty streak) IIa (progression-prone) IIb (progression-resistant)	Accumulation of lipoprotein in intima; lipid in macrophages and smooth muscle cells; visible to the naked eye as fatty streaks.	
Type III (preatheroma)	All type II features, plus multiple deposits of pooled extracellular lipid.	Progressive eccentric thickening of the intima; small zones of low reflectivity, >300 μm thick; occasional acoustic shadowing indicating calcification.
Type IV (atheroma)	All type III features, plus confluent mass of extracellular lipid (lipid core), with massive structural damage to the intima.	Eccentric thickening of the intima; zones of low (dark) reflectivity in the deeper media, adjacent to the part of the lesion with smooth borders.
Type Va (fibroatheroma)	All type IV features, plus development of marked collagen layers and increase in smooth muscle cells above lipid core.	Features as type IV; thinner zones of bright reflectivity between zone of low reflectivity and vessel lumen.
Vb (calcified lesion)	Any advanced type V lesion composed predominantly of calcium.	Lesion with eccentric or concentric thickening of the intima, with large zones of bright reflectivity and acoustic shadowing graded according to the angle of shadowing; reverberation may be present.
Vc (fibrotic lesion)	Any advanced type V lesion composed predominantly of collagen.	Eccentric or concentric lesions with bright reflectivity, with or without ultrasound attenuation, but no shadowing or reverberation.
Type VI (complicated lesion) VIa	Plaque ulceration.	Regular lesion configuration, with tear in a membrane covering a zone of low reflectivity; demostration of communication by contrast dye between vessel lumen and lesion under tear, located centrally or eccentrically.
VIb	Plaque hematoma/hemorrhage.	Intact endoluminal border; multiple zones with irregular borders; free-floating structures; change of shape during pulsation.
VIc	Plaque fissuring or rupture, with signs of mural or complete thrombus formation.	Lesion showing signs of single or multiple mural layering, with or without irregular endoluminal borders; free-floating structures; speckled reflective tissue; footprint left by catheters.

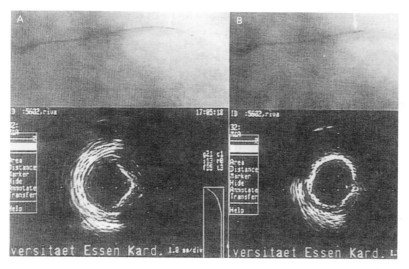

Figure 7-6. Type Vb lesions: Coronary angiograms without contrast injection, and IVUS images at corresponding sites (arrows) of the left anterior descending coronary artery. Even though IVUS shows severe calcification, as indicated by the acoustic shadowing produced by the very bright reflections between 12 and 6 o'clock in (A) and between 9 and 6 o'clock in (B), fluoroscopy shows only mildly enhanced radiographic shadowing.[19]

circumference, this limit has been found to be in the range of 60%.[34] This part of the natural history of plaques can also be studied by IVUS.[35-38] Normally, vessel size tapers off from the proximal to the distal part of the vessel. In areas of the vessel in which plaque formation takes place, vessel size increases instead of tapering off (Fig. 7-7). As was observed with the histological findings, the remodeling process can be assessed by IVUS, which shows that the critical limit is in the range of 45%.[35] Quantitatively, a plaque size of 10-14 mm² is the limit beyond which luminal narrowing occurs and it is found in patients with normal or nearly normal coronary angiograms. These findings correspond to the early preclinical stage of coronary artery disease and represent the upper limit of plaque size beyond which the remodeling process is exhausted.[35] In addition, saphenous vein bypass grafts with a diseased lumen also show vascular remodeling.[39, 40] Luminal narrowing has to be more than 90% before resting flow decreases.[41] Even in normal or nearly normal looking coronary arteries, the

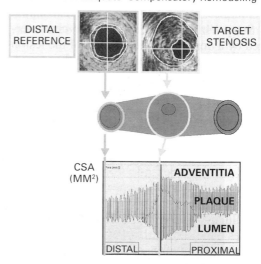

Lesion with Adequate Compensatory Remodeling

Figure 7-7. Positive remodeling demonstrated by IVUS imaging and 3-D reconstruction. The largest vessel diameter and area are present at the site of the smallest luminal diameter, indicating the presence of the largest plaque area between both lines. Y-axis area calculated, X-axis distance from distal to proximal segment during pull back IVUS imaging (0.5 mm/s).[55] Von Birgelen et al. Heart 1998; 79:137-43.

Table 7-2. Lesion Types and Clinical Manifestations in Patients with Significant Coronary Artery Disease

AHA clinical classification	Lesion type						
	IV (n = 22)	Va (n = 25)	Vb (n = 11)	Vc (n = 28)	VIa (n = 35)	VIb (n = 1)	VIc (n = 12)
Stable angina	14	12	11	27	10	1	5
Unstable angina	8	13	0	1	25	—	7
Area of stenosis (IVUS)%	65 ± 9	67 ± 8	70 ± 7	68 ± 8	56 ± 17	—	72 ± 14

plaque load can be enormous, as has been demonstrated in earlier anatomo-pathological studies.[5, 6, 42-47]

These findings confirm that coronary angiography cannot detect early signs of coronary arteriosclerosis.[5, 46, 47] Table 7-2 shows that advanced lesion types are detected by IVUS in the presence of a normal coronary angiogram. Accordingly, minimal luminal narrowing visualized by coronary angiography usually involves plaque loads of >45%.[35]

The remodeling process can also explain why even after successful coronary angioplasty with a residual coronary narrowing of less than 30%, IVUS still reveals a plaque load in the range of 60-70%.[48-51]

In more advanced stages of CAD, not only remodeling but also negative (Fig. 7-8), instead of positive, compensatory enlargement

Lesion with Inadequate Remodeling («Shrinkage»)

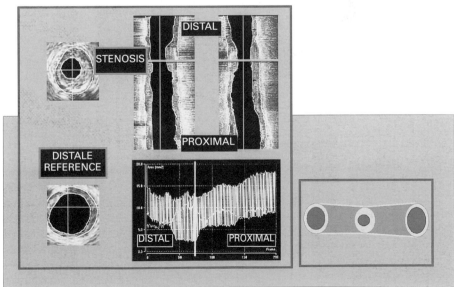

Figure 7-8. Negative remodeling, as indicated by the reduction in vessel area at the site of the smallest luminal area with the largest plaque burden. Analyzed by pull-back IVUS imaging from the distal to the proximal vessel segment. y-axis shows calculated areas, x-axis shows the distance in frames (0.5 mm/s).[55]. Von Birgelen et al. Heart 1998; 79:137-43.

is found.[52, 53, 54] *This is regarded as shrinkage of the coronary vessel, possibly induced by a plaque rupture-induced healing process that is similar to plaque repair.* The differentiation between positive and negative remodeling may be important when coronary interventions are performed.[55] Plaques showing Stary IV and Va lesions are particularly prominent in areas with positive remodeling and rarely found in vessels with negative remodeling, in which Stary Vb and Vc are much more frequently described.[55, 56]

PRECLINICAL DISEASE

Since coronary angiography (Fig. 7-3) cannot detect early signs of arteriosclerosis, many coronary angiograms are regarded as normal or nearly normal despite a large plaque load.[20, 35] This remains an important problem in daily practice, because in catheterization laboratories that have excellent screening protocols, 10-15% of studies are regarded as normal, while in other institutions up to 40% may be considered normal.[57] However, coronary morphology can be better studied using IVUS. In addition, intracoronary Doppler flow wire measurements can be used to assess coronary flow velocity and coronary blood flow. Coronary flow velocity reserve (CFVR) can be determined by injecting adenosine, 12 mg in the right coronary artery and 18 mg in the left coronary artery.[58-60] Newer studies have shown that even higher doses should be used to reach maximal coronary flow velocity,

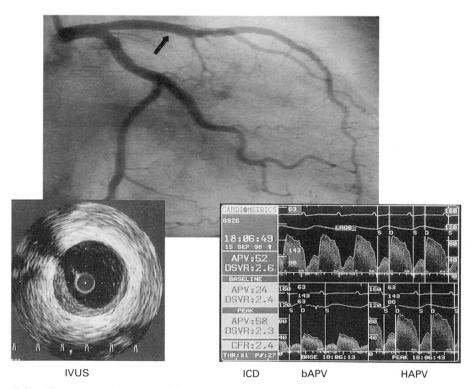

IVUS   ICD   bAPV   HAPV

Figure 7-9. Coronary angiogram with IVUS and intracoronary Doppler (ICD) analysis showing morphological and functional findings in coronary arteries. The injection of adenosine increases coronary flow velocity, which is automatically calculated as coronary velocity flow reserve (CFR). The diastolic/systolic velocity ratio is given (DSVR).

which is otherwise only found in the hyperemic stage after myocardial ischemia.[60]

A value of ≥ 3 for CFVR can be regarded as normal according to a literature review by Baumgart et al.[59] CFVR reaches ≥ 4 in patients in which plaque formation has been ruled out, the so-called true normals.[61] In order to elucidate coronary vasomotor activity, acetylcholine can be injected into the coronary artery to test endothelium-dependent vasodilation.[62] By quantitative coronary angiography, an increase in diameter of $\geq 25\%$ can be regarded as normal.[62] Coronary flow velocity reserve increases by ≥ 2.5. Using nitroglycerin, endothelium-independent vasodilation can also be tested, which results in an increase in CFVR of ≥ 2.5.[63] Using both techniques, patients with normal or nearly normal coronary angiograms can be better differentiated.[61]

Taking both techniques into account (Fig. 7-9), only 10 % of patients with angiographically normal coronary arteries can be regarded as truly normal.[61] Patients with reduced CFVR and no evidence of plaque formation must be regarded as syndrome X. Consequently, angina pectoris with normal coronary angiograms, as well as positive stress tests with signs of ischemia, can no longer be regarded as the gold standard for defining syndrome X. Nowadays, normal IVUS and normal intracoronary Doppler studies must also be considered when defining syndrome X.[61] In the future, this should help to better characterize this «chameleon-like» clinical picture, which is still not well understood and is very difficult to treat.[61]

Patients with normal coronary angiograms (Fig. 7-10) and signs of early arteriosclerosis can be differentiated into patients with reduc-

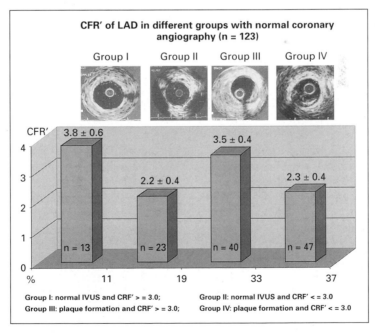

Figure 7-10. Results of IVUS and intracoronary Doppler analysis in patients with normal coronary angiograms but suspected coronary artery disease. Patients can be subdivided into 4 groups: I) True normal, meaning no plaque formation, normal coronary flow reserve (CFR'), II) Syndrome X, meaning angina, normal angiogram, signs of ischemia, reduced CFR' but normal IVUS, III) coronary artery disease, with plaque formation detected by IVUS and normal CFR', IV) coronary artery disease but reduced CFR', meaning that coronary artery disease can be present with a reduced CFR' but normal coronary angiograms.[64]

ed CFVR and patients without reduced CFVR. That means that some patients, possibly due to silent plaque rupture leading to atypical chest pain presenting as an isolated or repetitive periodic event, have developed microvascular dysfunction or epicardial endothelial injury as a result of the arteriosclerotic process, which leads to changes in microvascular function.[61, 64] This has been proposed by the findings of experimental studies.[65, 66] On the other hand, positive results in stress tests, single-photon emission tomography, or echocardiography may be referred to as true positive results, rather than as false positives, as long as CFVR has not been measured and IVUS studies have not been performed.[61]

Long-term follow-up studies in patients with apparently normal coronary angiograms have shown that the prognosis of patients is poor, not excellent as previously suggested.[67-69]. These results have inspired additional long-term follow-up studies using newer imaging techniques.

ACUTE CORONARY SYNDROMES

In Stary II-IV lesions, but particularly in the presence of Stary Va lesions, complications can occur due to vascular injury resulting in fissuring or even plaque rupture. Stary Va and IV lesions are known variously as «plaques at risk», «plaques prone to rupture,» or «vulnerable plaques.»[70-73] Histologically, patients usually have only one lesion in the whole coronary artery tree, showing plaque rupture.[73] However, multiple complicated lesions may be present in patients who are studied for acute coronary syndromes. We also need to consider that patients with these lesions are asymptomatic in the absence of flow-limiting stenosis, thanks to the remodeling process.[74, 75] This is supported by the observation that more than 50% of patients with acute myocardial infarction have no symptoms. Studies of coronary arteries prior to acute myocardial infarction have shown coronary narrowing of

less than 75% diameter stenosis in $\geq 90\%$ of cases.[75] The relation between lesion type and the clinical manifestations of the disease is shown in Table 7-2, which demonstrates that plaque rupture can be visualized even in patients with stable angina, and that not all patients with unstable angina have documented complicated lesions

Among the lesions that lead to ACS are:

1. Plaques with ulceration after rupture (Stary VIa).
2. Intramural hematomas (Stary VIb).
3. Thrombus formation superimposed on fissure formation or plaque rupture (Stary VIc).[10]

STARY VIa LESIONS

All three forms of complicated lesions must be considered in patients with ACS. Using coronary angiography, ruptured and ulcerated plaques appear as aneurysms and have been classified previously.[1-3] Using IVUS, complicated lesions can be clearly differentiated.[19, 24] Most aneurysms of the coronary artery reveal plaque ulceration, whereas true aneurysms are rarely seen.[76] Ulcerated plaques exhibit fibrous caps with tears (Fig. 7-11) that fill with contrast agent when coronary angiography is performed.[76, 77] The volume of the ulcer left after the lipid core washes out can be as much as 1 cc. This indicates that a huge amount of plaque material has embolized because the absence of local thrombus formation has failed to prevent the wash-out effect. Microembolization under such circumstances can cause chest pain that is unresponsive to nitroglycerin. It may be detected as a rise in troponin T or I level indicating the presence of microinfarction.[78, 79] These infarcts can further increase in size, as the arteriosclerotic tissue, with cholesterol crystals and other substances it contains, attracts further thrombus formation, particularly as a result of induction by the tissue factor present in this tissue. Histology findings indicate that these events may

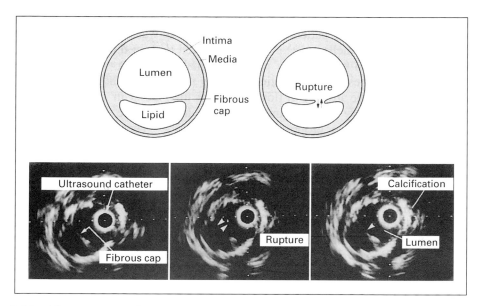

Figure 7-11.   Plaque rupture (Stary VIa) with tears in the ruptured fibrous cap detected by IVUS and illustrated by a schematic drawing.[24]

be repetitive and thus can lead to multiple microinfarctions, which can also induce ischemic cardiomyopathy and sudden death.[73]

In up to 10 % of the lesions, plaque rupture (Fig. 7-12) is found in the absence of the formation of a fibrous cap.[24] Such plaque rup-

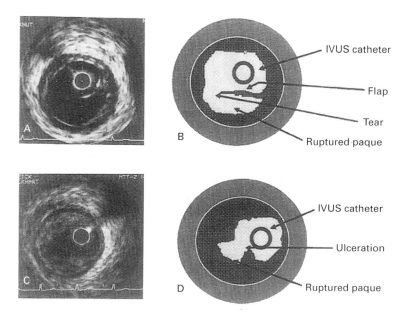

Figure 7-12.   Plaque ulceration without formation of a fibrous cap and tearing, as part of type VIa lesion in unstable angina.[24]

of the Working Group of Coronary Circulation and of the Subgroup on Intravascular Ultrasound of the Working Group on Echocardiography of the European Society of Cardiology. Clinical application and image interpretation in intracoronary ultrasound. *Eur Heart J* 1998; 19:207-229.

26. Hempel H. Lehrbuch der allgemeinen Pathologie und der pathologischen Anatomie. *Springer:* Berlin 1968.

27. Maehara A, Fitzgerald PJ. Coronary calcification: assessment by intravascular ultrasound imaging. *Z Kardiol* 2000; 2:112-6.

28. Wang J, Nomura M, Kurokawa H, Tachiki S, Ando T, Ishii J, Kinoshita M, Iwase M, Kondo T, Watanabe Y, Hishida H. Is pre-intervention intravascular ultrasound necessary in evaluating target lesion calcification in patients undergoing therapy? *Jpn Circ J* 1996; 8:567-74.

29. Mintz GS, Douek P, Pichard AD, Kent KM, Satler LF, Popma JJ, Leon MB. Target lesion calcification in coronary artery disease: an intravascular ultrasound study. *J Am Coll Cardiol* 1992; 20:1149-55.

30. Tuzcu EM, DeFranco AC, Goormastic M, et al. Dichotomous pattern of coronary atherosclerosis 1 to 9 years after transplantation: insights from systematic intravascular ultrasound imaging. *J Am Coll Cardiol* 1996; 27:839-846.

31. Mintz GS, Popma JJ, Pichard AD, et al. Limitations of angiography in the assessment of plaque distribution in coronary artery disease: a systematic study of target lesion eccentricity in 1446 lesions. *Circulation* 1996; 93:924-931.

32. Ge J, Erbel R. Characteristic plaque morphology. In: Erbel R, Roelandt JRTC, Ge J, Görge G (eds): *intravascular ultrasound* London: Martin Dunitz; 1998. 77-80.

33. Glagov S, Weisenberg E, Zarins C, et al. Compensatory enlargement of human atherosclerotic coronary arteries. *N Engl J Med* 1987; 316:1371-1375.

34. Zarins CK, Weisenberg E, Kolettis G, Stankunavicius R, Glagov S. Differential enlargement of artery segments in response to enlarging atherosclerotic plaques. *J Vasc Surg* 1988; 7:386-394.

35. Ge J, Erbel R, Zamorano J, Koch L, Kearny P, Görge G, et al. Coronary arterial remodeling in atherosclerotic disease: an intravascular ultrasound study in vivo. *Coron Artery Dis* 1993; 4:981-986.

36. Hermiller JB, Tenaglia AN, Kislo KB, et al. In vivo validation of compensatory enlargement of atherosclerotic coronary arteries. *Am J Cardiol* 1993; 71:665-668.

37. Losordo DW, Rosenfield K, Kaufman J, et al. Focal compensatory enlargement of human arteries in response to progressive atherosclerosis; in vivo documentation using intravascular ultrasound. *Circulation* 1994; 89:2570-2577.

38. Gerber TC, Erbel R, Görge G, Ge J, Rupprecht HJ, Meyer J. Extent of atherosclerosis and remodeling of the left main coronary artery determined by intravascular ultrasound. *Am J Cardiol* 1994; 73:666-671.

39. Ge J, Liu F, Bhate R, Haude M, Görge G, Baumgart D, Sack S, Erbel R. Does remodeling occur in the diseased human saphenous vein bypass grafts? An intravascular ultrasound study. *Intern J Card Imag* 1999; 15:295-300.

40. Hong MK, Mintz GS, Hong MK, Abizaid AS, Pichard AD, Satler LF, Kent KM, Leon MB. Intravascular ultrasound assessment of the presence of vascular remodeling in diseased human saphenous vein bypass grafts. *Am J Cardiol* 1999; 84:992-998.

41. Gould KL, Lipscomb K, Harrison GW. Physiological basis for assessing critical coronary stenosis. *Am J Cardiol* 1974; 33: 87-94.

42. Stiel GM, Stiel LSG, Schofer J, Donath K, Mathey DG. Impact of compensatory enlargement of atherosclerotic coronary arteries on angiographic assessment of coronary artery disease. *Circulation* 1989; 80: 1603-1609.

43. Sahn DJ, Copeland JG, Temkin LP, Wirt DP, Mammana R, Glenn W. Anatomic-ultrasound correlations for intraoperative, open chest imaging of coronary artery atherosclerotic lesions in human beings. *J Am Coll Cardiol* 1984; 3:1169-1177.

44. McPherson DD, Armstrong M, Rose E, Kieso RA, Megan M, Hunt M, et al. High-

frequency epicardial echocardiography for coronary artery evaluation: *in vitro* and *in vivo* validation of arterial lumen and wall thickness measurements. *J Am Coll Cardiol* 1986; 8:600-606.

45. Arnett EN, Isner JM, Redwook CR, et al. Coronary artery narrowing in coronary heart disease: comparison of cineangiographic and necropsy findings. *Ann Intern Med* 1979; 91:350-356.

46. Grodin CM, Dydra I, Pastgernac A, et al. Discrepancies between cineangiographic and postmortem findings in patients with coronary artery disease and recent myocardial revascularization. *Circulation* 1974; 49:703-709.

47. Vlodaver Z, Frech R, van Tassel RA, et al. Correlation of the antemortem coronary angiogram and the postmortem specimen. *Circulation* 1973; 47:162-168.

48. Tobis JM, Mallery JA, Gessert J, et al. Intravascular ultrasound cross-sectional arterial imaging before and after balloon angioplasty in vitro. *Circulation* 1989; 80: 873-882.

49. Nissen SE, Gurley JC, Grines CL, et al. Intravascular ultrasound assessment of lumen size and wall morphology in normal subjects and patients with coronary artery disease. *Circulation* 1991; 84:1087-1099.

50. Gerber TC, Erbel R, Görge G, Ge J, Rupprecht HJ, Meyer J. Classification of morphologic effects of percutaneous transluminal coronary angioplasty assessed by intravascular ultrasound. *Am J Cardiol* 1992; 70:1546-1554.

51. Baptista J, Di Mario C, Ozaki Y, Escaned J, Gil R, De Feyter P, Roelandt JRTC, Serruys PW. Impact of plaque morphology and composition on the mechanisms of lumen enlargement using intracoronary ultrasound and quantitative angiography after balloon angioplasty. *Am J Cardiol* 1996; 77:115-121.

52. Nishiola T, Luo H, Eigler NL, Berglund H, Lim CJ, Siegel RJ. Contribution of inadequate compensatory enlargement to development of human coronary artery stenosis: an in vivo intravascular ultrasound study. *J Am Coll Cardiol* 1996; 27:1571-1576.

53. Pasterkamp G, Schoneveld AH, van der Wal AC, Haudenschild CC, Clarijs RJ,

Becker AE, Hillen B, Borst C. Relation of arterial geometry to luminal narrowing and histologic markers for plaque vulnerability: the remodeling paradox. *J Am Coll Cardiol* 1998; 32:655-62.

54. Shoenhagen P, Ziada K, Kapadia SR, Crowe TD, Nissen SE, Tuzcu EM. Extent and direction of arterial remodeling in stable versus unstable coronary syndromes: an intravascular ultrasound study. *Circulation* 2000; 101:598-603.

55. von Birgelen C, Klinkhart W, Mintz GS, et al. Size of emptied plaque cavity following spontaneous rupture is related to coronary dimensions, not to the degree of lumen narrowing. A study with intravascular ultrasound in vivo. *Heart* 2000; 84:483-8.

56. Davies MJ. Glagovian remodeling, plaque composition, and stenosis generation. *Heart* 2000; 84:461-462.

57. Kern MJ. Syndrome X: understanding and evaluating the patient with chest pain and normal coronary arteriograms. *Heart Dis Stroke* 1992; 1:299-302.

58. Wieneke H, Haude M, Ge J, Altmann C, Kaiser S, Baumgart D, von Birgelen C, Welge D, Erbel R. Corrected coronary flow velocity reserve: a new concept for assessing coronary perfusion. *J Am Coll Cardiol* 2000; 35:1713- 20.

59. Baumgart D, Haude M, Liu F, Ge J, Görge G, Erbel R. Current concepts of coronary flow reserve for clinical decision making during cardiac catheterization. *Am Heart J* 1998; 136:136-49.

60. Jeremias A, Filardo SD, Whitbourn RJ, Kernoff RS, Yeung AC, Fitzgerald PJ, Yock PG. Effects of intravenous and intracoronary adenosine 5ñ-triphosphate as compared with adenosine on coronary flow and pressure dynamics. *Circulation* 2001; 103:E58.

61. Erbel R, Ge J, Bokisch A, Kearny P, Görge G, Haude M, Schümann D, Zamorano J, Rupprecht HJ, Meyer J. Value of intracoronary ultrasound and Doppler in the differentiation of angiographically normal coronary arteries: a prospective study in patients with angina pectoris. *Eur Heart J* 1996; 17:880-889.

62. Zeiher AM, Drexler H, Wollschläger H, Just H. Endothelial dysfunction of the cor-

onary microvasculature is associated with impaired coronary flow regulation in patients with early atherosclerosis. *Circulation* 1991; 84:1984-92.

63. Hasdai D, Lerman A. The assessment of endothelial function in the cardiac catheterization laboratory in patients with risk factors for atherosclerotic coronary disease. *Herz* 1999; 24:544-7.

64. Qian J, Ge J, Baumgart D, et al. Prevalence of microvascular disease in patients with significant coronary artery disease. *Herz* 1999; 24:548-57.

65. Merkus D, Chilian WM, Stepp DW. Functional characteristics of the coronary microcirculation. *Herz* 1999; 24:496-508.

66. Saitoh S, Saito T, Onogi F, et al. Effect of antiplatelet agents on microvascular remodeling induced by repetitive endothelial injury of epicardial coronary artery in pig. *Eur Heart J* 1998; 19:617.

67. Fichtlscherer S, Zeiher AM. Assessment of endothelial dysfunction in acute coronary syndromes. *Herz* 1999; 24:534-43.

68. Kelm M. Interaktion von koronarer Makro- und Mikrostrombahn. *Z Kardiol* 2001; 90: 946-952.

69. Kaiser H, Altmann Ch, Baumgart D, Haude M, Wieneke H, Erbel R (personal communication).

70. Ridolfi RL, Hutchins GM. The relationship between coronary artery lesions and myocardial infarcts: ulceration of atherosclerotic plaques precipitating coronary thrombosis. *Am Heart J* 1977; 93: 468-86.

71. Fuster V, Stein B, Ambrose JA, Badimon JJ, Chesebro JH. Atherosclerotic plaque rupture and thrombosis: evolving concepts. *Circulation* 1990; 82:47-59.

72. Davies MJ, Bland MJ, Hangartner WR, Angelini A, Thomas AC. Factors influencing the presence or absence of acute coronary thrombi in sudden ischemic death. *Eur Heart J* 1989; 10:203-8.

73. Falk E. Unstable angina with fatal outcome: dynamic coronary thrombosis leading to infarction and/or sudden death: autopsy evidence of recurrent mural thrombosis with peripheral embolization culminating in total vascular occlusion. *Circulation* 1985; 71:699-708.

74. Falk E. Plaque rupture with severe pre-existing stenosis precipitating coronary thrombosis. Characteristics of coronary atherosclerotic plaques underlying fatal occlusive thrombi. *Br Heart J* 1983; 50:127-34.

75. Falk E., Fuster V. Angina pectoris and disease progression. *Circulation* 1995; 92: 2058-65.

76. Ge J, Liu F, Kearny P, et al. Intravascular ultrasound approach to the diagnosis of coronary aneurysms. *Am Heart J* 1995; 130:765-71.

77. Zamorano J, Erbel R, Görge G, Kearny P, Koch L, Scholte A, Meyer J. Spontaneous plaque rupture visualized by intravascular ultrasound. *Eur Heart J* 1994; 15:131-133.

78. Erbel R, Heusch G. Spontaneous and iatrogenic microembolization: A new concept for the pathogenesis of coronary artery disease. *Herz* 1999; 24:493-5.

79. Heusch G, Schulz R, Baumgart D, Haude M, Erbel R. Coronary microembolization. *Prog Cardiovasc Dis* 2001; 44:217-230.

80. Davies MJ, Bland MJ, Hangartner WR, et al. Factors influencing the presence or absence of acute coronary thrombi in sudden ischemic death. *Eur Heart J* 1989; 10:203-8.

81. Baumgart D, Liu F, Haude M, et al. Acute plaque rupture and myocardial stunning in patient with normal coronary arteriography. *Lancet* 1995; 346:193-4.

82. Ambrose JA, Hjemdahl-Monsen CE. Arteriographic anatomy and mechanisms of myocardial ischemia in unstable angina. *J Am Coll Cardiology* 1987; 9:1397-402.

83. Abdelmeguid AE, Topol EJ. The myth of the myocardial infarctlet during percutaneous coronary revascularization procedures. *Circulation* 1996; 94:3369-75.

84. Davies M, Richardson P, Woolf N, et al. Risk of thrombosis in human atherosclerotic plaques: role of extracellular lipid, macrophage, and smooth muscle cell content. *Br Heart J* 1993; 69:377-81.

85. Schmermund A, Erbel R. Unstable coronary plaque and its relation to coronary calcium. *Circulation* 2001; 104:1682-1687.

86. Richardson PD, Davies M, Born GVR. Influence of plaque configuration and stress distribution on fissuring of coronary atherosclerotic plaques. *Lancet* 1989; 2: 941-4.

87. Burke A, Farb A, Malcom GT, Liang YH, Smialek JE, Virmani R. Plaque rupture and sudden death related to exertion in men with coronary artery disease. *JAMA* 1999; 281:921-926.

88. Burke A, Farb A, Malcom GT, Liang YH, Smialek JE, Virmani R. Coronary risk factors and plaque morphology in patients with coronary disease dying suddenly. *N Engl J Med* 1997; 336: 1276-1282.

89. Heidland UE, Strauer BE. Left ventricular muscle mass and elevated heart rate are associated with coronary plaque disruption. *Circulation* 2001; 104:1477-82

90. Kearney P, Erbel R, Rupprecht HJ, Ge J, Koch L, Voigtländer T, Stahr P, Görge G, Meyer J. Differences in the morphology of unstable and stable coronary lesions and their impact on the mechanisms of angioplasty. *Eur Heart J* 1996; 17:721-730.

91. Bocksch WG, Schartl M, Beckmann SH, Dreysse S. Intravascular ultrasound imaging in patients with acute myocardial infarction: comparison with chronic stable angina pectoris. *Coron Artery Dis* 1994; 5: 727-735.

92. Franzen D, Sechtem U, Höpp HW. Comparison of angioscopic intravascular ultrasonic and angiographic detection of thrombus in coronary stenosis. *Am J Cardiol* 1998; 82:1273-1275.

93. De Feyter PE, Ozaki Y, Baptista J, Escaned J, Di Mario C. Ischemia related lesion characteristics in patients with stable und unstable angina: a study with intracoronary angioscopy and ultrasound. *Circulation* 1995; 92:1408-1413.

94. Claudon D, Claudon D, Edwards J. Primary dissecting aneurysm of coronary artery: a cause of acute myocardial ischemia. *Circulation* 1972; 45:259-266.

95. Kearney P, Erbel R, Ge J, Zamorano J, Koch L, Görge G, Meyer J. Assessment of spontaneous coronary artery dissection by intravascular ultrasound in a patient with unstable angina. *Cathet and Cardiovasc Diagn* 1994; 32:58-61.

96. Ge J, Haude M, Görge G, Liu F, Erbel R. Silent healing of spontaneous plaque disruption demonstrated by intracoronary ultrasound. *Eur Heart J* 1995; 16:1149-1151.

97. Jeremias A, Ge J, Erbel R. New insight into plaque healing after plaque rupture with subsequent thrombus formation detected by intravascular ultrasound. *Heart* 1997; 77:293.

98. Bocksch W, Beckmann S, Dreysse S, Paeprer H, Schartl M. Morphological changes after PTCA in patients with chronic stable angina versus acute myocardial infarction. Intravascular ultrasound study. *Eur Heart J* 1993; 14:109.

99. Herrmann J, Haude M, Lerman A, Schulz R, Volbracht L, Ge J, Schmermund A, Wieneke H, von Birgelen C, Eggebrecht H, Baumgart D, Heusch G, Erbel R. Abnormal coronary flow velocity reserve after coronary intervention is associated with cardiac markers elevation. *Circulation* 2001; 103:2339-2345.

100. Meyer J, Schmitz H, Erbel R, Kiesslich T, Bocker-Josephs B, Krebs W, Braun PC, Bardos P, Minale C, Messer BJ, Effert S. Treatment of unstable angina pectoris with percutaneous transluminal coronary angioplasty (PTCA). *Cathet Cardiovasc Diagn* 1981; 7:361-71.

8

Three-Dimensional Reconstruction of Intravascular Ultrasound Images: From Technical Considerations to Practical Issues

CLEMENS VON BIRGELEN, MD
RAIMUND ERBEL, MD
JOUKE DIJKSTRA, MD

Introduction. 3D IVUS: Rationale and First Overview. Conventional Motorized IVUS Pullbacks. ECG-Gated Image Acquisition. Computer-Assisted Boundary Detection (Quantitative 3D Coronary Ultrasound). Validation of Quantitative 3D IVUS. On-line and Off-line Use of 3D IVUS. Quantitative 3D IVUS in Research and Clinical Practice. Three-Dimensional Reconstruction (Image Fusion). Outlook on Further Developments of 3D IVUS. References.

INTRODUCTION

The transmural cross-sectional image information about the lumen and vessel wall provided by intravascular ultrasound (IVUS)[1-5] goes far beyond what is displayed by coronary angiography, which portrays the silhouette of the lumen by dye injection.[6,7] The possibility offered by IVUS to meticulously evaluate coronary lesions of angiographically uncertain severity and perform serial IVUS examinations for purposes of guidance, device selection, and endpoint assessment of catheter-based interventions makes this a practical clinical tool.[4,8] However, conventional IVUS is a planar technique, which displays only a single tomographic slice of the coronary vessel at a time. Accordingly, in conventional IVUS there is a lack of an angiography-like longitudinal visualization of the coronary segment examined. Moreover, quantification by manual boundary tracing on IVUS images is relatively time-consuming and subjective.

3D IVUS: RATIONALE AND FIRST OVERVIEW

These limitations can only be overcome by three-dimensional (3D) reconstruction of IVUS images sequences, acquired with a known sample spacing.[3,9-17] Three-dimensional IVUS systems were initially used to visually assess the configuration of plaques, dissections (Fig. 8-1), and stents, and to perform basic measurements.

The option to longitudinally visualize an entire coronary segment has recently been integrated into standard IVUS systems (Fig. 8-2). The longitudinal display avoids the difficult mental conceptualization required when using conventional IVUS, provides more detailed insight into the complex

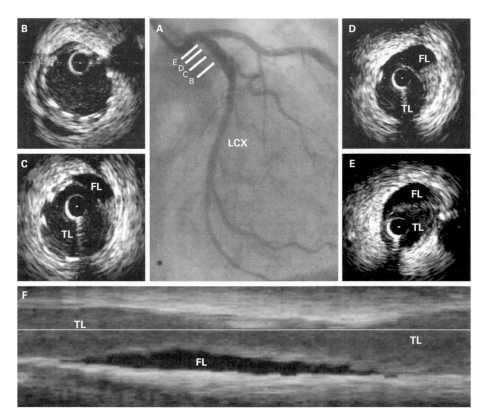

Figure 8-1. Incomplete stent-coverage of a dissection shown by 3D IVUS. Angiographic control (A) after stenting a proximal left circumflex (LCX) coronary artery suggested a satisfactory vessel patency. IVUS showed good distal stent expansion (B). At the proximal stent entry (C), the dissection flap was not completely covered by the stent and extended into the proximal vessel segment (D, E). The longitudinal reconstruction (F), derived from the «linear» 3D IVUS data set, provided detailed information on the full extent of the dissection and clearly showed the false lumen (FL) and true lumen (TL). Modified and reproduced with the kind permission of Eggebrecht et al. *J Intervent Cardiol* 1999; 12:519-520.[12]

plaque architecture, and facilitates serial IVUS studies.[16] All commercially available 3D IVUS systems provide (artificially) straightened 3D and longitudinal displays only, while highly sophisticated 3D systems can be used to obtain geometrically correct spatial 3D reconstructions.[16, 18-28]

In parallel with progress in quantitative angiographic techniques, which started with manual caliper assessment and eventually lead to the development of computer-assisted methods, dedicated systems for quantitative 3D IVUS analysis have been developed.[3, 29-43] These techniques reduce analysis time and the subjectivity of manual boundary tracing,[44] and permit careful evaluation and accurate quantitative assessment of coronary segments of interest using computer algorithms for the detection of vascular structures (Fig. 8-3).

The IVUS images need to be acquired during motorized pullback of the transducer,[3, 4, 16, 45-50] which can be performed at a uniform speed or in an ECG-triggered way. Image sampling and digitization can be performed on-line or off-line at a pre-defined image digitization rate or in an ECG-gated mode.

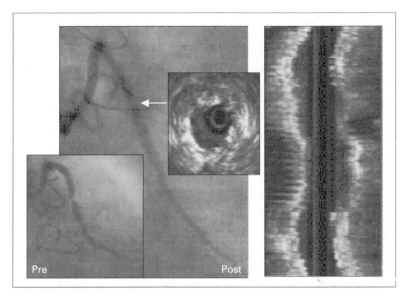

Figure 8-2. Cross-sectional and longitudinal IVUS views after the placement of two stents. In this patient we performed IVUS after stenting the mid and distal segment of an old, severely diseased, saphenous vein graft to the left circumflex coronary artery. On the longitudinally reconstructed IVUS view (right panel, Endosonics), the range of the stents is visualized.

For any quantitative analysis, the images have to be segmented. This step identifies structures of interest by applying dedicated algorithms, which discriminate between the blood-pool (= lumen), vessel wall, and adventitia. The quality of the reconstruction and accuracy of the quantitative analysis are highly influenced by the characteristics of the algorithm applied: the pioneering approach of «acoustic quantification» uses an algorithm for statistical pattern recognition,[8, 51-53] while «contour detection systems,»[3, 29-34, 41-43] apply a minimum cost algorithm to detect the lumen and external vessel boundary (= external elastic membrane, EEM).

Specific shading and rendering techniques can be used to give reconstructed views a spatial appearance when displayed on the computer screen[16] (Fig. 8-4), but for the time being, longitudinally reconstructed views without such rendering features are the most important reconstructed views.

CONVENTIONAL MOTORIZED IVUS PULLBACKS

Two main technical configurations of IVUS systems are currently used. A mechanical system has a flexible imaging cable that rotates a single transducer (at 1800 rpm, resulting in 30 frames/second) at its distal tip inside an echolucent distal sheath, which prevents any direct contact between the transducer and vessel wall, and avoids friction during the pullback of the imaging core. An electronic (solid-state) catheter system has multiple imaging elements (nowadays 64, also resulting in 30 frames/second) at its distal tip, providing cross-sectional images by sequentially activating the imaging elements in a circular way. With both systems, a motorized pullback device can be used for continuous (1.0 or 0.5 mm/s) retraction of the IVUS transducer (or the entire IVUS catheter, depending on the system used). During any IVUS pullback, injections of dye should

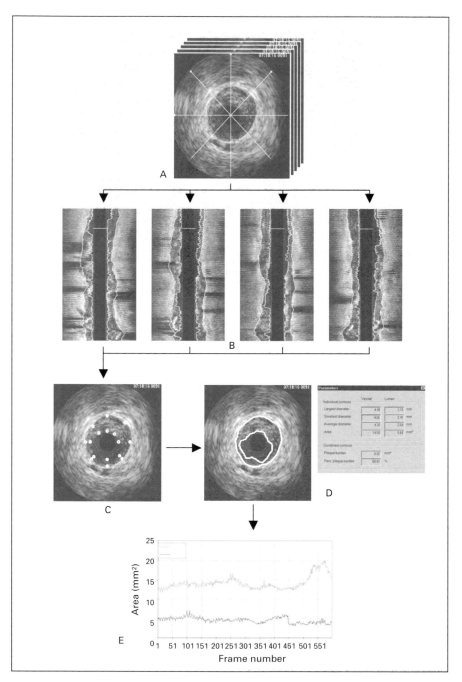

Figure 8-3. Computer-assisted boundary detection. Combination of transversal and longitudinal contour detection. (A) Generation of a user-defined number (here N = 4) of longitudinal images. (B) Detection of longitudinal vessel and lumen contours. (C) Generation of markers (attraction points) from the longitudinal contours in the transversal image. (D) Transversal lumen and vessel contour detection and example of derived parameters. (E) Plot presenting the vessel and lumen areas (vertical axis) for all frames (horizontal axis).

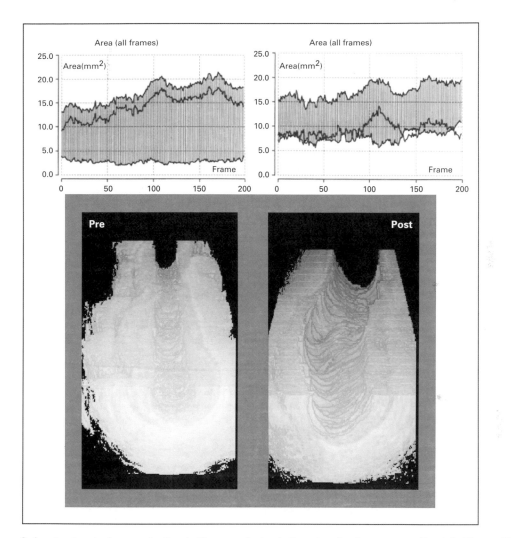

Figure 8-4. Lesion before and after balloon-optimized directional atherectomy. Spatial (linear 3D) views (lower panels) are reconstructed from the complete IVUS data sets, which are used for volumetric analysis. The upper panels show the cross-sectional area measurements, both before (left) and after the intervention (right). Linear functions of the vessel and lumen cross-sectional area form the upper and lower boundaries of the grayish area, which represents the plaque cross-sectional area measurementsfrom distal (left) to proximal (right). Alternatively, values of the plaque cross-sectional area can bederived directly from a linear function (single black line), which here mostly overlaps the grayish area. Modified and reproduced with the kind permission of von Birgelen et al. *Heart* 2000; 83:192-197.

be avoided. Note that during the first 5 to 10 mm of the pullback, the IVUS imaging core or catheter must be straightening before the correct length information (distance between particular images along the long vessel axis) can be obtained. Accordingly, the IVUS

transducer should (if possible) be positioned 5 to 10 mm distal to the actual segment of interest before motorized pullback is started. The entire IVUS examination should be recorded on super-VHS videotape and/or digitally for off-line assessment. In serial studies, side-branches or spots of calcium are used as topographic landmarks to ensure reliable comparison of the same coronary segment.[16]

ECG-GATED IMAGE ACQUISITION

During the cardiac cycle, the position of the IVUS catheter within the lumen may vary. Therefore, image acquisition from a continuous stream of IVUS images obtained during motorized pullback may result in longitudinal reconstructed views that show sawtooth image artifacts (Fig. 8-5) which hamper both visual interpretation and computer-assisted boundary detection.[16] In addition, longitudinal movement of the catheter may result in inaccuracies. Both mechanical and solid-state transducers can move as much as 5 mm between the end-diastole and systole, which may impair quantitative assessment of small vessel structures. Accurate determination of the stent edges may also be difficult.

ECG-gated image acquisition (during continuous or ECG-triggered stepped motorized pullback) can prevent such artifacts.[45-50, 54] Using a dynamic 3D reconstruction system, initially designed for 3D reconstruction of echocardiographic images (EchoScan, TomTec), the arterial segment can even be dynamically displayed, showing the motion of an entire cardiac cycle. The feasibility of using a dedicated ECG-triggered pullback device in humans *in vivo* was demonstrated in 30 coronary arteries;[32] ECG-gated image acquisition was successfully performed within approximately 4 ± 1.5 minutes and was well tolerated. Even online application of IVUS contour detection systems was possible following ECG-gated image acquisition.[50] Nevertheless, this approach requires buying additional technical equipment, training dedicated personnel in the catheterization laboratory, and spending significantly more time per procedure (for both preparation of the technical setup and image acquisition). Because of these limitations, which prevent general application, this interesting technical

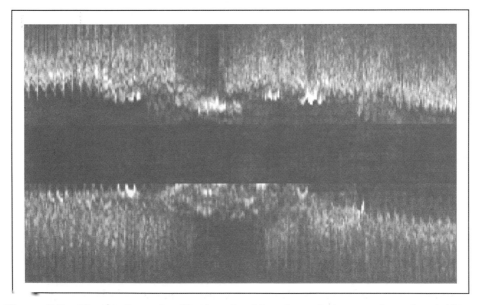

Figure 8-5. Non ECG-gated pullback series. Note the typical sawtooth motion artifacts.

approach has only been applied within some sophisticated scientific studies.

As an alternative to the gold standard of using a dynamic 3D reconstruction system to steer an ECG-triggered stepped motor-driven pullback device,[45, 46] frames from the same cardiac phase can be selected during loading (post hoc ECG-triggered sampling) if the ECG signal is stored along with the IVUS data. Nevertheless, this results in a relatively wide space between adjacent image frames (approximately 0.5 to 1 mm), while ECG-gated image acquisition with the dynamic 3D reconstruction system and a stepping pullback at 0.2 mm-steps allows complete scanning of the coronary vessel (at the price of a much longer image-acquisition time).

COMPUTER-ASSISTED BOUNDARY DETECTION (QUANTITATIVE 3D CORONARY ULTRASOUND)

Manual analysis of IVUS images, especially of long pullback sequences, is tedious, time-consuming, and suffers from high inter- and intra-observer variability.[44] To overcome these problems, different (semi-) automatic approaches have been developed.

Automated analysis of IVUS images offers several challenges caused by the low image resolution, non-uniform luminance and contrast, high noise content, and image artifacts like shadow regions behind calcified plaques, guide-wire artifacts and dropout regions.[37, 38] Fully automated segmentation generally demands a trade-off between accuracy and stability, in which higher algorithm sensitivity increases the risk of segmentation failure.[29] Development of the technique for automated analysis of 2D IVUS images started in the early 1990s. In most cases, single-frame 2D methods became the core of more complex 3D and 4D IVUS analysis methods. Several methods have been developed based on thresholding, statistical pattern recognition, and adaptive active contour models.[35, 39] Most successful techniques are based on contour detection techniques using minimal cost algorithm (MCA) approaches in a region of interest, which is either defined manually or by contours found in adjacent slices or in longitudinal images.[3, 29, 33, 34, 36, 38] The latter method is used in several commercially available software packages for the analysis of IVUS images.

Computer boundary detection basically uses the following methods (Fig. 8-3). It starts by stacking up individual slices in the computer memory. The source of the images can be analogue, from a VCR or IVUS acquisition device, or from a digital storage medium like a hard disc or CD-R. For the analogue signal a video acquisition device is needed. It should be considered that image quality degrades if the images are stored analogue on a videotape, even in case of the S-VHS format.

Next is the creation of longitudinal sections, two for the TomTec/Rotterdam system (TomTec, Munich, Germany)[32] and many more, typically 8 or 16, for the QCU-CMS®/Leyden system (MEDIS Medical Imaging Systems, Leyden, the Netherlands),[55] resulting in a straight (linear) reconstruction of the vessel segment. Since the longitudinal reconstruction may contain a lot of artifacts, e.g., due to cardiac motion, the longitudinal images are used to guide contour detection, not for quantitative purposes. To enhance the quantitative analysis, with the QCU-CMS system the user can identify a segment of interest (e.g., a stent), and a representative proximal and distal segment (e.g., to study vascular remodeling).

Then the vessel contours are detected in the longitudinal images using the minimal cost algorithm (MCA). This is a dynamic programming technique, which ensures that the most optimal solution will always be found for a contour, given the fact that the region of interest has been chosen correctly. Dynamic programming methods have been widely used in the field of medical image processing, particularly for contour detection in ultrasound images, because they are robust in terms of image noise. The method is based on the leading-edge strength (for lumen detection) and leading and trailing-edge combination strength (for vessel detection), which is determined for each individual point in the area of interest.

With the QCU-CMS system, in the longitudinal sections the vessel contours are detected simultaneously, which means that they have knowledge about each other's position. For example, the following situation may occur. At one side of the vessel in the longitudinal image, a clear vessel transition is present which would force the vessel contour detection to the left. On the other side of the vessel, multiple potentially vague vessel transitions in different directions are present. The simultaneous technique will now select the combination of strong transition at one side, and a transition on the other side that best matches the morphological continuity of the vessel and the shape and size of the vessel. This technique is especially useful for regions behind calcified plaques and in side branches, where there is little or no image information available to support contour detection. If a stent is present, the vessel contour will also be forced outside a previously detected stent.

Despite all additional models and knowledge, the detection results may still be influenced by image artifacts and speckle noise. Therefore, the results of contour detection are not always entirely correct and some manual interaction may be required. An important difference between the software packages available is the handling and flexibility of user-interaction. In the ideal situation, user-interaction is as efficient as possible, reducing the number of corrections and thus the time required for analysis. To overcome image artifacts, additional knowledge is incorporated, e.g., to remove the ring-down artifact, to avoid guide wire artifacts, and to use models to solve the problem of shadowed regions behind calcified plaques. As previously stated, the longitudinal contours are used for guidance and not for quantitative measurements.

Next, the contours are transferred to the transversal slices, where they result in guiding points for the region of interest in transversal contour detection (both the TomTec and QCU-CMS systems). The transversal contour detection of the boundaries of the vessel, lumen, and stent is based on the same principles as longitudinal detection. However, for transversal detection the images are transformed to a polar image, which is actually the native format of IVUS images. The final contours are transformed back to the normal view. Vessel, stent, and lumen parameters can be determined for each individual slice, based on the derived transversal contours. Cross-sectional areas (Fig. 8-6), average diameters, symmetry data, and various other derived parameters, which have recently been suggested,[56, 57] can be obtained.

In the QCU-CMS software, stent contour detection is performed in two steps in the transversal images. The first step is the global estimation of the location of the stent struts based on their intensity and location with respect to the catheter. It is more likely that bright stent struts are located closer to the catheter than calcified spots. Using the Minimum Cost Algorithm (MCA), candidate points are identified to create a model for the second, more locally directed, detection of strut location. This second detection uses the approximately circular shape of the stent and the strong leading edges of the stent struts. Stent detection can correct itself based on a 3D model in which the change in size and position of the stent contour is limited over a short distance. Even in slices with poorly defined stent struts, a meaningful stent contour can be found in this way. Stent detection is performed only in the transversal images, because in the longitudinal cross-sections the appearance of the stent struts is much less regular and sometimes the struts are not visible at all.

After detection of all contours in the segment of interest, volumetric parameters can be determined using information on the slice thickness. Generally, Simpson's rule is used for volumetric measurements. Also, other

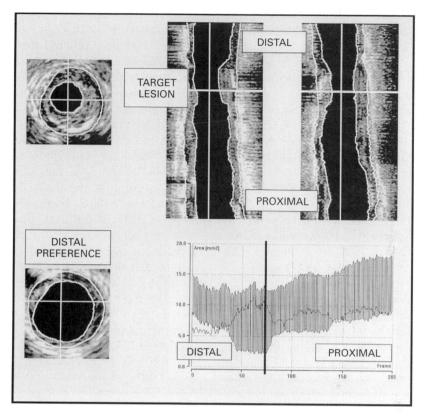

Figure 8-6. Coronary segment with inadequate compensatory vascular enlargement. This quantitative 3D analysis of a «shrinkage» lesion clearly shows the smallest vessel cross-sectional area at the target lesion site. Markers indicate that site on two reconstructed longitudinal views (upper right panels) and the display of the cross-sectional area measurements (lower right panel). Linear functions of the vessel and lumen cross-sectional area form the upper and lower boundaries of the grayish area, which represents theplaque cross-sectional area. Alternatively, the values of the plaque cross-sectional area can be derived directly from a linear function (single black line), which is here partly overlapping the grayish area. Reproducedwith the kind permission of von Birgelen et al. *Heart* 1998; 79:137-142.[58]

length-based measurements can be performed like measurements of stent length. The slice thickness (mm) can easily be calculated by dividing the pullback speed (mm/s) and number of frames per second.

VALIDATION OF QUANTITATIVE 3D IVUS

Quantitative 3D systems extend the measurement features of IVUS by longitudinal and volumetric measurements, and provide automated quantification of the plaque and/or lumen. These measurements are frequently used for scientific studies, as contour detection-based measurements in 3D image data sets are most accurate and ideal for core lab activities.[41-43,58-61] Accordingly, it was important to make a decent validation, which is summarized below for the TomTec/Rotterdam and the QCU-CMS/Leyden boundary detection systems.

The main in vitro validation of the *Tom-Tec/Rotterdam* system was performed in postmortem atherosclerotic human coronary arteries.[31] Cross-sectional area and volume measurements by 3D IVUS agreed well with the results obtained by manual tracing, showing low between-method differences with low standard deviations and high correlation coefficients (r $\geqslant$ 0.97); the 3D IVUS measurements also correlated well with the histomorphometric data.[31] Moreover, a validation study was performed in a tubular «lumen» phantom with segments of various luminal dimensions; the 3D IVUS contour detection showed good agreement and high correlations with the true values.[30]

The *in vivo* measurement variability of analyzing clinical 3D image sequences from continuous motorized transducer pullbacks was studied[30] and was found to be low (cross-sectional areas: $\leqslant$ 10.8 %, volumes: <2.8 %). However, in this study, IVUS sequences of coronary segments with excessive cyclical movement were not considered for analysis, as the systolic-diastolic sawtooth image artifacts on the longitudinally reconstructed sections hindered automated contour detection.

In ECG-gated 3D image sets of 30 patients, there was an excellent agreement between automated contour detection with conventional manual measurements on 200 randomly chosen IVUS images (differences $\leqslant$ 1.6 % with SD $\leqslant$ 9.1 %).[32] Although the coronary segments in this ECG-gated study[32] were non-selected and included calcified portions and some side branches, 3D contour analyses of the ECG-gated image sets showed a low measurement variability (for cross-sectional area measurements $\leqslant$ 7.2 %), which was considerably lower than that reported for the study with non-gated 3D image sets.[30] Volumetric measurements showed a particularly low measurement variability ($\leqslant$ 3.2 %), which reflects an averaging of the differences of the cross-sectional area measurements.[54]

The *QCU-CMS software* has also been carefully validated in different ways.[42, 43] An agar phantom with well-known vessel and lumen dimensions[62] was used to determine the systematic and random errors of the vessel and lumen detection. The real dimensions of the phantom were determined by photomacroscopy. The areas measured by the QCU-CMS software using images from a phased array acquisition system and the macroscopy show an excellent correlation for both the vessel and lumen dimensions (r = 0.99) with small mean differences.[43] The same phantom was also measured using a mechanical (rotating) catheter system. The differences in area measurements between images from a phased array system and a rotating catheter system were very small and not significant. When the contours of the automatic system were compared to the manually drawn contours in these phantom images, only an average diameter difference of 0.01 mm was found.

In another validation, the cross-sectional areas from manually traced and automatically detected boundaries in *in vivo* images (number of images) were compared and resulted in a correlation of 0.98-0.99 for both the vessel and lumen contour.

Furthermore, a set of 14 pullback sequences acquired *in vivo* with a mechanical rotating catheter were analyzed both by the QCU-CMS software and by the TomTec software. The coronary segments, which were analyzed with both systems, were identical. A total of 877 images were analyzed, resulting in a correlation coefficient of 0.98 between the lumen areas and 0.99 between the vessel areas of both systems. The overall difference between the QCU-CMS and TomTec system for the lumen area was -0.13 ± 0.70 mm^2, which is almost equal. For the lumen area it was 0.86 ± 0.57 mm^2. The IVUS experts felt that the difference in vessel area could be the result of a slight underestimation of vessel size by the TomTec system, as manually corrected contours on the TomTec system corresponded very well with the automatically detected contours on the QCU-CMS system.[43]

ON-LINE AND OFF-LINE USE OF 3D IVUS

The requirements for automatic contour detection of IVUS images are different for the on-line application in the catheterization laboratory during a catheterization procedure, and the off-line application for clinical research or methodological evaluation. For on-line application, the speed of operation is much more important than the exact volumetric data from the pullback image series. It is important to obtain an overview of plaque distribution and lumen dimensions. In addition, the location and parameters of the narrowest lumen site and the parameters of the reference slices should be detected. This should be done with as little user-interaction as possible to speed up the process and permit measurements in the catheterization laboratory by technicians or nurses. The operating cardiologist may still be responsible for final judgment, but will generally not perform measurements personally. For on-line application, extensive three-dimensional reconstruction (e.g., using biplane angiograms for correct reconstruction to improve the volumetric calculation) is neither necessary nor realistic. However, synchronization between IVUS images and a marker in the angiograms could theoretically be useful to combine locally derived information of IVUS with the global information of the X-ray images.

For off-line quantification, accurate contour detection and correct 3D reconstruction will improve the volumetric measurements,[26] which may be important for detecting small differences in plaque volume. However, in many small segments the volumetric calculation error due to curvature and torsion is small.[27] Off-line, the speed of operation is less critical and more user-interaction is allowed to correct for small misinterpretations.[42]

QUANTITATIVE 3D IVUS IN RESEARCH AND CLINICAL PRACTICE

Atherosclerotic plaque distribution and both lumen and vessel dimensions can be examined with IVUS along an entire coronary segment. Accordingly, vascular remodeling can be studied by comparing the lesion with the reference vessel dimensions.[1] Previous IVUS studies have demonstrated that many significant coronary lesions reflect the process of adaptive «Glagovian» remodeling (compensatory vascular enlargement with an increase in plaque burden), while other lesions show no or even inadequate compensatory vascular enlargement (or so-called «shrinkage,» Fig. 8-6).[58, 59, 63, 64] Computer-assisted boundary detection using 3D IVUS image sets is the most accurate and ideal method for IVUS studies of the progression and regression of atherosclerosis, percutaneous catheter-based coronary interventions, and pharmacological interventions.[65]

There are also various clinical scenarios, where longitudinal reconstruction and/or computer-assisted measurements can be clinically helpful. Information on dissection length-and hence the length of the stent that should cover it- can be derived from the time information of the motorized pullback. As a more elegant alternative, systems for three-dimensional reconstruction and quantification of IVUS images allow direct measurement of the length of a flap on longitudinally reconstructed images[16](Fig. 8-1).

Pre-intervention 3D examination of the coronary segment to be treated provides insight into the relation between plaque and side-branches, which may permit appropriate sizing of a stent (diameter and length). The spatial geometry of coronary stents can accurately be reconstructed, and automated measurement of stent area facilitates the detection of stent underexpansion, as changes of stent lumen area during motorized pullbacks are smooth, mostly gradual, and often difficult to recognize by the conventional use of IVUS.[17, 50] Volumetric IVUS evaluation[14] before and after the atherectomy procedure (Fig. 8-4) may be used to obtain a reliable quantification of both plaque ablation and luminal enlargement[59, 63] and thus, the efficacy of the intervention. But for the time being, this volumetric approach, which can also be used to assess the 6-months follow-up result of percutaneous coronary interventions (Fig. 8-7), is mostly restricted to core laboratory activities of clinical studies (Fig. 8-8) and/or research applications.

In addition, coronary brachytherapy for the prevention of restenosis is a potentially interesting field for the application of 3D IVUS. The rationale is as follows: Coronary lesions with an extreme difference in vascular remodeling following percutaneous interventions show a great difference in the distance between the center of the lumen and the external vessel boundary.[58] Beta-radiation shows a relatively steep dose-decline with increasing distance from the source. Therefore, lesions with very different vascular remodeling will show large differences in beta-radiation exposure to the external vessel boundary or the adjacent adventitia (Fig. 8-9). As IVUS is the only technique that allows the *in vivo* assessment of the true vessel dimensions and of vascular remodeling inside the cardiac catheterization laboratory, com-

puter-assisted boundary detection of 3D IVUS image sets may be an ideal tool for dosimetry of brachytherapy. Besides the potential application of IVUS for dosimetry (particularly of beta-emitting sources), IVUS is the ideal technique for evaluating the mechanisms of restenosis reduction by brachytherapy and its potential adverse consequences.[66-69]

True geometric 3D reconstruction of coronary vessels based on image fusion techniques provides further scientific insights and yields data on blood velocity profiles and local shear stresses.[70-72] The technical issues of such approaches and an outlook on future applications is presented in later sections of this chapter.

THREE-DIMENSIONAL RECONSTRUCTION (IMAGE FUSION)

Currently, IVUS images are stacked into a straight pipe, which is a simple and fast ap-

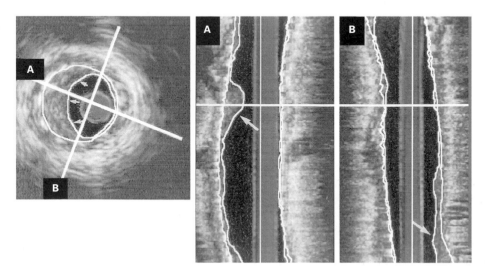

Figure 8-7. Analysis of in-stent neointimal proliferation. On 2 perpendicular longitudinal images (Aand B), reconstructed from the entire IVUS data set, the coronary lumen, stent struts, and neointimal ingrowth (arrowheads) can be well distinguished. The origin of the planar IVUS image on the left side is indicated by a horizontal cursor on the longitudinal images; it shows focal neointimal proliferation (smaller arrowheads). Reproduced with the kind permission of von Birgelen et al. *Am J Cardiol* 1998;82:129-134.[60]

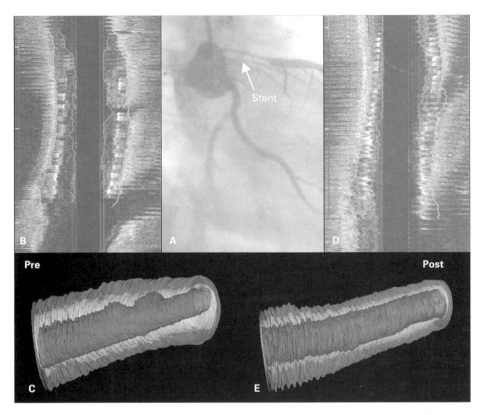

Figure 8-8. 3D quantitative IVUS to study lumen gain by directional atherectomy inside a restenotic stent. The pre-intervention angiographic image (A) shows a stent with in-stent restenosis. Also, the corresponding longitudinal IVUS image (B) shows the in-stent restenosis, which also can be visualized in 3D by the individual contours (the dark irregular cylinder is the remaining lumen, the brighter structure is the stent surrounded by the vessel contour). After the DCA procedure, the longitudinal IVUS image (D) shows a much wider lumen that is also visible in the 3D reconstruction (E). From the volumetriccalculations, it appeared that the amount of in-stent neointima volume was reduced from 128.5 mm^3 to 71.2 mm^3 while the minimal lumen diameter increased from 1.9 to 2.6 mm.

proach for 3D reconstruction and provides a useful overview of the IVUS information.[10-13] However, conventional straight stacking of the IVUS images does not result in entirely correct volumetric results.[25] More realistic 3D reconstruction methods have been described, which take into account the curved path of the transducer trajectory during a motorized pullback of the IVUS transducer. These methods reconstruct the 3D path from multiple biplanar X-ray images of successive transducer locations or use the vessel centerline as an approximation.[73, 74] These ap-

proaches still suffer from crucial reconstruction problems, related to the determination of the true orientation of the IVUS cross-sections and respiratory motion.

A powerful angiographic tool for morphological analyses of the vessel tree is spatial reconstruction of the vessels from biplane angiograms. From the known imaging geometry, and based on epipolar constraints, any point visible in both projections can be spatially reconstructed by retracing the projection rays back to the point of their intersection. However, due to slight reconstruc-

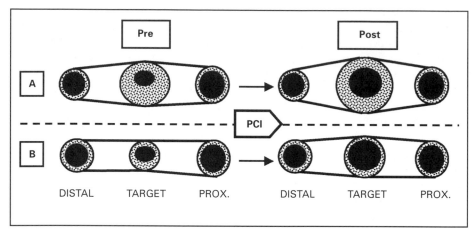

Figure 8-9. Rationale for the use of IVUS in brachytherapy. Lesions with compensatory (A) and inadequate «shrinkage» remodeling (B) show a considerable difference in the distance between the lumen center and the external vessel boundary, both before (left panels) and after (right panels) percutaneouscoronary interventions (PCI). In fact, IVUS is the only technique that allows *in vivo* assessment of the true vessel dimensions and remodeling state inside the catheterization laboratory. This information may be most useful in the context of beta-radiation and could be used for dosimetry.

tion or calibration errors, these intersection points may not be found and therefore their closest location is estimated. For the volumetric analysis of the vessel and lumen, a very high accuracy of reconstruction is required. The imaging process of angiograms introduces numerous geometrical distortions and, together with distorted axial rotations and shifts, a lot of errors are introduced. Newer reconstruction techniques try to overcome these shortcomings. Different additional methods have been described for calibration and correction, like lead markers on the image intensifier, calibration balls[25] or

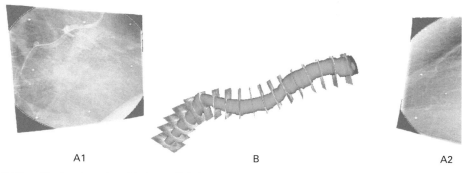

A1   B   A2

Figure 8-10. Fusion imaging. Fusion of biplane angiographic image (A1 and A2) in which the catheter and vessel contour are detected. Next, the 3D trajectory of the catheter is determined, the orientation is determined, and torsion is compensated, resulting in, e.g., the visualization of the geometrically correct lumen contour (B) on which original IVUS slices are superimposed. Many ways of visualization exist, even a fly-through.

the use of a calibration cube, which is filmed after the procedure.[26]

The 3D reconstruction starts with the extraction of the 3D catheter trajectory from a biplanar set of end-diastolic frames, which optimally show the IVUS catheter and contrast-filled lumen. Also, in these angiographic images the lumen borders are detected using standard QCA approaches.

After the lumen contours in the IVUS images have been detected using the methods described earlier, the IVUS cross-sections are distributed at equidistant intervals on the reconstructed catheter path (Fig. 8-10). The imaging planes are positioned perpendicular to the catheter path and then rotated angularly, based on the following principles. First, an arbitrary rotation for the distal IVUS image is chosen and the rotation of each consecutive plane is derived by a discrete implementation of the Frenet-Serret formulas.[18] This algorithm corrects for the catheter-twist that occurs when the catheter passes through helical curves, resulting in the rotation of the IVUS images. This approach, however, only describes the relation between adjacent slices relative to each other. What remains to be determined is the absolute orientation of the set of images.

A method for achieving a correct overall match of the IVUS and angiographic data is to use anatomic landmarks like side-branches. However, the location and orientation of the branches often cannot be determined accurately enough in both the angiographic and IVUS images.[21] Another approach is to use the vessel outline in the angiographic image as reference.[18, 23, 26] The lumen from the reconstructed IVUS pullback stack is projected back into the biplane angiograms. By rotating the reconstructed IVUS image stack, the best match for the distance between the catheter and the lumen in both the IVUS images and the angiogram can then be determined. Varying the angular rotation of the IVUS stack causes the reconstruction to rotate around the catheter trajectory until it fits «like a sock on a foot».

Therefore, another method uses the out-of-center position relative to the lumen, which is visible in both the angiographic and IVUS images. The angiographic lumen is reconstructed as an elliptical contour based on the contours from the original biplane images. The IVUS data is mapped into 3D using the initial orientation along with the relative twist. For each frame location, the out-of-center strength and the difference angles in the angiographic versus IVUS reconstruction are determined. Based mainly on the strongest out-of-center positions, a single correction angle is determined and applied to all IVUS frames to come to the absolute orientation.[22, 25]

The output of these geometrically correct (true) three-dimensional reconstructions can be used for correct volume estimation, length measurements, and curvature measurements, thus overcoming the limitations of linear stacking of the frames.

OUTLOOK ON FURTHER DEVELOPMENTS OF 3D IVUS

Longitudinally reconstructed IVUS views can now be used in clinical practice. The possibility to meticulously evaluate coronary lesions and to perform serial IVUS examinations for the assessment of catheter-based or pharmacological interventions including brachytherapy makes «Quantitative 3D Coronary Ultrasound» a powerful tool in clinical research.

The output of three-dimensional reconstructions can be used for 3D visualization of the vessel wall (including virtual angioscopy), determination of the plaque distribution on the inner and outer curves, determination of the change in vessel geometry after an intervention or overtime,[75] and for computational fluid dynamics (CFD) calculations, since the correct geometry of the vessel is known together with detailed information on wall morphology provided by IVUS. Computational fluid dynamics is a general term for numerical techniques to calculate the pressure and velocity of fluid elements at each location in a studied geometry, solving the incompressible Navier-Stokes equations. The Navier-Stokes equations are 3D non-linear differential equations which describe the movement of fluid elements based on conservation of energy and mass. Numerical techniques are needed to solve them. From these calculations, the velocity profiles, pressure differences, and shear stresses can be derived. The initiation, localization, growth, composition, and rupture[1] of intracoronary atheromatous plaques-factors that define the natural history of coronary artery disease are all dependent on inhomogeneities and irregularities of intracoronary local blood flow and wall shear stress. Low shear stress leads to plaque development and progression. High shear stress contributes significantly to plaque rupture. Recent research has combined three-dimensional reconstructed IVUS with CFD and obtained valuable insights into the interrelation of (re)stenosis and local shear stress.[70, 71] A next step may be to include time in the 3D reconstruction process, which results in 4D models of the coronary artery.[28]

REFERENCES

1. von Birgelen C, Klinkhart W, Mintz GS, et al. Plaque distribution and vascular remodeling of ruptured and nonruptured coronary plaques in the same vessel: an intravascular ultrasound study in vivo. *J Am Coll Cardiol* 2001; 37:1864-1870.

2. Erbel R, Ge J, Bockisch A, et al. Value of intracoronary ultrasound and Doppler in the differentiation of angiographically normal coronary arteries: a prospective study in patients with angina pectoris. *Eur Heart J* 1996; 17:880-889.

3. Dijkstra J, Wahle A, Koning G, Reiber JHC, Sonka M. Quantitative coronary ultrasound: state of the art. In: Reiber JHC, van der Wall EE (editors). What's new in Cardiovascular Imaging. *Dordrecht: Kluwer Academic Publishers,* 1998; 79-94.

4. Mintz GS, Pichard AD, Kovach JA, et al. Impact of preintervention intravascular ultrasound imaging on transcatheter treatment strategies in coronary artery disease. *Am J Cardiol* 1994; 73:423-430.

5. von Birgelen C, Airiian SG, Mintz GS, et al. Variations of remodeling in response to left main atherosclerosis assessed with intravascular ultrasound in vivo. *Am J Cardiol* 1997; 80:1408-1413.

6. Escaned J, Baptista J, Di Mario C, et al. Significance of automated stenosis detection during quantitative angiography: insights gained from intracoronary ultrasound. *Circulation* 1996; 94:966-972.

7. von Birgelen C, Kutryk MJB, Gil R, et al. Quantification of the minimal luminal cross-sectional area after coronary stenting: two- and three-dimensional intravascular ultrasound versus edge detection and videodensitometry. *Am J Cardiol* 1996; 78:520-525.

8. Oesterle Limpijankit T, Yeung AC, et al. Ultrasound logic: the value of intracoronary imaging for the interventionalist. *Cathet Cardiovasc Intervent* 1999; 47:475-490.

9. Kitney R, Moura L, Straughan K. 3-D visualization of arterial structures using ultrasound and voxel modelling. *Int J Cardiac Imag* 1989; 4:135-143.

10. Rosenfield K, Losordo DW, Ramaswamy K, Isner JM. Three-dimensional reconstruction of human coronary and peripheral arteries from images recorded during two-dimensional intravascular ultrasound examination. *Circulation* 1991; 84:1938-1956.

11. Mintz GS, Pichard AD, Satler LF, Popma JJ, Kent KM, Leon MB. Three-dimensional intravascular ultrasonography: reconstruction of endovascular stents in vitro and in vivo. *Clin Ultrasound* 1993; 21:609-615.

12. Eggebrecht H, Baumgart D, von Birgelen C, et al. Assessment of postangioplasty coronary dissection by three-dimensional intravascular ultrasound. *J Intervent Cardiol* 1999; 12:519-520.

13. Roelandt, JRTC, Di Mario C, Pandian NG, et al. Three-dimensional reconstruction of intracoronary ultrasound images: Rationale, approaches, problems and directions. *Circulation* 1994; 90:1044-1055.

14. von Birgelen C, Slager CJ, Di Mario C, de Feyter PJ, Serruys PW. Volumetric in-

tracoronary ultrasound: a new maximum confidence approach for the quantitative assessment of progression/regression of atherosclerosis? *Atherosclerosis* 1995; 118 (Suppl.): S103-S113.

15. Di Mario C, von Birgelen C, Prati F, et al. Three-dimensional reconstruction of two-dimensional intracoronary ultrasound: clinical or research tool? *Br Heart J* 1995; 73(Suppl. 2): 26-32.

16. von Birgelen C, Mintz GS, de Feyter PJ, et al. Reconstruction and quantification with three-dimensional intracoronary ultrasound: an update on techniques, challenges, and future directions. *Eur Heart J* 1997; 18:1056-1067.

17. von Birgelen C, Kutryk MJB, Serruys PW. Three-dimensional intravascular ultrasound analysis of coronary stent deployment and in-stent neointimal volume: current clinical practice and the concepts of TRAPIST, ERASER, and ITALICS. *J Invas Cardiol* 1998; 10:17-26.

18. Laban M, Oomen JA, Slager CJ, et al. ANGUS: a new approach to three-dimensional reconstruction of coronary vessels by combined use of angiography and intravascular ultrasound. In: Computers in Cardiology 1995, Vienna, AT: *IEEE Computer Society Press,* 1995; 325-328.

19. Evans JL, Ng KH, Wiet SG, et al. Accurate three-dimensional reconstruction of intravascular ultrasound data: spatially correct three-dimensional reconstructions. *Circulation* 1996; 93:567-576.

20. Slager CJ, Wentzel JJ, Oomen JA, et al. True reconstruction of vessel geometry from combined X-ray angiographic and intracoronary ultrasound data. Semin Interv *Cardiol* 1997; 2:43-47.

21. Prause GPM, DeJong SC, MacKay SA, Sonka M. Semi-automated segmentation and 3-D reconstruction of coronary biplane angiography and intravascular ultrasound data fusion. In: Medical Imaging 1996: Physiology and function from multidimensional images, Newport Beach, CA: *SPIE,* 1996; 82-92.

22. Prause GPM, DeJong SC, McKay CR, Sonka M. Towards a geometrically correct 3-D reconstruction of tortuous coronary arteries based on biplane angiography and in-

travascular ultrasound. *Int J Card Imag* 1997; 13:451-462.

23. Shekhar R, Cothren RM, Vince DG, et al. Three-dimensional segmentation of luminal and adventitial borders in serial intravascular ultrasound images. *Comput Med Imaging Graph* 1999; 23:299-309.

24. Wahle A, Prause G, von Birgelen C, Erbel R, Sonka M. Fusion of angiography and intravascular ultrasound in vivo: establishing the absolute 3-D frame orientation. *IEEE Trans Biomed Eng* 1999; 46:1176-1180.

25. Wahle A, Prause GPM, DeJong SC, Sonka M. Geometrically correct 3-D reconstruction of intravascular ultrasound images by fusion with biplane angiography - Methods and validation. *IEEE Trans On Medical Imaging* 1999; 18:686-699.

26. Slager CJ, Wentzel JJ, Schuurbiers JC, et al. True 3-dimensional reconstruction of coronary arteries in patients by fusion of angiography and IVUS (ANGUS) and its quantitative validation. *Circulation 2000;* 102:511-516.

27. Schuurbiers JCH, von Birgelen C, Wentzel JJ, et al. On the IVUS plaque volume error in coronary arteries when neglecting curvature. *Ultrasound Med Biol* 2001; 26:1403-1411.

28. Wahle A, Mitchell SC, Ramaswamy SD, Chandran KB, Sonka M. Virtual angioscopy in human coronary arteries with visualization of computational hemodynamics. In: Medical Imaging 2001: Physiology and Function from Multidimensional Images San Diego, CA: *SPIE Proceedings,* 2001; 32-43.

29. Li W, von Birgelen C, Di Mario C, et al. Semi-automatic contour detection for volumetric quantification of intracoronary ultrasound. In: Computers in Cardiology 1994. Los Alamitos, CA: *IEEE Computer Society Press,* 1994; 277-280.

30. von Birgelen C, Di Mario C, Li W, et al. Morphometric analysis in three-dimensional intracoronary ultrasound: an in-vitro and invivo study using a novel system for the contour detection of lumen and plaque. *Am Heart J* 1996; 132:516-527.

31. von Birgelen C, van der Lugt A, Nicosia A, et al. Computerized assessment of coronary lumen and atherosclerotic plaque dimen-

sions in three-dimensional intravascular ultrasound correlated with histomorphometry. *Am J Cardiol* 1996; 78:1202-1209.

32. von Birgelen C, de Vrey EA, Mintz GS, et al. ECG-gated three-dimensional intravascular ultrasound: feasibility and reproducibility of an automated analysis of coronary lumen and atherosclerotic plaque dimensions in humans. *Circulation* 1997; 96:2944-2952.

33. Sonka M, Liang W, Zhang X, De Jong S, Collins SM, McKay CR. Three-dimensional automated segmentation of coronary wall and plaque from intravascular ultrasound pullback sequences. In: Computers in Cardiology 1995. Los Alamitos, CA: *IEEE Computer Society Press,* 1995; 637-640.

34. Sonka M, Zhang X, Siebes M, et al. Segmentation of intravascular ultrasound images: A knowledge-based approach. *IEEE Trans on medical imaging* 1995; 14:719-732.

35. Matar FA, Mintz GS, Douek P, et al. Coronary artery lumen volume measurement using three-dimensional intravascular ultrasound: validation of a new technique. *Cathet Cardiovasc Diagn* 1994; 33:214-220.

36. Herrington DM, Johnson T, Santago P, Snyder WE. Semi-automated boundary detection for intravascular ultrasound. In: Computers in Cardiology 1992 Durham, NC: *IEEE Computer Society Press,* 1992; 103-106.

37. Maurincomme E, Finet G, Reiber JHC, Savalle L, Magnin I. Quantitative intravascular ultrasound imaging: evaluation of an automated approach. *J Am Coll Cardiol* 1995; 25(Suppl.):354A.

38. Meier DS, Cothren RM, Vince DG, Cornhill JF Automated morphometry of coronary arteries with digital image analysis of intravascular ultrasound. *Am Heart J* 1997; 133:681-690.

39. Klingensmith JD, Shekhar R, Vince DG, et al. Evaluation of three-dimensional segmentation algorithms for the identification of luminal and medial-adventitial borders in intravascular ultrasound images. *IEEE Trans Med Imaging* 2000; 19:996-1011.

40. van der Lugt A, Hartlooper A, van Essen JA, et al. Reliability and reproducibility of automated contour analysis in intravascular ultrasound images of femoropopliteal arteries. *Ultrasound Med Biol* 1998; 24:43-50.

41. Koning G, Dijkstra J, von Birgelen C, et al. Improved contour detection for three-dimensional intravascular ultrasound: an invivo validation study. *J Am Coll Cardiol* 2000; 35(Suppl.):47A.

42. Dijkstra J, Koning G, Tuinenburg JC, Oemrawsingh PV, Reiber JHC. Automated Border Detection in IntraVascular Ultrasound Images for Quantitative: Measurements of the Vessel, Lumen and Stent Parameters. In: Computers in Cardiology 2001 Rotterdam, NL: *IEEE Computer Society Press,* 2001; 25-28.

43. Koning G, Dijkstra J, von Birgelen C, et al. Advanced Contour Detection for Three-Dimensional Intracoronary Ultrasound: A Validation —*in vitro* and *in vivo*. *Int J Card Imag*— *in press.*

44. Peters RJG, Kok WEM, Rijsterborgh H, et al. Reproducibility of quantitative measurements from intracoronary ultrasound images. *Eur Heart J* 1996; 17:1593-1599.

45. Bruining N, von Birgelen C, Di Mario C, et al. Dynamic three-dimensional reconstruction of ICUS images based on an ECG gated pull-back device. In: Computers in Cardiology 1995, Los Alamitos: *IEEE Computer Society Press,* 1995; 633-636.

46. Bruining N, von Birgelen C, Mallus M, et al. ECG-gated ICUS image acquisition combined with a semi-automated contour detection provides accurate analysis of vessel dimensions. *Computers in Cardiology* 1996; 53-56.

47. Bruining N, von Birgelen C, de Feyter PJ, Ligthart J, Serruys PW, Roelandt JRTC. Dynamic imaging of coronary stent structures: an ECG-gated three-dimensional intracoronary ultrasound study in humans. *Ultrasound Med Biol* 1998; 24:631-637.

48. Bruining N, von Birgelen C, de Feyter PJ, Roelandt JRTC, Serruys PW. Ultrasound appearances of coronary stents as obtained by three-dimensional intracoronary ultrasound imaging in vitro. *J Invas Cardiol* 1998; 10:332-338.

49. Bruining N, von Birgelen C, de Feyter PJ, et al. ECG-gated versus non-gated three-dimensional intracoronary ultrasound analy-

sis: implications for volumetric measurements. *Cathet Cardiovasc Diagn* 1998; 43:254-260.

50. von Birgelen C, Mintz GS, Nicosia A, et al. Electrocardiogram-gated intravascular ultrasound image acquisition after coronary stent deployment facilitates on-line three-dimensional reconstruction and automated lumen quantification. *J Am Coll Cardiol* 1997; 30:436-443.

51. Gil R, von Birgelen C, Prati F, Di Mario C, Ligthart J, Serruys PW. Usefulness of three-dimensional reconstruction for interpretation and quantitative analysis of intracoronary ultrasound during stent deployment. *Am J Cardiol* 1996;77:761-764.

52. Prati F, Di Mario C, Gil R, von Birgelen C, et al. Usefulness of on-line three-dimensional reconstruction of intracoronary ultrasound for guidance of stent deployment. *Am J Cardiol* 1996; 77:455-461.

53. von Birgelen C, Gil R, Ruygrok P, et al. Optimized expansion of the Wallstent compared with the Palmaz-Schatz stent: online observations with two- and three-dimensional intracoronary ultrasound after angiographic guidance. *Am Heart J* 1996; 131:1067-1075.

54. von Birgelen C, de Feyter PJ, de Vrey EA, et al. Simpson's rule for the volumetric ultrasound assessment of atherosclerotic coronary arteries: a study with ECG-gated three-dimensional intravascular ultrasound. *Coron Artery Dis* 1997; 8:363-369.

55. Reiber JHC, Koning G, Dijkstra J, et al. Angiography and Intravascular Ultrasound. In: Sonka M, Fitzpatrick JM, (editors). Handbook of Medical Imaging —Volume 2: Medical Image Processing and Analysis. *Belligham, WA.: SPIE,* 2000; 711-808.

56. Di Mario C, Görge G, Peters R, et al. Clinical application and image interpretation in intracoronary ultrasound. *Eur Heart J* 1998; 19:207-229.

57. Mintz GS, Nissen SE, Anderson WD, et al. American College of Cardiology Clinical Expert Consensus Document on Standards for Acquisition, Measurement and Reporting of Intravascular Ultrasound Studies (IVUS). A report of the American College of Cardiology Task Force on Clinical Expert Consensus Documents. *J Am Coll Cardiol* 2001; 37:1478-1492.

58. von Birgelen C, Mintz GS, de Vrey EA, et al. Atherosclerotic coronary lesions with inadequate compensatory enlargement have smaller plaque and vessel volumes: observations with three-dimensional intravascular ultrasound in vivo. *Heart* 1998; 79:137-143.

59. von Birgelen C, Mintz GS, de Vrey EA, et al. Preintervention lesion remodeling affects operative mechanisms of balloon-optimized directional atherectomy procedures: a volumetric study with three-dimensional intravascular ultrasound. *Heart* 2000; 83:192-197.

60. von Birgelen C, Airiian SG, de Feyter PJ, et al. Coronary Wallstents show significant late, post-procedural expansion despite implantation with adjunct high-pressure balloon inflations. *Am J Cardiol* 1998; 82:129-134.

61. de Vrey EA, Mintz GS, von Birgelen C, et al. Serial volumetric (three-dimensional) intravascular ultrasound analysis of restenosis after directional coronary atherectomy. *J Am Coll Cardiol* 1998; 32:1874-1880.

62. Brunette J, Mongrain R, Cloutier G, et al. A novel realistic three-layer phantom for intravascular ultrasound (IVUS) imaging. Int *J Card Imaging* 2001; 17:371-381.

63. von Birgelen C, Mintz GS, de Vrey EA, et al. Successful directional atherectomy of de novo coronary lesions assessed with three-dimensional intravascular ultrasound and angiographic follow-up. *Am J Cardiol* 1997; 80:1540-1545.

64. von Birgelen C, Di Mario C, Serruys PW. Structural and functional characterization of an intermediate stenosis with intracoronary ultrasound and Doppler: A case of «reverse Glagovian modeling». *Am Heart J* 1996; 132:694-696.

65. Schartl M, Bocksch W, Koschyk DH, et al. for the GAIN-Study Investigators. Use of intravascular ultrasound to compare effects of different strategies of lipid-lowering therapy on plaque volume and composition in patients with coronary artery disease. *Circulation* 2001; 104:387-392.

66. Sabate M, Serruys PW, van der Giessen WJ, et al. Geometric vascular remodeling after balloon angioplasty and betaradiation therapy: a three-dimensional intravascular ultrasound study. *Circulation* 1999; 100:1182-1188.

67. Sabate M, Marijnissen JPA, Carlier SG, et al. Residual plaque burden, delivered dose and tissue composition predict 6-month outcome after balloon angioplasty and beta-radiation therapy. *Circulation* 2000; 101: 2472-2477.

68. Carlier SG, Marijnissen JPA, Coen VLMA, et al. Guidance of intracoronary radiation therapy based on dose-volume histograms derived from quantitative intravascular ultrasound. *IEEE Trans Med Imaging* 1998; 17:772-778.

69. Carlier SG, Marijnissen JPA, Coen VLMA, et al. Comparison of brachytherapy strategies based on dose-volume histograms derived from quantitative intravascular ultrasound. *Cardiovasc Radiat Med* 1999; 1:115-124.

70. Wentzel JJ, Krams R, Schuurbiers JC, et al. Relationship between neointimal thickness and shear stress after Wallstent implantation in human coronary arteries. *Circulation* 2001; 103:1740-1745.

71. Wentzel JJ, Kloet J, Andhyiswara I, et al. Shear-stress and wall-stress regulation of vascular remodeling after balloon angioplasty: effect of matrix metalloproteinase inhibition. *Circulation* 2001; 104:91-96.

72. Wentzel JJ, Whelan DM, van der Giessen WJ, et al. Coronary stent implantation changes 3-D vessel geometry and 3-D shear stress distribution. *J Biomech* 2000; 33:1287-1295.

73. Koch L, Kearney P, Erbel R, et al. Three dimensional reconstruction of intracoronary ultrasound images: roadmapping with simultaneously digitized coronary angiograms. In: Computers in Cardiology 1993, Los Alamitos: *IEEE Computer Society Press* 1993; 89-91.

74. Ge J, Koch T, Görge G, et al. Three-dimensional reconstruction and quantification of intracoronary ultrasound images under guidance of biplane fluoroscopy. *Herz* 1995; 20:263-276.

75. Gyongyosi M, Yang P, Khorsand A, Glogar D. Longitudinal straightening effect of stents is an additional predictor for major adverse cardiac events. Austrian Wiktor Stent Study Group and European Paragon Stent Investigators. *J Am Coll Cardiol* 2000; 35:1580-1589.

9

Cardiac Allograft Vasculopathy

Samir R. Kapadia, MD

E. Murat Tuzcu, MD

Introduction. Rationale for Using IVUS to Study Transplant CAD. Imaging Protocols. IVUS Analysis of Transplant Coronary Artery Disease. Safety of IVUS Examination. Insights into Transplant Coronary Artery Disease. Donor Disease. Transplant Vasculopathy. Remodeling in Transplant CAD. Summary. References.

INTRODUCTION

Cardiac transplantation is an important therapeutic alternative for patients with severe irreversible congestive heart failure. Transplant vasculopathy continues to be a troublesome long-term complication of heart transplantation. It is the major cause of death in patients surviving 1 year after transplantation.[1,2]

Coronary angiography, despite its well-recognized limitations, has served as an important tool to investigate coronary anatomy in normal and diseased states.[3] Rapid progress in technology has led to the emergence of intravascular ultrasound (IVUS) as a widely utilized tool to study a number of morphological and developmental questions regarding transplant coronary artery disease (CAD).[4] The major advantage of IVUS imaging is its ability to visualize the vessel wall *in vivo*, whereas angiography can only discern the effects of the disease process on the vessel lumen.[3]

RATIONALE FOR USING IVUS TO STUDY TRANSPLANT CAD

Transplant coronary artery disease (CAD) includes atherosclerosis lesions transmitted from donors and newly developed vasculopathy lesions (Fig. 9-1). The early lesions of transplant CAD are difficult to study with angiography because they are small, eccentric lesions that frequently do not encroach upon the lumen due to arterial remodeling. Further, these early lesions are clinically silent and do not produce ischemia on stress testing.[5,6] By the time vasculopathy manifests as ischemia on noninvasive functional studies, the disease process is usually well advanced.

Multiple studies using isotopes of thallium or technetium have been reported to investigate transplant vasculopathy. Stress testing with exercise can identify patients with severe transplant vasculopathy. Although these studies show poor sensitivity and high specificity,[7] they seem to predict long-term outcome after heart transplantation.[8] Studies using higher doses of dipyridamole may help to improve sensitivity.[9] Further, non-homogeneous distribution of isotopes has been shown to be associated with the presence of transplant vasculopathy.[10] In one study, a lung/heart ratio ≥ 0.40 on dipyridamole thallium testing was shown to be a sensitive predictor of coronary events after heart transplantation.[11]

Stress echocardiography has also shown promise in identifying patients with signifi-

B   Transplant Vasculopathy

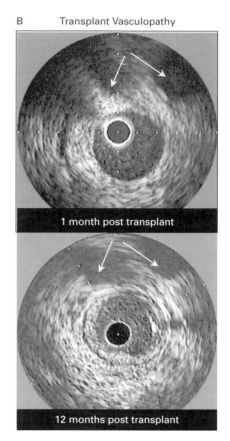

1 month post transplant

12 months post transplant

A   Donor Atherosclerosis

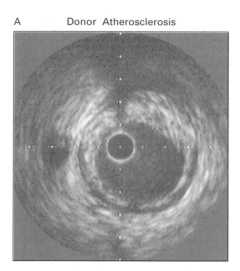

Figure 9-1. Transplant coronary artery disease comprises transmitted donor atherosclerosis lesions and transplant vasculopathy lesions that develop after transplantation. Panel A shows an IVUS image of a proximal LAD captured 30 days after cardiac transplantation. This eccentric lesion is an example of donor-transmitted atherosclerosis. Panel B shows a site in the LAD imaged 1 month (top) and 1 year (bottom) after cardiac transplantation. Site matching is accomplished by identifying ultrasound (arrows) and angiographic landmarks. This is an example of transplant vasculopathy lesion because the lesion developed at a previously normal site. These examples also underscore the importance of an early baseline study with serial follow-up for the accurate identification of donor atherosclerosis and transplant vasculopathy lesions.

cant transplant vasculopathy and poor long-term outcome.[12-14] Recent studies have tried to identify patients with transplant vasculopathy using a combination of echocardiography and nuclear imaging.[9] These studies have been encouraging but do not allow detection of early transplant vasculopathy. Another approach to detecting allograft vasculopathy has been to identify endothelial dysfunction soon after transplantation. This functional impairment correlates with early morphological changes.[15-17] Invasive techniques with assessment of coronary flow in response to vasodilators have been used to determine endothelial function. The ability of noninvasive studies to detect endothelial dysfunction and to accurately predict morphological changes remains unknown.[18] IVUS imaging, due to its ability to visualize arterial wall structure *in vivo*, provides a sensitive tool for studying early transplant vasculopathy lesions.

IMAGING PROTOCOLS

Different imaging protocols have been used in various institutions to study transplant coronary artery disease. Many institutions use yearly surveillance angiography to assess transplant coronary artery diseases, but the utility of this measure has been questioned recently.[19] Investigators have combined the use of intravascular ultrasound imaging with annual angiography to study the onset and progression of the disease process. Few centers have used intravascular ultrasound soon after transplantation to determine prevalence of donor-transmitted atherosclerosis. Besides the timing of the imaging, the extent of imaging and method of imaging (motorized pullback vs. manual pullback) also vary in published reports. Most centers have used single-vessel imaging as a representative sample for assessing the disease process in the entire coronary tree. Further, only the proximal coronary segments are routinely visualized in many institutions. Interestingly, it has been demonstrated that three-vessel imaging with inclu-

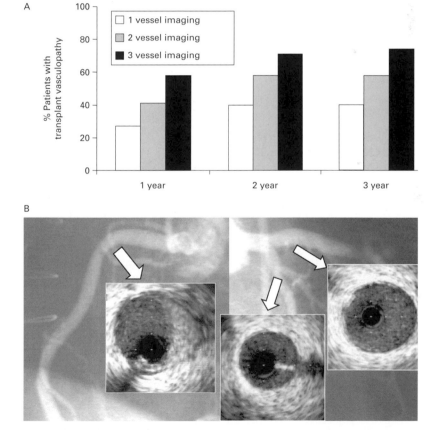

Figure 9-2. Panel A shows the prevalence of transplant vasculopathy depending on whether 1, 2, or 3 vessels were imaged. Three-vessel imaging identifies more patients with transplant vasculopathy. This holds true even when vessels are imaged 1, 2, and 3 years after transplantation. Panel B shows an example of a patient in which the LAD and LCX showed no evidence of any lesions, but a lesion was present in the RCA. If only the LAD or LCX had been imaged, the patient would have been classified as not having transplant coronary artery disease. Sensitivity of identifying transplant coronary disease increases with 3-vessel imaging. (Adapted from Kapadia et al).[20]

sion of distal segments leads to better and more accurate quantification of disease processes.[20] Single-vessel imaging frequently underestimates disease prevalence (Fig. 9-2). Initial studies were performed with manual pullback of the transducer, which does not permit accurate determination of the length of a lesion. Various sampling methods have been described to overcome this limitation (*see below*). However, more recent study protocols have employed motorized pullback with accurate determination of lesion length and plaque volume. Motorized pullback also facilitates the matching of coronary segments in serial studies investigating plaque progression or regression.

IVUS ANALYSIS OF TRANSPLANT CORONARY ARTERY DISEASE

Definition of a Lesion

Limited data are available to describe the range of normal intimal thickness in humans. Using vessels that were not pressure-fixed, a necropsy study showed an age-related increase in intimal thickness. The average intimal thickness was 0.21 mm for ages 21 to 25, increasing slightly to 0.25 mm for ages 36 to 40.[21] Other small studies report normal intimal thickness ranging from 0.1 mm to 0.35 mm and medial thickness from 0.15 mm

to 0.25 mm.[21-23] A comparative intravascular ultrasound and necropsy study reported that histologic measurements were reduced by an average of 19% following tissue processing.[24] Further, the measurement of intimal thickness by intravascular ultrasound includes the thickness of the media as well. Therefore, the «intimal» thickness in intravascular ultrasound studies is more precisely «intima + media» thickness. In a study of 262 subjects using intravascular ultrasound within 2 months of transplantation, at least one site with an «intimal» thickness <0.5 mm was identifiable. Furthermore, all patients <40 years of age had at least one site with «intimal» thickness <0.3 mm. Therefore, an «intimal» thickness of 0.3-0.5 mm has been used as a threshold to identify early atherosclerosis (Fig. 9-3). However, it is important to recognize that intimal thickness is a continuous variable and defining atherosclerosis as a categorical variable has limitations.[25]

Lesion Morphology

There are no standard definitions for describing the morphology of lesions in transplant coronary artery disease. The longitudinal extent (focal vs. diffuse) of disease can be described using the classification of coronary artery segments as defined in Coron-

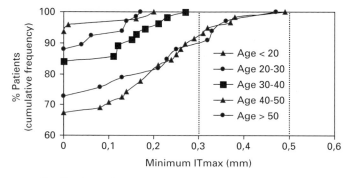

Figure 9-3. Frequency distribution of «normal» intimal thickness (ITmax) in different age groups. In populations less than 40 years old, the «normal» intimal thickness is less than 0.3 mm. For the entire population it was less than 0.5 mm. These *in vivo* findings provide justification for using 0.3-0.5 mm as a threshold to define a lesion. (From Tuzcu et al).[25]

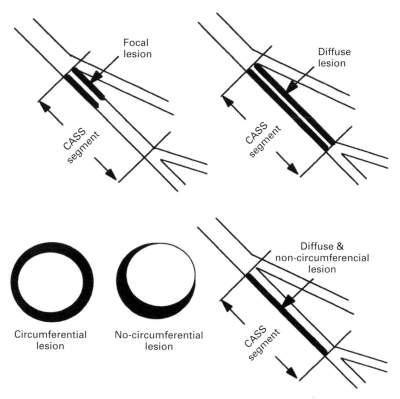

Figure 9-4. An example of definitions of the morphological characteristics of a lesion of transplant coronary artery disease used in a study. If the lesion did not affect the entire coronary artery segment, it was defined as focal, and if it involved the entire circumference, it was defined as circumferential. (From Kapadia et al).[41]

ary Artery Surgery Study. A lesion can be defined as focal if there is at least one normal site in the same CASS segment. A lesion is diffuse when it involves the entire segment.[26] A lesion is circumferential if it involves the entire circumference of a vessel and non-circumferential if any arc of the vessel wall is free of disease (Fig. 9-4).

Quantitative IVUS Analysis

The basic principles of intravascular ultrasound measurement of lesions in transplant vasculopathy are similar to those used with other techniques.[27] Intimal thickness is defined as the distance from the intimal leading edge to the external elastic membrane (ad-

ventitial leading edge) (Fig. 9-5). As pointed out earlier, the measurement of the intima therefore includes the media. Lumen cross-sectional area (Lcsa), external elastic membrane cross-sectional area (EEMcsa), or vessel area, maximal intimal thickness (ITmax), and minimal intimal thickness (ITmin) are commonly measured at the sites of interest. Intimal (or plaque) cross-sectional area (ITcsa) is calculated from the difference of EEMcsa and Lcsa. The maximal intimal thickness is a commonly used measure to describe the severity of lesions. A standardized classification for the extent of transplant vasculopathy has been proposed using the severity of intimal thickening and the degree of circumferential involvement (Table 9-1).[28]

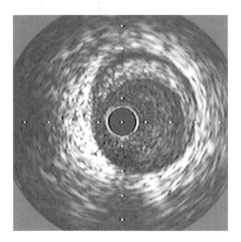 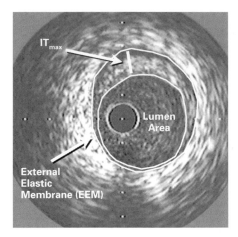

Figure 9-5. An example to illustrate the correct method for measurement of an IVUS image. The lumen is defined by the interface between blood and intima. Intimal thickness is measured from lumen to external elastic lamina and includes the media (the echolucent zone) in the measurement.

Although IVUS examination of a single coronary artery yields thousands of cross-sectional images, some of these have to be selected for measurement in order to express this information quantitatively. Various approaches for sampling of the sites have been proposed. One approach is to select multiple sites, at least 1 cm apart, from the proximal coronary segments to represent the entire coronary tree. The sample is neither derived according to predefined criteria, nor is it randomly selected, so it is subject to selection bias. An alternative method is to select sites according to predefined criteria where two sites, one with the least intimal thickness and another with the greatest intimal thickness, are selected from each segment of a coronary artery. The third approach, morphometry, allows three-dimensional information to be obtained from data collected in two dimensions using mathematical modeling.[29] The pullback sequence of a coronary artery of interest is divided into approximately equal time intervals and a site is randomly selected closest to the time of interest. Volumes are calculated using mathematical modeling.

Table 9-1.   Grading of Transplant Vasculopathy Lesions

Class	Grade	Initial thickness (mm)	Vessel circumference
0		None	None
I	Minimal	<0.3	<180°
II	Mild	<0.3	>180°
III	Moderate	0.3-0.5	<180°
IV	Severe	>0.5 or >1.0 in any area	>180°

However, volumes can be precisely calculated by performing automated pullback at a known pullback speed. For this, lumen and intimal areas are measured at sites that are 1-2 mm apart. The volumes are calculated using Simpson's formula. All these approaches have been employed in cross-sectional and serial study designs.

In a serial study design, a comparison is made of various measurements of certain segments of a coronary artery from the analysis of ultrasound examinations performed at two or more different time points. The variability of measurements varies in reports depending on the protocol of imaging and analysis.[30,31] Different methods are used to match sites or segments under investigation. Site-matching on serial studies can be accomplished by utilizing angiographic and intravascular ultrasound landmarks. Even after careful site-matching using verbal annotations, and angiographic and ultrasound landmarks, serial measurements may have significant variations due to differences in vessel tone, blood pressure (distention pressure), transducer location in the vessel lumen and variation induced by cardiac cycle.[31] Volumetric analysis of the entire segment of a coronary artery can help to eliminate the need for individual site-matching. However, this requires motorized pullback for image acquisition and measurement of multiple equidistant sites from a well-defined fiduciary point.

Tissue Characterization

It was originally expected that IVUS imaging would allow characterization of the tissue components of atherosclerosis on the basis of their characteristic intensity pattern.[32,33] Subsequent studies, however, have demonstrated significant limitations in tissue characterization by IVUS intensity patterns alone, especially in discriminating fibrous and fatty tissues.[34] In some studies, unprocessed ultrasound radiofrequency (RF) signal analysis has been shown to distinguish different tissue structures more reliably than gray-scale interpretation of conventional ultrasound images. In an animal model of aortic transplantation, RF analysis was able to detect the changes of rejection more effectively compared to visual or quantitative gray-scale analysis.[35] However, human studies for tissue characterization in transplant vasculopathy are lacking.

SAFETY OF IVUS EXAMINATION

The safety of intravascular ultrasound imaging has been well documented, with rare complications. The most frequently encountered complication is a focal coronary spasm (2-5% of cases), which usually responds rapidly to intracoronary nitroglycerin. Data from multiple European centers performing IVUS examinations reported a 1.1%complication (spasm, vessel dissection, or guide wire entrapment) rate in a total of 718 examinations. All complications occurred in patients with atherosclerotic coronary disease undergoing percutaneous intervention.[36] In another multi-center report from 28 centers on 2207 IVUS studies, where 505 (23 %) studies were performed in heart transplant recipients and 1702 (77 %) in non-transplant patients, spasm was reported in 63 (2.9 %) patients. None of the transplant patients had any other complication in this series.[37] In another safety report from intracoronary ultrasound in 170 cardiac transplant recipients (240 intracoronary studies) from a single center, there was no reported clinical morbidity, however, there was an 8.3% (20 patients) incidence of angiographically evident coronary spasm despite pretreatment with nitroglycerin. In all the cases, this was reversed by additional nitroglycerin. Furthermore, the angiographic measurements in the previously instrumented and non-instrumented vessels at 1 year of follow-up were similar, indicating no accelerated progression of angiographically quantifiable coronary artery disease.[38] With a better profile of the newer catheter systems now available, the incidence of vasospasm appears to be even lower than reported in these early experiences. The long-term safety of this procedure has also been studied in transplant patients. It has been shown that instrumentation of the coronary arteries does not lead to development or progression of transplant vasculopathy.[39]

INSIGHTS INTO TRANSPLANT CORONARY ARTERY DISEASE

As previously indicated, transplant coronary artery disease includes transmitted lesions of donor atherosclerosis and newly developed lesions of transplant vasculopathy. The lesions of transplant vasculopathy have different characteristics compared to the lesions of donor atherosclerosis (Table 9-2).[40] However, due to the vast heterogeneity in the morphology of both these lesion types, it is impossible to ascertain the origin of each lesion by morphology alone.[41] Lesions of atherosclerosis tend to be more eccentric and focal but there are many lesions of transplant vasculopathy that are eccentric and focal. The only certain way to identify lesions of donor atherosclerosis is to perform intravascular ultrasound examin-

ation soon after transplantation. The lesions identified on IVUS examinations made within 2 months of heart transplantation represent donor atherosclerosis rather than transplant vasculopathy. Serial IVUS examinations performed thereafter can spot newly developing lesions of transplant vasculopathy.

DONOR DISEASE

Lesions seen on IVUS examination performed within the first 2 months after transplantation are thought to represent donor atherosclerosis because the prevalence and severity of these lesions are dependent on donor age, gender, and donor atherosclerosis risk factors and *not* on recipient characteristics.[25]

Despite the young donor age, atherosclerosis is detected in more than 50% of transplanted patients (Fig. 9-6).[25] Age and male gender of donor are the most important predictors of atherosclerosis. Not surprisingly, most of these lesions are angiographically silent.[23] Donor atherosclerosis lesions are frequently focal, non-circumferential and involve proximal coronary artery segments with a predilection for bifurcations (Table 9-3).[26]

The long-term natural history of donor atherosclerosis lesions after transplantation

Table 9-2. Comparison of Transplant Vasculopathy with Conventional Atherosclersosis

Characteristics	Transplant Vasculopathy	Donor Atherosclerosis
Intimal proliferation	Circumferential	Non-circumferential
Internal elastic lamina	Intact	Disrupted
Calcium deposition	Absent	Frequently present
Intra-myocardial vessels	Involved	Spared
Inflammation	Infrequent	Never
Rate of development	Months	Years

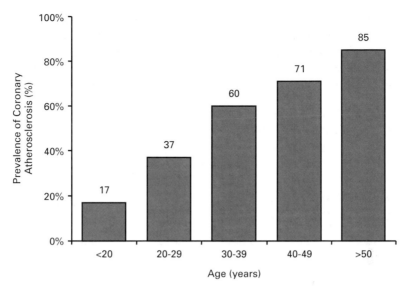

Figure 9-6. Prevalence of lesions of coronary atherosclerosis according to age (donor age) distribution. This study imaged coronary arteries with IVUS within 2 months of transplantation and used 0.5 mm as a threshold to define a lesion. (From Tuzcu et al).[25]

remains largely unknown. In a serial study, donor disease progression, defined as $\geqslant 0.3$ mm increase in maximal intimal thickness, was seen in 42% of patients during the first year after transplantation.[26] Interestingly, the progression of the donor lesions was insignificant between the first and second year after transplantation.[29] This «progression» may represent transplant vasculopathy

lesions developing over atherosclerosis or actual progression of atherosclerosis. Rarely, regression of donor atherosclerosis has also been documented.

Factors determining the progression of donor lesions have not been adequately studied. A small study of 36 patients with donor lesions investigated the role of conventional atherosclerosis risk factors on the pro-

Table 9-3. Morphology of Lesions

Distribution of Analyzed Sites	Donor Lesions (Baseline), n = 89				*De Novo* Lesions (1 y), n = 107			
	Prox n = 323	Mid n = 172	Distal n = 122	Total n = 617	Prox n = 323	Mid n = 172	Distal n = 122	Total n = 617
Circumferential lesions	32 (51%)	8 (38%)	0 (0%)	40 (45%)	41 (62%)	25 (78%)	8 (89%)	74 (69%)
Focal lesions	44 (70%)	17 (81%)	5 (100%)	66 (74%)	32 (48%)	11 (34%)	3 (33%)	46 (43%)

The percentage under each number represents the proportion of lesions in each distribution (proximal, mid, or distal) exhibiting the designated morphological pattern (circumferential or focal). Donor lesions were significantly more focal ($P = 0.0009$) and more non-circumferential ($P = 0.005$) than *de novo* lesions.

gression of these lesions. In the multivariate analysis, recipient pre-transplant body mass index and post-transplant serum triglyceride level were significant predictors for the progression of donor atherosclerosis. Older recipient age showed a trend in predicting the progression of lesions; however donor age did not affect disease progression.[42]

The scarcity of organs has led to more frequent acceptance of older donors, which in turn has increased the prevalence of donor atherosclerosis in transplanted hearts. Fortunately, careful selection of older donors does not affect graft survival adversely.[43] Even the incidence of angiographically detectable transplant CAD on 5-years follow-up is similar in recipients of older hearts compared to younger donors.[43] This finding is in accordance with the observation that evidence of atherosclerosis on IVUS examination is not associated with more frequent or severe transplant vasculopathy.

TRANSPLANT VASCULOPATHY

The incidence of angiographically detected transplant vasculopathy ranges from 10-20% at 1 year and up to 50% by 5 years. This is an underestimation of the true disease prevalence as vasculopathy lesions are detected in almost 50% of the patients after 1 year of transplantation with multi-vessel IVUS imaging.[26]

Vasculopathy lesions are defined as lesions appearing at previously normal sites, underscoring the value of baseline examination soon after transplantation. Without a baseline study, accurate identification of vasculopathy lesions is not feasible because these lesions cannot be confidently differentiated from early atherosclerosis by morphology alone. The early lesions of vasculopathy are frequently located in the proximal segments and commonly involve vessel bifurcation. The predilection for bifurcations suggests a role of shear stress in the generation of transplant vasculopathy.[44] These lesions

are more frequently diffuse and circumferential compared to the donor lesions.[26]

The natural history of transplant vasculopathy has been investigated in cross-sectional studies where only one IVUS examination is performed after a variable time interval from transplantation. In such studies, it has been shown that the intimal thickness and intimal area increase progressively with time. Interestingly, in a serial study of a relatively small number of patients, it appears that lesion severity does not increase rapidly after the first year of transplantation but new lesions continue to develop at previously normal sites.[29] This finding underscores the importance for continued surveillance for transplant vasculopathy.

IVUS imaging has been used to evaluate factors affecting the development of vasculopathy lesions. In a study by Mehra et al, significant independent predictors of severe intimal hyperplasia included donor age >35 years, first-year mean biopsy score >1 and hypertriglyceridemia. Additionally, subjects with severe intimal thickening had a fourfold higher cardiac event rate than those without severe intimal proliferation on IVUS.[45] In another study of patients with evidence of rejection, the rate of progression of transplant vasculopathy correlated with the severity of rejection.[46] Escobar et al. reported total cholesterol, low-density lipoprotein cholesterol, triglyceride levels, obesity indexes, donor age, and years following cardiac transplantation to be independent predictors of the severity of cardiac allograft vasculopathy.[47] Similarly, a study by Rickenbacher et al demonstrated a significant correlation between fasting plasma triglyceride level and weight with severity of intimal thickening.[48] Further, male recipients of a female allograft have worse vasculopathy compared with either male or female recipients of a male allograft at 1 year of heart transplantation.[49]

IVUS imaging has also provided insight into the effectiveness of various therapies influencing transplant vasculopathy. A subgroup analysis from a randomized trial showed that the decrease in cholesterol levels and improvement in survival with pravastatin therapy was associated with a decrease in the rate of progression of vasculopathy lesions.[50] Another small study reported a reduction in intimal thickness with treatment utilizing diltiazem, ACE inhibitors, or both.[51] In a retrospective study, conventional atherosclerosis risk factors do not predict the development of allograft vasculopathy, but a greater change in serum LDL cholesterol level during the first year after transplant is associated with more severe vasculopathy. This may suggest that the maintenance of LDL cholesterol as close to pre-transplant values as possible may help to limit the rate of progression of acquired allograft vasculopathy.[42]

The findings of IVUS imaging are shown to predict long-term clinical outcome. In a study of 74 patients, patients with severe intimal thickening (>0.5mm) had more events (death, MI, and re-transplantation) at approximately 4 years of follow-up.[52] Wiedermann et al reported that patients with intimal thickness >1 mm had worst survival.[53] On the other hand, Rickenbacher et al.[54] have reported increased cardiac event rate in patients with a mean intimal thickening of >0.3 mm in 145 heart transplant recipients at 48 months of follow-up. The experience at Cleveland Clinic Foundation from 100 patients with approximately 4 years of follow-up also demonstrated a higher event rate with rapidly progressive intimal thickening in the first year of transplantation.[29] Whether or not aggressive immuno-suppression changes outcomes in patients with evidence of early transplant vasculopathy has not been adequately studied. In one such non-randomized series, a favorable response to aggressive immunosuppression was seen in patients with pulse steroid therapy.[55]

In some patients, percutaneous interventions, including vascular brachytherapy, have been used for revascularization in severe focal epicardial cases of transplant coronary artery disease.[56] Intravascular ultrasound examination can potentially help to guide these procedures. IVUS can be used in this situation to assess vessel size, extent of disease, and the result of that intervention and to help manage the complications of the intervention.[57,58]

REMODELING IN TRANSPLANT CAD

Glagov et al originally described coronary artery remodeling in a necropsy study of left main coronary arteries as a compensatory enlargement of vessels to prevent lumen loss in early stages of atherosclerosis. In recent years, histopathological and IVUS studies have demonstrated that at some lesion sites the vessel may shrink in size and contribute to, rather than compensate for, the degree of luminal stenosis, a phenomenon described as negative remodeling or arterial shrinkage. Both these phenomena have been studied in transplantation populations using serial and cross-sectional study designs.

In a cross-sectional study design, remodeling can be studied by means of a comparison of lesion sites with reference sites. Serial measurements of lumen, plaque, and vessel areas at the lesion site can provide the most rigorous evidence for remodeling, but the logistics of this type of studies, variability of measurements, and practical difficulties in identifying the same exact site on follow-up examinations limit the usefulness of this methodology.[29] Positive and negative remodeling have been demonstrated in cross-sectional and serial studies in transplant patients.[59] The rate of remodeling has been shown to be dependent on the time interval from transplantation.[3] Ziada et al. have reported differences in the rate of remodeling of donor lesions compared with that of vasculopathy lesions in a 3-year serial follow-up. Further, vessel remodeling appears to be more pronounced in eccentric lesions than in concentric lesions.[60] Negative remodeling may be important in large coronary segments because it appeared to be a major contributor to lumen loss in the first year after transplantation in one study.[61] However, in a study with 5-year follow-up, a biphasic response, consisting of early expansion and late constriction, was seen.[62]

SUMMARY

IVUS imaging is a safe, feasible and sensitive method for investigating transplant CAD. It can be used to identify patients with rapidly progressive vasculopathy in whom timely aggressive measures may help to prolong graft survival. Further, serial IVUS information can be used to judge response to therapy. IVUS examination may provide useful surrogate endpoints for the long-term survival of transplant recipients in future trials using newer immunosuppressive therapies and other measures to halt transplant vasculopathy.

REFERENCES

1. UNOS. Annual report of the U.S. Scientific Registry for Organ Transplantation and the Organ Procurement and Transplantation Network. *U S Department of Health and Human Services* 1990.
2. Bieber CP, Hunt SA, Schwinn DA, Jamieson SA, Reitz BA, Oyer PE, Shumway NE, Stinson EB. Complications in long-term survivors of cardiac transplantation. *Transplantation Proceedings* 1981; 13:207-211.
3. Ziada KM, Kapadia SR, Tuzcu EM, Nissen SE. The current status of intravascular ultrasound imaging. *Curr Probl Cardiol* 1999; 24:541-66.
4. Nissen SE, Yock P. Intravascular ultrasound: novel pathophysiological insights and current clinical applications. *Circulation* 2001; 103:604-16.
5. Stark RP, McGinn AL, Wilson RF. Chest pain in cardiac-transplant recipients. Evidence of sensory reinnervation after cardiac transplantation [see comments]. *New Eng-*

6. land Journal of Medicine* 1991; 324:1791-1794.
6. Schroeder JS, Hunt SA. Chest pain in heart-transplant recipients [editorial; comment]. *New England Journal of Medicine* 1991; 324:1805-1807.
7. Smart FW, Ballantyne CM, Cocanougher B, Farmer JA, Sekela ME, Noon, GP, Young JB. Insensitivity of noninvasive tests to detect coronary artery vasculopathy after heart transplant. *American Journal of Cardiology* 1991; 67:243-247.
8. Verhoeven PP, Lee FA, Ramahi TM, Franco KL, Mendes de Leon C, Amatruda J, Gorham NA, Mattera JA, Wackers FJ. Prognostic value of noninvasive testing one year after orthotopic cardiac transplantation. *J Am Coll Cardiol* 1996; 28:183-9.
9. Ciliberto GR, Ruffini L, Mangiavacchi M, Parolini M, Sara R, Massa D, De Maria R, Gronda E, Vitali E, Parodi O. Resting echocardiography and quantitative dipyridamole technetium-99m sestamibi tomography in the identification of cardiac allograft vasculopathy and the prediction of long-term prognosis after heart transplantation. *Eur Heart J* 2001; 22:964-71.
10. Yen RF, Ho YL, Chou NK, Hsu RB, Huang PJ. Inhomogeneity of myocardial perfusion in heart transplant recipients: evaluation with dobutamine thallium-201 SPECT. *Nucl Med Commun* 2001; 22:1015-9.
11. Lenihan DJ, Rosenbaum AF, Burwinkel P, Tseng CY, Bhat G, Wagoner L, Walsh RA, Gerson MC. Prediction of human transplantation arteriopathy and coronary events with lung/heart count ratios during intravenous dipyridamole thallium-201 imaging. *Am Heart J* 1999; 137:942-8.
12. Spes CH, Klauss V, Mudra H, Schnaack SD, Tammen AR, Rieber J, Siebert U, Henneke KH, Uberfuhr P, Reichart B, Theisen K, Angermann CE. Diagnostic and prognostic value of serial dobutamine stress echocardiography for noninvasive assessment of cardiac allograft vasculopathy: a comparison with coronary angiography and intravascular ultrasound. *Circulation* 1999; 100:509-15.
13. Spes CH, Mudra H, Schnaack SD, Klauss V, Reichle FM, Uberfuhr P, Theisen K, Angermann CE. Dobutamine stress echocardiog-

raphy for noninvasive diagnosis of cardiac allograft vasculopathy: a comparison with angiography and intravascular ultrasound. *American Journal of Cardiology* 1996; 78:168-74.

14. Derumeaux G, Redonnet M, Soyer R, Cribier A, Letac B. Assessment of the progression of cardiac allograft vasculopathy by dobutamine stress echocardiography. *J Heart Lung Transplant* 1998; 17:259-67.

15. Weis M, Wildhirt SM, Schulze C, Rieder G, Wilbert-Lampen U, Wolf WP, Arendt RM, Enders G, Meiser BM, von Scheidt W. Endothelin in coronary endothelial dysfunction early after human heart transplantation. *J Heart Lung Transplant* 1999; 18:1071-9.

16. Mugge A, Brandes RP, Heublein B, Nolte C, Haverich A, Lichtlen PR. Endothelial dysfunction in heart transplanted patients with graft vasculopathy. *Eur Heart J* 1995; 16 Suppl J:78-83.

17. Mills RM, Jr., Billett JM, Nichols WW. Endothelial dysfunction early after heart transplantation. Assessment with intravascular ultrasound and Doppler. *Circulation* 1992; 86:1171-4.

18. Allen-Auerbach M, Schoder H, Johnson J, Kofoed K, Einhorn K, Phelps ME, Kobashigawa J, Czernin J. Relationship between coronary function by positron emission tomography and temporal changes in morphology by intravascular ultrasound (IVUS) in transplant recipients. *J Heart Lung Transplant* 1999; 18:211-9.

19. Clague JR, Cox ID, Murday AJ, Charokopos N, Madden BP. Low clinical utility of routine angiographic surveillance in the detection and management of cardiac allograft vasculopathy in transplant recipients. *Clin Cardiol* 2001; 24:459-62.

20. Kapadia SR, Ziada KM, L'Allier PL, Crowe TD, Rincon G, Hobbs RE, Bott-Silverman C, Young JB, Nissen SE, Tuzcu EM. Intravascular ultrasound imaging after cardiac transplantation: advantage of multi-vessel imaging. *J Heart Lung Transplant* 2000; 19:167-72.

21. Velican D, Velican C. Comparative study on age-related changes and atherosclerotic involvement of the coronary arteries of male and female subjects up to 40 years of age. *Atherosclerosis* 1981; 38:39-50.

22. Wong M, Edelstein J, Wollman J, Bond MG. Ultrasonic-pathological comparison of the human arterial wall. Verification of intima-media thickness. *Arteriosclerosis & Thrombosis* 1993; 13:482-6.

23. Tuzcu EM, Hobbs RE, Rincon G, Bott-Silverman C, De Franco AC, Robinson K, McCarthy PM, Stewart RW, Guyer S, Nissen SE. Occult and frequent transmission of atherosclerotic coronary disease with cardiac transplantation. Insights from intravascular ultrasound. *Circulation* 1995; 91: 1706-1713.

24. Potkin BN, Bartorelli AL, Gessert JM, Neville RF, Almagor Y, Roberts WC, Leon MB. Coronary artery imaging with intravascular high-frequency ultrasound. *Circulation* 1990; 81:1575-1585.

25. Tuzcu EM, Kapadia SR, Tutar E, Ziada KM, Hobbs RE, McCarthy PM, Young JB, Nissen SE. High prevalence of coronary atherosclerosis in asymptomatic teenagers and young adults: evidence from intravascular ultrasound. *Circulation* 2001; 103: 2705-10.

26. Kapadia SR, Nissen SE, Ziada KM, Guetta V, Crowe TD, Hobbs RE, Starling RC, Young JB, Tuzcu EM. Development of transplantation vasculopathy and progression of donor-transmitted atherosclerosis: comparison by serial intravascular ultrasound imaging. *Circulation* 1998; 98:2672-8.

27. Mintz GS, Nissen SE, Anderson WD, Bailey SR, Erbel R, Fitzgerald PJ, Pinto FJ, Rosenfield K, Siegel RJ, Tuzcu EM, Yock PG. American College of Cardiology Clinical Expert Consensus Document on Standards for Acquisition, Measurement and Reporting of Intravascular Ultrasound Studies (IVUS). A report of the American College of Cardiology Task Force on Clinical Expert Consensus Documents. *J Am Coll Cardiol* 2001; 37:1478-92.

28. Botas J, Pinto FJ, Chenzbraun A, Liang D, Schroeder JS, Oesterle SN, Alderman EL, Popp RL, Yeung AC. Influence of preexistent donor coronary artery disease on the progression of transplant vasculopathy. An intravascular ultrasound study. *Circulation* 1995; 92:1126-32.

29. Kapadia SR, Nissen SE, Tuzcu EM. Impact of intravascular ultrasound in understanding

transplant coronary artery disease. *Curr Opin Cardiol* 1999; 14:140-50.

30. Bocksch W, Wellnhofer E, Schartl M, Dreysse S, Klimek W, Franke R, Musci M, Hetzer R, Fleck E. Reproducibility of serial intravascular ultrasound measurements in patients with angiographically silent coronary artery disease after heart transplantation. *Coron Artery Dis* 2000; 11:555-62.

31. Kapadia SR, Ziada KM, Crowe TD, Kim MH, Guetta V, Nissen SE, Tuzcu EM. Time Related Variation in the Size of the Coronary Arteries: A Confounding Factor in Interpretation of Coronary Remodeling. *Circulation* 1996; 96:Supp I: I-79, abs 434.

32. Gussenhoven EJ, Essed CE, Lancee CT, Mastik F, Frietman P, van Egmond FC, Reiber J, Bosch H, van Urk H, Roelandt J, et al. Arterial wall characteristics determined by intravascular ultrasound imaging: an in vitro study. *J Am Coll Cardiol* 1989; 14:947-52.

33. Tobis JM, Mallery J, Mahon D, Lehmann K, Zalesky P, Griffith J, Gessert J, Moriuchi M, McRae M, Dwyer ML, et al. Intravascular ultrasound imaging of human coronary arteries in vivo. Analysis of tissue characterizations with comparison to in vitro histological specimens. *Circulation* 1991; 83:913-926.

34. Kimura BJ, Bhargava V, DeMaria AN. Value and limitations of intravascular ultrasound imaging in characterizing coronary atherosclerotic plaque. *American Heart Journal* 1995; 130:386-396.

35. Jeremias A, Kolz ML, Ikonen TS, Gummert JF, Oshima A, Hayase M, Honda Y, Komiyama N, Berry GJ, Morris RE, Yock PG, Fitzgerald PJ. Feasibility of in vivo intravascular ultrasound tissue characterization in the detection of early vascular transplant rejection. *Circulation* 1999; 100:2127-30.

36. Batkoff BW, Linker DT. Safety of intracoronary ultrasound: data from a Multicenter European Registry. *Cathet Cardiovasc Diagn* 1996; 38:238-41.

37. Hausmann D, Erbel R, Alibelli-Chemarin MJ, Boksch W, Caracciolo E, Cohn JM, Culp SC, Daniel WG, De Scheerder I, DiMario C, et al. The safety of intracoronary ultrasound. A multicenter survey of 2207 examinations. *Circulation* 1995; 91:623-630.

38. Pinto FJ, St.Goar FG, Gao SZ, Chenzbraun A, Fischell TA, Alderman EL, Schroeder JS, Popp RL. Immediate and one-year safety of intracoronary ultrasonic imaging. Evaluation with serial quantitative angiography. *Circulation* 1993; 88:1709-1714.

39. Son R, Tobis JM, Yeatman LA, Johnson JA, Wener LS, Kobashigawa JA. Does use of intravascular ultrasound accelerate arteriopathy in heart transplant recipients? *Am Heart J* 1999; 138:358-63.

40. Billingham ME. Histopathology of graft coronary disease. *Journal of Heart &Lung Transplantation* 1992; 11:S38- 44.

41. Kapadia SR, Nissen SE, Ziada KM, Guetta V, Crowe TD, Hobbs RE, Starling RC, Young JB, Tuzcu EM. Development of transplantation vasculopathy and progression of donor-transmitted atherosclerosis: comparison by serial intravascular ultrasound imaging. *Circulation* 1998; 98:2672-8.

42. Kapadia SR, Nissen SE, Ziada KM, Rincon G, Crowe TD, Boparai N, Young JB, Tuzcu EM. Impact of lipid abnormalities in development and progression of transplant coronary disease: a serial intravascular ultrasound study. *J Am Coll Cardiol* 2001; 38:206-13.

43. Drinkwater DC, Laks H, Blitz A, Kobashigawa J, Sabad A, Moriguchi J, Hamilton M. Outcomes of patients undergoing transplantation with older donor hearts. *Journal of Heart &Lung Transplantation* 1996; 15:684-91.

44. Pethig K, Kofidis T, Heublein B, Westphal A, Haverich A. Impact of vascular branching sites on focal progression of allograft vasculopathy in transplanted hearts. *Atherosclerosis* 2001; 158:155-60.

45. Mehra MR, Ventura HO, Chambers R, Collins TJ, Ramee SR, Kates MA, Smart FW, Stapleton DD. Predictive model to assess risk for cardiac allograft vasculopathy: an intravascular ultrasound study. *Journal of the American College of Cardiology* 1995; 26:1537-44.

46. Jimenez J, Kapadia SR, Yamani MH, Platt L, Hobbs RE, Rincon G, Botts-Silverman C, Starling RC, Young JB, Nissen SE, Tuzcu M. Cellular rejection and rate of progression of transplant vasculopathy: a 3-year serial intravascular ultrasound study. *J Heart Lung Transplant* 2001; 20:393-8.

47. Escobar A, Ventura HO, Stapleton DD, Mehra MR, Ramee SR, Collins TJ, Jain SP, Smart FW, White CJ. Cardiac allograft vasculopathy assessed by intravascular ultrasonography and nonimmunologic risk factors. *American Journal of Cardiology* 1994; 74:1042-1046.

48. Rickenbacher PR, Kemna MS, Pinto FJ, Hunt SA, Alderman EL, Schroeder JS, Stinson EB, Popp RL, Chen I, Reaven G, Valantine HA. Coronary artery intimal thickening in the transplanted heart. An in vivo intracoronary ultrasound study of immunologic and metabolic risk factors. *Transplantation* 1996; 61:46-53.

49. Mehra MR, Stapleton DD, Ventura HO, Escobar A, Cassidy CA, Smart FW, Collins TJ, Ramee SR, White CJ. Influence of donor and recipient gender on cardiac allograft vasculopathy. An intravascular ultrasound study. *Circulation* 1994; 90:II78-82.

50. Kobashigawa JA, Katznelson S, Laks H, Johnson JA, Yeatman L, Wang XM, Chia D, Terasaki PI, Sabad A, Cogert GA, et al. Effect of pravastatin on outcomes after cardiac transplantation [see comments]. *N Engl J Med* 1995; 333:621-7.

51. Mehra MR, Ventura HO, Smart FW, Collins TJ, Ramee SR, Stapleton DD. An intravascular ultrasound study of the influence of angiotensin-converting enzyme inhibitors and calcium entry blockers on the development of cardiac allograft vasculopathy. *American Journal of Cardiology* 1995; 75:853-854.

52. Mehra MR, Ventura HO, Stapleton DD, Smart FW, Collins TC, Ramee SR. Presence of severe intimal thickening by intravascular ultrasonography predicts cardiac events in cardiac allograft vasculopathy. *J Heart Lung Transplant* 1995; 14:632-9.

53. Wiedermann JG, Wasserman HS, Weinberger JZ. Severe intimal thickening by intravascular ultrasonography predicts early death in cardiac transplant recipients. *Circulation* 1994; 90:I93.

54. Rickenbacher PR, Pinto FJ, Lewis NP, Hunt SA, Alderman EL, Schroeder JS, Stinson EB, Brown BW, Valentine HA. Prognostic importance of intimal thickness as measured by intracoronary ultrasound after cardiac transplantation. *Circulation* 1995; 92:3445-52.

55. Lamich R, Ballester M, Marti V, Brossa V, Aymat R, Carrio I, Berna L, Camprecios M, Puig M, Estorch M, Flotats A, Bordes R, Garcia J, Auge, Padro JM, Caralps JM, Narula J. Efficacy of augmented immunosuppressive therapy for early vasculopathy in heart transplantation. *J Am Coll Cardiol* 1998; 32:413-9.

56. Klauss V, Stempfle H, Theisen K, Kantlehner R, Poellinger B, Reichart B, Schiele TM. Vascular brachytherapy for treatment of cardiac allograft vasculopathy. *J Heart Lung Transplant* 2001; 20:792-4.

57. Chan AW, Carere RG, Khatri S, Della Siega A, Ignaszewski AP, Webb JG. Unprotected left main coronary artery stenting for cardiac allograft vasculopathy. *J Heart Lung Transplant* 2001; 20:776-80.

58. Kong W, Le May MR, Labinaz M, Davies RA. Stenting of an unprotected left main coronary artery stenosis in a cardiac transplant patient. *Can J Cardiol* 1999; 15: 1131-5.

59. Lim TT, Liang DH, Botas J, Schroeder JS, Oesterle SN, Yeung AC. Role of compensatory enlargement and shrinkage in transplant coronary artery disease. Serial intravascular ultrasound study. *Circulation* 1997; 95:855-9.

60. Schwarzacher SP, Uren NG, Ward MR, Schwarzkopf A, Giannetti N, Hunt S, Fitzgerald PJ, Oesterle SN, Yeung AC. Determinants of coronary remodeling in transplant coronary disease: a simultaneous intravascular ultrasound and Doppler flow study. *Circulation* 2000; 101:1384-9.

61. Wong C, Ganz P, Miller L, Kobashigawa J, Schwarzkopf A, Valentine von Kaeper H, Wilensky R, Ventura H, Yeung AC. Role of vascular remodeling in the pathogenesis of early transplant coronary artery disease: a multicenter prospective intravascular ultrasound study. *J Heart Lung Transplant* 2001; 20:385-92.

62. Tsutsui H, Ziada KM, Schoenhagen P, Iyisoy A, Magyar WA, Crowe TD, Klingensmith JD, Vince DG, Rincon G, Hobbs RE, Yamagishi M, Nissen SE, Tuzcu EM. Lumen loss in transplant coronary artery disease is a biphasic process involving early intimal thickening and late constrictive remodeling: results from a 5-year serial intravascular ultrasound study. *Circulation* 2001; 104:653-7.

10

Intravascular Ultrasound Assessment of Lesion Severity: from Anatomy to Physiology

Fernando Alfonso, MD

Perspective. Insights Provided by Intravascular Ultrasound. Intravascular Ultrasound versus Quantitative Coronary Angiography. Intravascular Ultrasound vs Intracoronary Physiological Assessment. Clinical Validation of Intravascular Ultrasound Parameters. References.

PERSPECTIVE

Intravascular ultrasound (IVUS) is a tomographic technique with the unique ability to provide direct visualization of the atherosclerotic plaque and residual coronary lumen *in vivo*.[1-4] In addition, the echoreflectivity of the plaque can be used as a surrogate to determine its underlying histology.[3] This comprehensive information represents a major breakthrough in our understanding of coronary artery disease, a disease of the vessel wall.[1-4] Until very recently, selective coronary angiography was the only available technique to study coronary anatomy in the clinical setting. Discrete lumen stenoses are readily detected by angiography, a technique well suited for depicting the coronary lumen silhouette as a shadowgram image.[1-5] Comparing the minimal lumen diameter of the target lesion with the adjacent, *angiographically normal* reference segment provides a valid estimate of relative lumen narrowing. This, in turn, has been classically considered a valid surrogate of stenosis severity. As a matter of fact, in most patients clinical manifestations of coronary artery disease only arise when plaque burden is large enough to impinge on the coronary lumen and narrow it

to some extent. However, nowadays the limitations of conventional angiography are well established.[5-74] Despite a thorough angiographic examination, we often encounter lesions that elude accurate characterization (Fig. 10-1). The paradigm of considering coronary angiography as the «gold standard» for the diagnosis of the extent and severity of coronary artery disease has been critically challenged during the last decade.[1-4, 5-7] Angiography provides a rough estimate of the physiologic implications of coronary lesions, but fails to provide critical anatomic insights to predict lesion-related flow limitations.[5-8] This has affected not only its acceptance as a reliable research tool, but also its so far undisputed utility for clinical decision-making. This is relevant because, our previous preoccupation with «coronary luminology»[5] has recently turned into concerns on how to gauge precise physiological insights in the catheterization laboratory.[8] Currently, assessment of stenosis severity constitutes a critical issue in decisions about coronary interventions.

IVUS is currently unsurpassed in providing precise direct measurements of lumen and vessel diameters and areas.[1-4] This is of major clinical relevance because IVUS studies

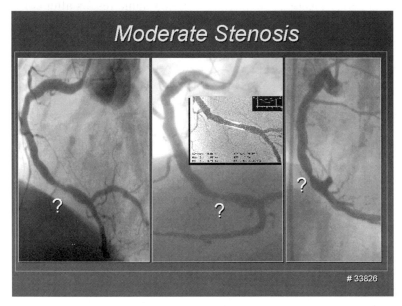

Figure 10-1. Moderate lesion in the distal right coronary artery. Despite the use of multiple views, lesion severity was difficult to establish. Quantitative coronary angiography also yielded borderline results with regard to the percent diameter stenosis although minimal lumen diameter was 2 mm. The lesion was not treated.

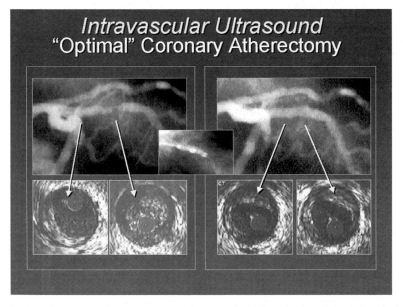

Figure 10-2. Left: Discrete angiographic stenosis in the middle section of the left anterior descending coronary artery. On intravascular ultrasound there was significant disease of the angiographically normal reference segment and a soft plaque at the lesion site where the imaging catheter was occlusive. Right: After directional atherectomy, an optimal angiographic result was obtained. Nevertheless, intravascular ultrasound revealed the presence of significant residual atheroma at the treated site.

have confirmed previous anatomopathologic observations, suggesting that angiography underestimates the extent and severity of coronary artery disease (Fig. 10-2).[1-4] The angiographically normal reference segment is universally involved in the atheromatous process and most lesions exhibit positive remodeling, explaining underestimation of lesion severity by angiography.[1-4] Theoretically speaking, direct measurements from tomographic IVUS images will provide the method of choice to accurately determine coronary lumen area both at the reference segment and lesion site.[9] In addition, lesion length may be accurately measured.[10-11] The 1999 ACC/AHA coronary angiography guidelines[12] characterized as a Class IIa Recommendation the use of IVUS to evaluate lesion severity at vessel locations difficult to image by angiography in a patient with a positive functional study and a suspected flow-limiting stenosis (Level of evidence = C). Likewise a Class IIa Recommendation was given for the assessment of suboptimal angiographic results after coronary interventions.[12]

In this chapter we will discuss the available evidence concerning the use of IVUS to gather further insights on the physiological significance of coronary lesions. With this aim, we will review: 1) IVUS findings with important physiological implications, 2) Correlation between IVUS and quantitative coronary angiography, and 3) Correlation between IVUS findings and intracoronary techniques specifically designed to assess coronary physiology. Finally, we will discuss the potential clinical implications of IVUS-derived physiological information.

INSIGHTS PROVIDED BY INTRAVASCULAR ULTRASOUND

The physiological consequences of coronary lesions depend largely on the extent and

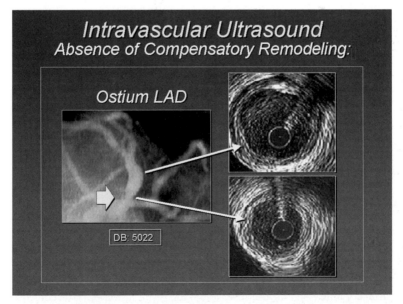

Figure 10-3. Left: Angiographic narrowing located at the ostium of the left anterior descending coronary artery (LAD) that eluded precise anatomical characterization. Right: Intravascular ultrasound was able to demonstrate that the residual lumen was large and that the narrowing was in fact caused by negative remodeling or vessel shrinkage without significant plaque deposition (in fact, the plaque area at this site was smaller than that seen at the distal reference segment where moderate lumen dilation could be appreciated).

severity of lumen narrowing and lesion length, but little on the amount of plaque burden.[8, 13-15] Before addressing the physiological implications of lumen narrowing, uniform IVUS terminology should be used to assess the severity of coronary stenosis. In the ACC clinical expert consensus document on IVUS,[13] a «*lesion*» is defined as an accumulation of atherosclerotic plaque compared with a predefined reference. Conversely, a «*stenosis*» is defined as a lesion that compromises the lumen by at least 50 % of cross-sectional area (compared with a reference segment lumen) (Figure 10-3). The worst stenosis is obviously the stenosis with the smallest lumen size. This site, however, may not necessarily have the largest atheroma and may slightly differ from its angiographic counterpart.[1] «*Minimal lumen diameter*» is the shorter diameter through the center of the lumen.[13] Furthermore, it is important to rec-

ognize that IVUS measurements (as in any ultrasound-based technique), should be performed at the leading edge of boundaries, never the trailing edge. Accordingly, lumen measurements should be performed using the interface between the lumen and the leading edge of the intima.[13] Finally, it should also be kept in mind that lumen area changes during the cardiac cycle and that the maximal lumen area occurs in mid-systole.[13-15] Although this lumen pulsatility accounts for a significant change in lumen area (up to 20 %) in normal segments, this phenomenon is nearly absent at sites with severe stenosis.[16, 17]

Direct measurements from tomographic IVUS images provide the method of choice to accurately determine coronary lumen area[1-4, 8, 13-15] (Fig. 10-4). IVUS-derived minimal luminal area has a better correlation with the physiological consequences of coronary lesions (using the pressure-derived fractional

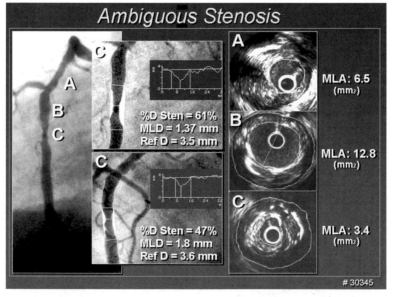

Figure 10-4. Value of intravascular ultrasound in assessing minimal lumen area (MLA). Left: This proximal right coronary artery had diffuse disease but the distal lesion (C) was considered to be significant on visual assessment. Middle: Edge-detection QCA of the C lesion revealed a minimal lumen diameter (MLD) ranging from 1.3 to 1.8 mm and a % diameter stenosis from 61% to 47% (orthogonal views). Right: Intravascular ultrasound revealed a massive plaque burden at the proximal lesion (A) with a MLA of 6.5 mm², a significant plaque burden at the reference segment (B), and a severe lesion at the distal narrowing (C), where MLA was only 3.4 mm².

flow reserve as the reference) than quantitative angiography.[18-19] The measurement of lumen diameters also remains an important diagnostic application.[13-15] Cross-sectional lumen narrowing may be directly calculated by standard planimetry or sophisticated automatic computer-based algorithms.[13-15, 20] Although IVUS currently provides the most precise tool for measuring vessel lumen area, this technique also has some specific problems and inherent limitations,[9, 13-15] as summarized in Table 10-1. In some circumstances IVUS tends to overestimate lumen area. Non-uniform rotational distortion (NURD) artifact, typical of mechanical catheters, arises from an uneven rotation of the transducer due to friction. NURD generates image distortion, with stretched and compacted sectors, that can affect lumen size. Transducer oscillations generate the ring-down artifacts that obscure the near field and may suggest an acoustic catheter size larger than its physical size. In fact, although the physical size of currently available catheters has improved to a large extent, this still represents a problem while measuring severe stenoses.[21, 22] Nevertheless, this is not a real problem in medium-sized to large vessels, where wedging of the imaging catheter always indicates a tight stenosis[9] (Fig. 10-5). Finally, the off-axis position of the IVUS catheter may produce geometric distortion and elliptical vessel shapes leading to overestimation of lumen area.[23] Again, although this can produce misleading measurements in reference segments, it does not influence measurements at the lesion site. Careful interrogation to identify the image slide with the smallest lumen may be challenging, especially in focal stenosis or when only a manual pullback has been performed. Finally, poor image quality may cause the true minimal lumen area to be missed and lesion severity to be underestimated[9, 13, 13-15] (Table 10-1).

Table 10-1.   Potential Problems/Pitfalls in Lumen Area Measurements with IVUS

Situation	Resulting phenomena
Before intervention:	
1. Failure to pass severe lesions.	Data unavailable.
2. Wedging of IVUS catheter.	Dotter effect (lesion dilation).
3. Wedging of IVUS catheter.	Catheter size itself limits minimal lumen area.
4. Ring-down artifact.	Hampers measurement of residual lumen area.
5. Slow-flow (tight lesions).	Poor definition of the lumen-intima interface.
After intervention:	
1. Poor catheter preparation.	Ambiguous delineation of the lumen-intima interface.
2. Poor dynamic range/faint plaque reflectivity.	Intimal drop-out (overestimation of lumen area).
3. Non Uniform Rotation Distortion (NURD).	Unreliable measurements (mechanical systems).
4. Taking back of dissections by catheter.	Artifact leading to overestimation of lumen area.
5. Catheter angulation or eccentric position.	Ovoid, distorted lumen shape.
6. Manual pullback recordings.	Failure to detect site of minimal lumen area and lesion length.
7. 2-D motorized pullback.	Problems to identify minimal lumen area (vs 3-D reconstruction).
8. ECG-triggered image acquisition not used.	Sawtooth artifact related to the cardiac cycle.

IVUS=Intravascular ultrasound. Adapted from Alfonso et al. reference #9

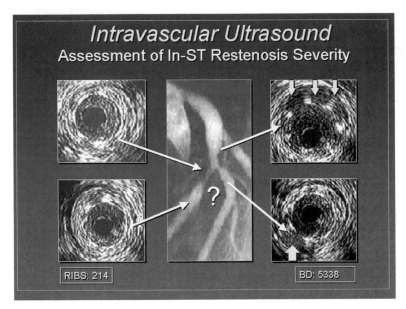

Figure 10-5.   Value of intravascular ultrasound in patients with in-stent restenosis. This lesion in the middle left anterior coronary artery was considered to be the result of in-stent restenosis, although this could not be clearly defined angiographically because the stent could not be visualized. In addition, this was the only view where the stenosis appears as severe. Intravascular ultrasound revealed that the lesion was, in fact, severe (top left), with wedging of the imaging catheter. The stent was jailing a major diagonal branch (bottom right). Furthermore, the most proximal part of the stent was not apposed against the vessel wall (top right). All this information proved very useful during the subsequent coronary intervention.

From the practical perspective, lumen detection may be facilitated by observing the dynamic changes in the speckle pattern typical of flowing blood.[15] In cases with complex lumen shapes (for instance after interventions), a bolus injection of contrast or saline may help to define boundaries during real-time imaging although final measurements should not be performed during this maneuver.[15] Finally, a special anatomic situation is *the left main coronary artery*. This segment represents a diagnostic challenge for angiography.[4, 24, 25.] However, assessment of left main lesions with IVUS also deserves particular attention. An eccentric catheter position may be particularly difficult to avoid in some patients; inducing elliptic configurations of the lumen. NURD artifacts are also relatively common at this site. Care should also be taken to disengage the guide catheter so that a complete IVUS interrogation of the left main (up to the aortic-coronary junction) is performed. Last but not least, special care should be taken to prevent potential ischemic consequences of prolonged IVUS interrogation at this critical coronary segment.

Another indication of IVUS is the evaluation of coronary «pseudostenosis»[26] (Figs. 10-7 and 10-8). In some patients, the use of stiff guidewires induces an artificial straightening of the vessels. In angled coronary segments, this facilitates the appearance of intimal wrinkles or coronary intussusception, which creates a functional stenosis. Physiological study of these «pseudostenoses» reveals that they can indeed cause flow obstruction.[27] However, this phenomenon (also called the «accordion effect» or «crumpled coronary artery») is benign, spon-

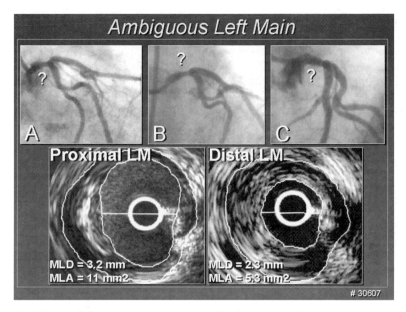

Figure 10-6. Ambiguous left main coronary artery. Doubts persisted concerning lesion severity at the distal trunk despite the use of multiple angulated views. Intravascular ultrasound, however, revealed a severe lesion located in the distal left main coronary artery.

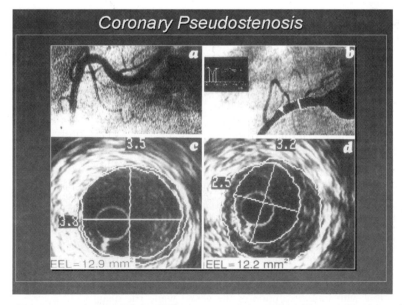

Figure 10-7. Coronary angiogram of the right coronary artery, before intervention (a) and after advancing a stiff guidewire (b), showing the appearance of a lumen narrowing. At the stenotic site (d), intravascular ultrasound visualized a faint hypoechogenic semilunar image causing lumen narrowing but without vessel remodeling. (c) Distal reference segment. Adapted from Alfonso F et al Ref#26.

taneously resolving after the procedure, but requires appropriate diagnosis and management. IVUS can readily detect the asymmetric lumen associated with the typical image of intussusception and exclude a significant atheroma burden or residual dissection at sites with misleading angiographic images[26] (Figs. 10-7 and 10-8).

On the other hand, lesion length may also be accurately measured from motorized IVUS-pullback recordings.[10-11, 13-15] Different studies have established the accuracy of lumen length measurements either directly from the automatic pullbacks or after three-dimensional reconstruction. Therefore, the major players involved in the physiological behavior of coronary lesions (minimal lumen area, percent lumen area stenosis, and lesion length) can be precisely evaluated with IVUS. Overall, as we will discuss later, this anatomic information provides a valid estimate of lesion severity as compared with direct intracoronary physiologic measurements.

Nevertheless, other anatomic factors, such as stenosis morphology and entrance and exit angles may potentially affect flow dynamics. These factors are currently investigated by IVUS using sophisticated three-dimensional reconstruction models of vessel lumen, but are still difficult to incorporate in the clinical setting.[28] Moreover, factors such as the mechanical characteristics of the vessel wall, including coronary distensibility, may also be studied with simultaneous IVUS and intracoronary pressure analysis[16-17, 29] or, more recently, with elastography,[30] but again, they have still not been incorporated into detailed analysis of lesion severity. Finally, other complex factors, such as coefficients of viscous friction and separation, together with the status of the microvascular bed, are also

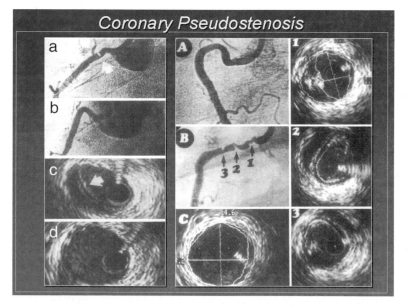

Figure 10-8. Left: (a) Severe focal narrowing of the proximal right coronary artery that disappeared after the removal of the guidewire (b). Intravascular ultrasound demonstrated (c) the elliptic lumen with an image compatible with intussusception of the vessel wall. The distal right coronary artery (d) was normal. Right: Multiple pseudostenoses caused by a stiff wire advanced into a right coronary artery with a shepherd's crook configuration. The typical images of wrinkles (flattened intimal thickening associated with a posterior echo-free space, but without significant plaque burden) were visualized on intravascular ultrasound (2 and 3). Adapted from Alfonso F et al. Reference #26.

implicated in the resistance to flow but cannot be measured with IVUS.[8] However, the incorporation of flow resistance caused by microvascular derangement into the physiological assessment may actually be a limitation instead of an asset (for instance with Doppler) when the only pertinent decision involves treating or deferring a patient with an ambiguous angiographic lesion.[8]

To summarize, most relevant determinants of the flow resistance caused by relatively discrete epicardial narrowing (that is, lesions that can be treated by percutaneous coronary interventions) can be thoroughly analyzed with IVUS. In two large classical studies, IVUS findings pre-intervention changed the management strategy in up to 20 % of patients.[31, 32] Now we know that in angiographically ambiguous or indeterminate coronary lesions IVUS may be helpful not only in the decision of performing or deferring the intervention but also in selecting the interventional device of choice and optimizing procedural results.[13-15] Currently, IVUS is used in many cardiac catheterization laboratories around the world to help in the clinical decision making process involved in coronary interventions. This roughly represents 8 % of all coronary interventions currently performed in the United States although its use is somewhat less in Europe.[14]

INTRASCULAR ULTRASOUND VS QUANTITATIVE CORONARY ANGIOGRAPHY

Visual assessment of coronary stenosis is convenient and rapid, but is associated with large inter and intraobserver variability. Therefore, quantitative coronary angiography (QCA) has been used during the last decade whenever accurate measurements of lumen diameters and stenosis severity were needed.[33] In fact, multicenter clinical trials have systematically required this technique which eventually has become a standard for clinical research.[33] In the clinical setting,

however, many limitations of conventional angiography also apply to QCA.[9, 33] Unrecognized disease at the reference segments remains a common limitation of any angiographic technique, potentially leading to underestimation of lesion severity.[1-4, 13-15] Vessel foreshortening and overlapping side-branches also remain practical limitations of QCA.[5-10] In addition, despite the use of multiple views, angiography may misrepresent the extent of luminal narrowing in eccentric lesions. Ostial lesions and bifurcated lesions are particularly challenging.[13-15] Coronary dissections that appear after the procedure may also have important physiological implications, and are much better detected by IVUS than by angiography.[9] Finally, other radiological factors such as inadequate contrast opacification, cardiac motion, veiling glare or pincushion distortion may prevent precise measurements with QCA.[34]

Preliminary studies used calipers to provide an objective assessment of lesion severity. These measurements showed a relatively poor agreement with IVUS data, mainly after coronary interventions. Nakamura et al.[35] suggested that plaque fracture with passage of contrast material through a dissection plane caused overestimation of minimal lumen diameter by angiography. They studied 91 lesions after balloon angioplasty with IVUS and quantitative angiography using digital calipers. In 44 lesions with a pattern of superficial injury on IVUS (no plaque fracture or just a superficial tear), there was a good correlation between IVUS and angiography for minimal lumen diameter (r = 0.67) and lumen area (r = 0.69). However, in the 47 lesions that presented deep plaque fracture (reaching the media) the correlation between IVUS and angiography for minimal lumen diameter (r = 0.05) and lumen area (r = 0.28) was very poor.

More recently, the automated measurements of computerized systems of QCA have proved to be a valuable tool in providing reliable and reproducible measurements, alleviating the subjectivity and variability of visual assessment.[33] Experimental studies have validated the performance (accuracy and precision) of QCA-derived measurements against true values obtained from phantom stenoses.[36] Nevertheless, debate still exists regarding the relative merits of the two QCA techniques most frequently used, namely edge-detection QCA and videodensitometry.[36-40] In edge-detection QCA, the boundaries of the selected coronary segment are automatically detected by a threshold method, an algorithm using the weighted sum of the first and second derivative functions of the brightness profile. Smoothing procedures and minimal cost algorithms are usually applied to detect lumen contours. The reference segment is either selected by the operator or automatically interpolated by the system. The catheter, used as a scaling device, allows absolute measurements. Eventually, lumen cross-sectional areas are «*calculated*» from orthogonal projections (assuming an elliptic model) or from the worst view (as a circle).[36-40] Conversely, videodensitometry is based on the relation between the optical density of the contrast-filled lumen and absolute vessel dimensions. The cross-sectional area function is obtained from brightness values calibrated for the amount of X-ray absorption after subtracting the background contribution. Calibration of videodensitometric images is performed by equalizing the reference area to that calculated from the edge-detection algorithm.[36-40] Therefore, this technique measures vessel dimensions more independently of lesion contour and luminal shape. It requires, however, complete homogeneous opacification of the lumen and may be less reliable in calcified vessels or after the deployment of radiopaque stents. Whereas edge-detection QCA has gained widespread acceptance, the clinical value videodensitometry remains controversial.

Therefore, the advantages of IVUS (direct measurement) versus quantitative angiography (estimation or calculation) in the assess-

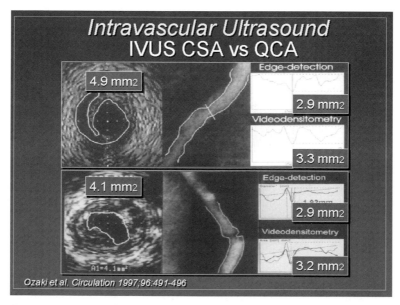

Figure 10-9. Differences in cross sectional minimal lumen area (CSA) according to the method of analysis [Edge-detection quantitative coronary angiography (QCA), Videodensitometry and intravascular ultrasound (IVUS)]. Adapted from Ozaki et al. Reference #39.

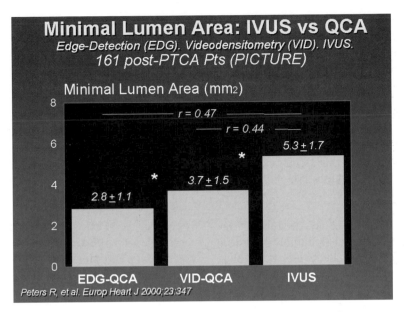

Figure 10-10. Differences in minimal lumen area according to the method of measurement. Videodensitometry provides information closer to the intravascular ultrasound data. Adapted from Peters et al. reference #40.

ment of physiologically important values such as minimal lumen area appear self-evident. However, as several factors (Table 10-1) explain why IVUS is still not universally accepted as the gold standard for lumen dimension measurements, in the absence of known true values, the Bland and Altman method is still required as an index of agreement between techniques. Most initial studies found a relatively good correlation between angiography and IVUS in normal looking segments and in simple lesions, whereas the correlation deteriorated in complex lesions or following intervention.[4, 36-40] In a detailed study, Ozaki et al.[39] suggested that lesions with complex morphology and those studied after interventions (haziness, dissections), account to a great extent for the discrepancies between the two QCA techniques (Fig. 10-9). It was concluded that the agreement between IVUS and QCA progressively deteriorated according to the degree of vessel damage, but this finding was less evident with videodensitometry.[39] In

fact, the correlation coefficient between videodensitometric QCA and IVUS increased after intervention. These observations concurred with previous data from von Birgelen et al.[37] showing that agreement between edge-detection QCA and videodensitometry was good after rotational atherectomy because the intervention yielded smooth, symmetrical lumens. However, dispersion increased after adjunctive balloon angioplasty, which generated more irregular lumens.[37] Finally, after stent deployment, and despite the device's metallic struts, a particularly good agreement was found between IVUS and videodensitometry, whereas correlation between IVUS and edge-detection QCA remained slightly behind, probably due to some asymmetric stent configurations.[38] Peters et al.[40] recently evaluated the correlations between edge-detection QCA, videodensitometric QCA and IVUS in 161 patients after successful balloon angioplasty in the PICTURE study. IVUS-derived lumen dimensions corresponded more closely to videodensitometry than to edge-detection QCA measurements (Fig. 10-10). However, the minimal lumen area obtained by IVUS was significantly larger than that measured by videodensitometry, which, in turn, was significantly larger than that obtained by edge-detection QCA. These relatively large differences may seem difficult to explain but confirm data from previous studies.[4, 9, 36-39] Ultimately, the concept that IVUS and video-densitometry are projection-independent appears to be a key factor in explaining these findings.[9, 36-40]

More recently, the development of the gradient field transform, including a *shortest path* algorithm rather than the traditional *smoothing* algorithm, renders eccentric and complex lesions more amenable to reliable edge-detection QCA analysis. Further studies, ideally using 3-D reconstruction of ECG-gated IVUS images simultaneously with the pressure wire, are required to provide more comprehensive and definitive insights into the relative merits of each QCA technique in the assessment of lesion severity.[9]

IVUS VS INTRACORONARY PHYSIOLOGICAL ASSESSMENT

How can we use IVUS-derived anatomic information to detect when a given epicardial stenosis is producing a significant resistance to flow? Since the pioneering research of Gould et al.[41, 42] three decades ago, which critically analyzed the relationship between the anatomic severity of a stenosis and its flow resistance, an ongoing and stimulating debate persists on this rapidly evolving field both from the academic standpoint and also from a practical perspective during clinical decision-making. In animal models, Gould et al.[43] demonstrated, using coronary constrictors, that coronary flow reserve deteriorates when lumen diameter stenosis exceeds 50%. Current technological refinements allow the assessment of the pressure-flow relationship distal to a target coronary stenosis during

routine clinical practice.[8, 18, 19] Here we will discuss the correlation between the previously described IVUS parameters and physiological data obtained with either intracoronary Doppler or the pressure wire.

Intracoronary Doppler

In most patients with stable angina, symptoms result principally from the ability of the stenosis to blunt increases to blood flow in response to metabolic demands. This phenomenon is well characterized with the analysis of coronary flow reserve. Intracoronary Doppler may be used to estimate relative changes in blood flow secondary to the administration of a coronary vasodilator.

In a preliminary study, Moses et al.[44] studied the relation between single tomographic IVUS parameters and intracoronary Doppler flow velocity in 41 patients with intermediately severe coronary artery stenoses. They found that IVUS reference segment area and lumen area were significantly larger in lesions with a coronary reserve ≥ 1.8 compared with those with a coronary reserve <1.8. However, there was only a weak correlation between IVUS-measured minimal lumen diameter and post-stenotic coronary reserve (r = 0.31, p = 0.045) determined by intracoronary Doppler. Of interest, the correlation between quantitative angiography and coronary reserve was even poorer. Kern et al.[45] and Ge et al.[46] also showed that after coronary interventions coronary flow reserve improved and correlated with the severity of residual stenosis as determined with IVUS.

In contrast, Abizaid et al.[47] demonstrated that IVUS-determined minimal cross-sectional area strongly correlated (r = 0.83, p < 0.0001) with Doppler-derived coronary flow reserve. In addition, a minimum lumen cross-sectional area pre-intervention >4 mm^2 had a diagnostic accuracy of 92% in predicting a coronary flow reserve ≥ 2. Moreover, a minimal lumen diameter ≥ 2 on IVUS also had a diagnostic accuracy of 89% in identifying a coronary flow reserve ≥ 2. In this study, the correlation between minimum lumen area and coronary reserve persisted, although attenuated, after balloon angioplasty (r = 0.51, p = 0.006) and after stent implantation (r = 0.62, p = 0.03). Using multivariate linear regression analysis, independent determinants of coronary flow reserve included IVUS minimal lumen cross-sectional area, angiographic lesion length and diabetes mellitus. As we will describe later on, the IVUS cut-off value of 4 mm^2 also appears to keep a good correlation with clinical outcome.

Finally, some commercially available phased-array IVUS catheters allow intracoronary flow visualization. The red signal of flow, superimposed on the coronary lumen, may be useful to further delineate lumen boundaries in patients with complex anatomy or coronary dissections. Preliminary data also suggest that flow quantification may be obtained from analysis of the rate of decorrelation of digitized radiofrequency ultrasound echo signals.[48, 49] Subsequently, flow information could be superimposed on the IVUS image using a color scale. Integration of the blood velocity components normal to the scan plane permits calculation of the volume flow. Preliminary validation of this method in animal models appears very promising.[48, 49]

Pressure Wire

Fractional flow reserve is an elegant physiological index, specific for the conductance of the epicardial coronary artery, that may be readily obtained with the pressure wire during maximal hyperemia.[50] Therefore comparison of IVUS findings with this index, currently considered the «gold-standard» for the functional evaluation of epicardial coronary stenosis severity has generated great interest. The correlation between the two techniques before coronary intervention has been well established confirms, once again, the validity of IVUS-derived physio-

logical assessment. However, the advantages and disadvantages of each technique after catheter-based interventions still remains an issue of debate where further research is needed.

Takagi et al.[18] studied 51 coronary lesions with IVUS and pressure wire. Minimal lumen area showed a positive correlation (r^2 = 0.62, p < 0.0001) and % area stenosis an inverse correlation (r^2 = 0.60, p < 0.0001) with fractional flow reserve values. In this study QCA parameters, including lesion length and severity, were also of value in predicting an abnormal fractional flow reserve (minimal lumen diameter <1.5 [sensitivity 92 %, specificity 92 %] and % diameter stenosis [sensitivity 88 %, specificity 89 %]). On IVUS, minimal lumen area <3 mm^2 (sensitivity 83 %, specificity 92 %) and % area stenosis >60 % (sensitivity 92 %, specificity 89 %) were the best thresholds to maximize sensitivity and specificity. The percent area stenosis by IVUS was the strongest independent determinant of fractional flow reserve values. Interestingly, these investigators demonstrated that an IVUS minimal lumen cross-sectional area <3 mm^2 associated with an area stenosis ≥ 60 % had a 100 % predictive accuracy for a pressure-wire derived fractional flow reserve of <0.75 (the ischemic threshold).

More recently Takayama et al.[51] used three-dimensional IVUS to predict the physiological significance of coronary stenosis. IVUS minimal lumen area correlated with fractional flow reserve (r^2 = 0.55, p = 0.003) and pressure gradient (r^2 = 0.52, p = 0.003). In addition, lesion length also had a positive correlation with the pressure gradient (r^2 = 0.45, p = 0.0007). On multivariate analysis, the only independent predictor of the fractional flow reserve was the ratio of minimal lumen area/ lesion length as determined by IVUS. Moreover, the IVUS-predicted pressure gradient correlated well with gradient values measured directly. They concluded that the physiological severity of coronary lesions is mainly determined by lumen area and lesion length, which can be readily obtained from 3-dimensional IVUS.

Briguori et al.[52] also compared IVUS findings with values of fractional flow reserve in 53 lesions causing intermediate coronary artery stenoses on angiography. Using ROC curves, they identified area stenosis >70 % (sensitivity 100 %, specificity 68 %), minimal lumen diameter <1.8 mm (sensitivity 100 %, specificity 66 %), minimal lumen area <4 mm^2 (sensitivity 92 %, specificity 56 %) and lesion length >10 mm (sensitivity 41 %, specificity 80 %) to be the best cut-off values to fit with a fractional flow reserve <0.75. All lesions with a plaque area stenosis <70 % had a fractional flow reserve >0.75. In addition, the combined evaluation of both percent area stenosis and minimal lumen diameter increased the value of IVUS to determine the functional significance of coronary artery stenoses. In this study there was no correlation whatsoever between IVUS-determined plaque area, or the remodeling pattern, and fractional flow reserve, indicating that this index determined the luminal compromise rather than the atherosclerotic plaque burden on the vessel wall. Brosh et al.[53] recently stressed the importance of lesion length as the main factor accounting for the apparent discrepancies between anatomic data obtained at the lesion site and physiologic parameters.

Finally, other studies have tried to identify the relative value of IVUS and pressure wire studies in the assessment of optimal stent deployment. This is important because many studies have demonstrated that IVUS minimal stent areas are more powerful predictors of restenosis than the angiographic parameters.[54-56] Results may differ depending on the type of stent used (coiled stent versus slotted-tube stent). In the study of Hanekamp et al.,[19] a fractional flow reserve >0.94 (ROC analysis) after coronary stenting with coil stents showed a concordance of 94 % with established IVUS criteria for optimal stent implantation. Interestingly, this value corresponds to the lower limit of the normal range of fractional flow reserve. Of 81 paired IVUS

and coronary pressure measurements, 91 % were concordant. On the contrary, QCA showed a low concordance rate with IVUS (concordance 48 %) and fractional flow reserve (concordance 46 %). Once again, this study confirms the value of IVUS for optimizing stent deployment and illustrates how QCA alone is insufficient for this purpose.

In the study of Katritsis et al.,[57] using slotted-tube stents, there was a good concordance between IVUS and pressure wire data when fractional flow reserve values were less than 0.91 or more than 0.94. However, fractional flow reserve values between 0.91 and 0.94 were more difficult to interpret. Finally, in a recent multicenter study, Fearon et al.[58] demonstrated that a fractional flow reserve <0.96 predicted suboptimal stent results (also with slotted-tube stents) based on validated IVUS criteria (negative predictive value of 88 %). However, a fractional flow reserve >0.96 did not reliably predict an optimal result (predictive accuracy 62 %). In other words, there was a significant number of patients in whom fractional flow reserve was optimal (>0.96) but IVUS results remained suboptimal (yielding a specificity of only 58 %). In addition, this study raised concerns regarding potential overestimation of fractional flow reserve in patients who may require higher than reported doses of intracoronary adenosine to achieve complete vasodilation of the microvasculature. It is especially important to maximize hyperemia after stenting because detection of very small gradients is necessary to distinguish between optimal and suboptimal stent deployment. In addition, obstructions occurring outside the stent and insufficient sensitivity of the fractional flow reserve to detect minimal obstruction to flow may also be involved.

Limitations and Technical Considerations

Limitations and technical considerations involved in the interpretation of IVUS and QCA correlations have already been described. Some of the technical considerations inherent to currently available tools for the study of coronary physiology also need to be emphasized to put correlations with IVUS findings into perspective. Doppler-derived coronary flow reserve detects the resistance to flow caused by epicardial stenosis as well as the resistance of the microcirculation.[44-47] An abnormal coronary reserve may just be the result of microvascular circulation compromised by diabetes, left ventricular hypertrophy, or altered rheological status. Although this drawback can be obviated by calculating relative flow reserve, using another major normal epicardial vessel as a reference (assuming that microcirculatory abnormalities are evenly distributed throughout the myocardium), this increases the complexity of the procedure when the relevant clinical question is assessing the severity of a given coronary stenosis. In addition, microcirculatory abnormalities are assumed to be uniform throughout the entire myocardium, so patients with a previous myocardial infarction should be excluded. Diffuse epicardial atherosclerosis, myocardial stunning, or small-vessel disease may also complicate the interpretation of Doppler findings.[8,44-47] In addition, increased baseline coronary flow may reduce the coronary flow reserve value despite excellent immediate results after intervention. In this regard, fractional flow reserve has gained popularity because its value is relatively independent of driving pressure, heart rate, and status of the microvasculature.[50] Pijls et al.[50] demonstrated that the hyperemic absolute distal coronary pressure, rather than the resting pressure gradient, was closely related to the potential of a given coronary stenosis to induce ischemia and reflects both antegrade and collateral blood flow. Therefore, this is a very attractive lesion-specific parameter for interventional cardiologists. However, a critical step in the assessment of coronary physiology with either Doppler or the pressure wire relies on obtaining complete and maximal vasodilation of the microvasculature (minimal resis-

tance of the microvascular bed). Technical and anatomic factors need to be taken into consideration to avoid theoretical concerns and ambiguity about the status of the microcirculation. This is important because only when maximal vasodilation of the microvascular bed is achieved can a close correlation between pressure and flow be assumed. Only in this situation does the curvilinear pressure-flow relationship produced by a significant coronary stenosis fall into a relatively straight segment that allows an accurate measurement of pressure loss, volumetric flow, and vessel resistance.[41-43] Probably this is the main potential practical limitation of the physiological information currently available since incomplete hyperemia overestimates the fractional flow reserve and underestimates lesion severity. Another problem of fractional flow reserve is assessing the hemodynamic significance of serial coronary artery stenoses. Diffuse disease or multiple stenoses may hinder interpretation of pressure wire findings because each stenosis influences the hemodynamic effects of the others, leading to underestimation of lesion severity (which is more pronounced for proximal lesions) unless complex stenosis interaction is accounted for.[59] Treating a severe distal lesion will unmask the true severity of the proximal lesion. In addition, in patients showing normal side branches between serial stenoses, flow through the distal stenoses can be reduced by diverting flow to the low-resistance branch. IVUS, however, may readily characterize the severity of each individual narrowing irrespective of the presence of major side-branches between the stenoses. All these potential limitations of currently available physiological techniques should be kept in mind during the interpretation of correlations with IVUS.

CLINICAL VALIDATION OF IVUS PARAMETERS

Some theoretical concerns persist regarding the potential limitations of using IVUS-

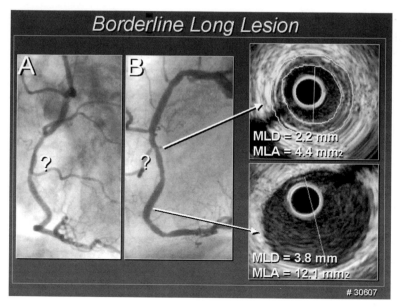

Figure 10-11. Intravascular ultrasound assessment of a long lesion in the middle right coronary artery. Although minimal lumen area was over 4 mm², the lesion length was 25 mm on the motorized pullback. Eventually this lesion was left untreated.

derived anatomic information as a valid alternative to direct physiological assessment. However, the clinical validation of using IVUS, not only in the decision to treat and as guidance for coronary interventions, but also in the decision to defer them, supports its clinical use in the catheterization laboratory. We will now describe some correlations of IVUS findings with non-invasive tests to detect ischemia and the clinical results obtained when IVUS findings are used to defer coronary revascularization (Fig. 10-11).

Non-invasive Detection of Ischemia

Nishioka et al.[60] compared IVUS-derived indices of lesion severity with the results of stress myocardial perfusion imaging. When SPECT myocardial perfusion imaging was considered the gold standard, lesion lumen area <4 mm² was a simple and highly accurate criterion (sensitivity 88%, specificity 90%) for significant coronary narrowing.

Exclusion of patients with microvascular abnormalities, which potentially affect SPECT results, increased sensitivity to 91% and specificity to 95%. Other indices, such as lesion percent area stenosis and lumen percent area stenosis were also good predictors (sensitivity and specificity above 80%) of the functional significance of coronary stenoses. Interestingly, an area stenosis >73% by IVUS had 81% sensitivity and 84% sensitivity for ischemia. These parameters can be used to complement the simplest measurement of minimal lumen area 1) in patients with borderline lumen area values, 2) when the luminal contour is poorly visualized, and 3) in relatively large or small vessels. However, it is important to emphasize once again that some patients may have + SPECT despite mild lumen narrowing due to the presence of microcirculatory alterations. Other non-invasive techniques such as stress echocardiography are also largely dependent on the status of the microvascular bed and therefore may overstimate the severity of epicardial coronary stenosis. Conversely, IVUS measurements are not influenced by the status of microcirculation and constitute a robust imaging modality for independently assessing the severity of epicardial coronary stenoses.

Long-term Clinical Outcome

Several studies have used IVUS to reach the decision to perform or defer coronary interventions. Abizaid et al.[61] used IVUS to study 300 patients (357 intermediate coronary stenoses), in which coronary intervention was deferred based on IVUS findings. Eligible «uncertain» stenoses included <70 % diameter stenoses on visual assessment. After a follow-up of 13 months, an event rate (death, myocardial infarction or target vessel revascularization) of 8 % was documented. In this study, no angiographic measurement was predictive of events at follow-up. It is noteworthy that the only independent pre-

dictors of events (after adjusting for clinical and angiographic variables) were IVUS minimal lumen area and percent area stenosis as detected by IVUS. In addition, the only independent predictors of target lesion revascularization were diabetes mellitus, IVUS minimal lumen area, and IVUS percent area stenosis. In 248 lesions with a minimal lumen area ≥ 4 mm^2, the requirement for revascularization during follow-up was only 2.8 %. They concluded that IVUS imaging was a valuable alternative to physiological assessment in patients with intermediate coronary lesions on angiography. In addition, the long-term follow-up after IVUS-guided deferred interventions was similar to that previously reported after direct physiological lesion assessment.[62-64] Therefore, the clinical usefulness of this cut-off value (>4 mm^2) appears well validated for IVUS-based deferred interventions. A potential limitation of this parameter is the assessment of lesions in small or secondary vessels. Few of these

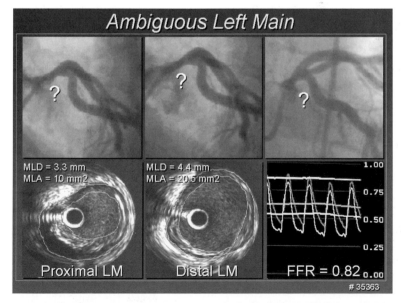

Figure 10-12. Ambiguous left main (LM) coronary artery. Lesion severity was difficult to ascertain due to a short left main coronary artery. Intravascular ultrasound allowed precise recognition of the anatomy of the lesion causing the narrowing with a minimal lumen diameter (MLD) of 3.3 mm and a minimal lumen area (MLA) of 10 mm^2. This information was reassuring and in keeping with the results of the guidewire which demonstrated a fractional flow reserve (FFR) of more than 0.80.

vessels were included in previous studies, so one may speculate that the percent area stenosis may be more useful in this subset of patients.

Finally, the angiographic assessment of the severity of disease in the left main coronary artery remains elusive in many patients (Fig. 10-12). In fact, the correlation between angiography and postmortem findings has been particularly poor at this site.[65,66] IVUS may overcome these angiographic limitations although still there is no consensus regarding the cross sectional area at which the left main disease should be considered significant. However, an area stenosis >50 % or an absolute minimal lumen area <9 mm^2 have been proposed as criteria for revascularization.[14] In the study of Abizaib,[25] 122 patients with moderate left main disease and ambiguous angiograms were evaluated with IVUS and subsequently did not undergo coronary revascularization. During a clinical follow-up of 1 year, 4 patients died, 3 required coronary interventions on the left main coronary, and 11 underwent by-pass surgery (total event rate of 14 %). Using logistic regression analysis, diabetes mellitus, an untreated vessel, and IVUS-derived minimal lumen diameter were independent predictors of cardiac events. The event rate was 3 % for the cohort of patients with minimal lumen diameter >3 mm. It is important to emphasize that in the entire patient cohort QCA data (including minimal lumen diameter and % diameter stenosis) correlated poorly with IVUS measurements and were not predictive of events.

We can conclude by saying that IVUS-derived information correlates closely with direct intracoronary physiological assessment. Ultimately, the clinical value of deferring coronary intervention for intermediate stenosis based on IVUS-derived anatomic information is remarkably consistent with that obtained from physiology-based techniques.[62-64] Furthermore, this review illustrates that IVUS parameters, Doppler data, and fractional flow reserve are complementary in the evaluation of lesion severity. Therefore, the use of each technique (clinical or research purposes) should be dictated by the primary aim of the study.

REFERENCES

1. Nissen SE, Gurley JC, Grines CL, Booth DC, McClure R, Berk M, Fisher CH, DeMaria AN. Intravascular ultrasound assessment of lumen size and wall morphology in normal subjects and patients with coronary artery disease. *Circulation* 1991; 84:1087-1099.

2. Tobis JM, Mallery J, Mahon D, et al. Intravascular ultrasound imaging of human coronary arteries in vivo. Analysis of tissue characterizations with comparison to in vitro histological specimens. *Circulation* 1991; 83:913-926.

3. Mintz GS, Kent KM, Pichard AD, Satler LF, Popma JJ, Leon MB. Contribution of inadequate arterial remodeling to the development of focal coronary artery stenoses. An intravascular ultrasound study. *Circulation* 1997; 95:1791-1798.

4. Alfonso F, Macaya C, Goicolea J, Iñiguez A, Hernandez R, Zamorano J, Pérez-Vizcayno MJ, Zarco P. Intravascular ultrasound imaging of angiographically normal coronary segments in patients with coronary artery disease. *Am Heart J* 1994; 127:536-544.

5. Topol TJ, Nissen SE. Our preoccupation with coronary luminology: the dissociation between clinical and angiographic findings in ischemic heart disease. *Circulation* 1995; 92:2333-2342.

6. Grondin CM, Dyrda I, Pasternac A, Campeau L, Bourassa MG, Lesperance J. Discrepancies between cineangiographic and postmortem findings in patients with coronary artery disease and recent coronary revascularization. *Circulation* 1974; 49: 703-708.

7. Arnett EN, Isner JN, Redwood DR, Kent KM, Baker WP, Ackerstein H, Roberts WC. Coronary artery narrowing in coronary heart disease: comparison of cineangiographic and necropsy findings. *Ann Intern Med* 1979; 91:350-356.

8. Kern MJ. Coronary physiology revisited. Practical insights from the cardiac catheterization laboratory. *Circulation* 2000; 101:1344-1351.

9. Alfonso F. Videodensitometric versus edge-detection quantitative angiography. Insights from intravascular ultrasound imaging. *Europ Heart J* 2000; 21:604-607.

10. Fuessl RT, Mintz GS, Pichard AD, Kent KM, Satler LF, Popma JJ, Leon MB. In vivo validation of intravascular ultrasound length measurements using a motorized transducer pull-back system. *Am J Cardiol* 1996; 77:1115-1158.

11. Rosenfield K, Losordo W, Ramaswany K et al. Three-dimensional reconstruction of human coronary and peripheral arteries from images recorded during two-dimensional intravascular ultrasound examinations. *Circulation* 1991: 84:1938-1956.

12. Scanlon PJ, Faxon DP, Audet AM, et al. ACC/AHA guidelines for coronary angiography. A report from the American College of Cardiology/American Heart Association Task Force on practice guidelines (Committee on coronary angiography). *J Am Coll Cardiol* 1999; 33:1756-1824.

13. Mintz GS, Nissen SE, Anderson WD, Bailey SR, Erbel R, Fitzgerald PJ, Pinto F, Rosenfield K, Siegel RJ, Tuzcu EM, Yock PG. American College of Cardiology clinical expert consensus document on standards for acquisition, measurement and reporting of intravascular ultrasound studies (IVUS). *J Am Coll Cardiol* 2001; 37:1478-1492.

14. Nissen SE, Yock P. Intravascular ultrasound: novel pathophysiological insights and current clinical applications. *Circulation* 2001; 103:604-616.

15. Di Mario C, Görge R, Peters R, Kearney P, Pinto D, Hausmann D, von Biergelen C, Colombo A, Mudra H, Roelandt J, Erbel R, on behalf of the working group of echocardiography of the European Society of Cardiology. Clinical application and image interpretation in intracoronary ultrasound. *Europ Heart J* 1998; 19:207-229.

16. Alfonso F, Macaya C, Goicolea J, Hernandez R, Segovia J, Zamorano J, Bañuelos C, Zarco P. Determinants of coronary compliance in patients with coronary artery disease: an intravascular ultrasound study. *J Am Coll Cardiol* 1994; 23:879-884.

17. Nakatani S, Yamagishi M, Tamai J, Goto Y, Umeno T, Kawaguchi A, Yutani C, Miyatake K. Assessment of coronary artery distensibility by intravascular ultrasound. Application of simultaneous measurements of luminal area and pressure. *Circulation* 1995; 91:2904-2910.

18. Takagi A, Tsurumi Y, Ishii Y, Suzuki K, Kawana M, Kasanuki H. Clinical potential of intravascular ultrasound for physiological assessment of coronary stenosis. Relationship between quantitative ultrasound tomography and pressure-derived fractional flow reserve. *Circulation* 1999; 100:250-255.

19. Hanekamp CEE, Koolen JJ, Pijls NHJ, Michels HR, Bonnier HJRM. Comparison of quantitative angiography, intravascular ultrasound and coronary pressure measurement to assess optimum stent deployment. *Circulation* 1999; 99:1015-1021.

20. Hausmann D, Friedrich G, Soni B, Daniel WG, Fitzgerald PJ, Yock PG. Validation of automatic border detection in intravascular ultrasound images. *Echocardiography* 1996; 6:599-608.

21. Alfonso F, Macaya C, Goicolea J, Hernandez R, Bañuelos C, Iñiguez A, Zamorano J, Zarco P. Angiographic changes (Dotter effect) produced by intravascular ultrasound imaging before coronary angioplasty. *Am Heart J* 1994; 128:244-251.

22. Alfonso F, Goicolea J, Perez, Vizcaíno MJ, Hernández R, Segovia J, Fernandez-Ortiz A, Bañuelos C, Macaya C. Intracoronary ultrasound before coronary interventions: a prospective comparison of two different catheters. *Cath Cardiovasc Diagn* 1997; 40:33-39.

23. Di Mario C, Madretsma S, Linker D, The SH, Bom N, Serruys PW, Gussenhoven EJ, Roelandt JR. The angle of incidence of ultrasonic beam: a critical factor for image quality in intravascular ultrasonography. *Am Heart J* 1993; 125:442-448.

24. Isner JM, Kishel J, Kent KM, Ronan JA, Ross AM, Roberts WC. Accuracy of angiographic determination of left main coronary arterial narrowing: angiographic-histologic correlative analysis in 28 patients. *Circulation* 1981; 63:1056-1064.

25. Abizaid AS, Mintz GS, Abizaid A, Mehran R, Lansky AJ, Pichard AD, Satler LF, Wu H, Kent KM, Leon MB. One-year follow-up after intravascular ultrasound assessment of moderate left main coronary artery disease in patients with ambiguous angiograms. *J Am Coll Cardiol* 1999; 34:707-715.

26. Alfonso F, Delgado A, Magalhaes D, Goicolea J, Hernandez R, Fernández-Ortíz A, Escaned J, Bañuelos C, Cortés J, Flores A, Macaya C. Value of intravascular ultrasound in the assessment of coronary pseudostenosis during coronary interventions. *Cathet Cardiovasc Diagn* 1999; 46:327-332.

27. Escaned J, Flores A, García P, Hernandez R, Alfonso F, Fernandez-Ortíz A, Sabaté M, Bañuelos C, Macaya C. Guidewire-induced coronary pseudostenosis as a source of error during physiological guidance of stent deployment. *Cathet Cardiovasc Intervent* 2000; 51:91-94.

28. von Birgelen C, de Vrey EA, Mintz GS, Nicosia A, Bruining N, Li W, Roeland JR, Serruys PW, de Feyter PJ. ECG-gated three-dimensional intravascular ultrasound: feasibility and reproducibility of automated analysis of coronary lumen and atherosclerotic plaque dimensions in humans. *Circulation* 1997; 96:2944-2952.

29. Botas J, Clark DA, Pinto F, Chenzbraun A, Fischell TA. Balloon angioplasty results in increasing segmental coronary distensibility: a likely mechanism of percutaneous transluminal coronary angioplasty. *J Am Coll Cardiol* 1994; 23:1043-1052.

30. de Korte CL, Pasterkamp G, van der Steen AF, Woutman HA, Bom N. Characterization of plaque components with intravascular ultrasound elastography in human femoral coronary arteries in vitro. *Circulation* 2000; 102:617-623.

31. Lee DY, Eigler N, Luo H, et al. Effect of intracoronary ultrasound imaging on clinical decision making. *Am Heart J* 1995; 129:1084-1093.

32. Mintz GS, Pichard AD, Kovach JA, et al. Impact of preintervention intravascular ultrasound imaging on transcatheter treatment strategies in coronary artery disease. *Am J Cardiol* 1994; 73:423-430.

33. Mancini GBJ. Quantitative coronary arteriographic methods in the interventional catheterization laboratory: an update and perspective. *J Am Coll Cardiol* 1991; 17:23B-33B.

34. Takahashi T, Honda Y, Russo RJ, Fitzgerald PJ. Intravascular ultrasound and quantitative coronary angiography. *Cathet Cardiovasc Diagn* 2002; 55:118-128.

35. Nakamura S, Mahon DJ, Maheswaran B, Gutfinger DE, Colombo A, Tobis JM. An explanation for discrepancy between angiographic and intravascular ultrasound measurements after percutaneous transluminal coronary angioplasty. *J Am Coll Cardiol* 1995; 25:633-639.

36. Keane D, Haase J, Slager CJ, van Swijndregt EM, Lehmann KG, Ozaki Y, di Mario C, Kirkeeide R, Serruys PW. Comparative validation of quantitative coronary angiography systems. Results and implications from a multicenter study using a standardized approach. *Circulation* 1995; 91:2147-2183.

37. von Birgelen C, Umans VA, di Mario C, Keane D, Gil R, Prati F, de Feyter P, Serruys PW. Mechanisms of highspeed rotational atherectomy and adjunctive balloon angioplasty revisited by quantitative coronary angiography: edge-detection versus videodensitometry. *Am Heart J* 1995; 130:405-412.

38. von Birgelen C, Kutryk MJB, Gil R, Ozaki Y, Di Mario C, Roelandt JRTC, de Feyter PJ, Serruys PW. Quantification of the minimal luminal cross-sectional area after coronary stenting by two- and three-dimensional intravascular ultrasound versus edge-detection and videodensitometry. *Am J Cardiol* 1996; 78:520-525.

39. Ozaki Y, Violaris AG, Kobayashi T, Keane D, Camenzind E, Di Mario C, de Feyter P, Roelandt JRTC, Serruys PW. Comparison of coronary luminal quantification obtained from intracoronary ultrasound and both geometric and videodensitometric quantitative angiography before and after balloon angioplasty and directional atherectomy. *Circulation* 1997; 96:491-499.

40. Peters RJG, Kok WEM, Pasterkamp G, von Birgelen C, Prins M, Serruys PPW, on behalf of the PICTURE study group. Videodensitometric quantitative angiography after

coronary balloon angioplasty, compared to edge-detection quantitative angiography and intracoronary ultrasound imaging. *Europ Heart J* 2000; 21:654-661.

41. Gould KL, Lipscomb K, Hamilton GW. Physiology basis for assessing critical coronary stenosis: instantaneous flow response and regional distribution during coronary hyperemia as measures of coronary flow reserve. *Am J Cardiol* 1974;33:87-94.

42. Gould KL, Kirkeeide RL, Buchi M. Coronary flow reserve as a physiological measure of stenosis severity. *J Am Coll Cardiol* 1990; 15:459-474.

43. Gould KL. Quantification of coronary artery stenosis in vivo. *Cir Res* 1985; 57:341-353.

44. Moses JW, Undermir C, Strain JE, Kreps EM, Higgins JE, Glein GW, Kern MJ. Relation between single tomographic intravascular ultrasound image parameters and intracoronary Doppler flow velocity in patients with intermediately severe coronary stenoses. *Am Heart J* 1998; 135:988-994.

45. Kern MJ, Dupouy P, Drury JH, Aguirre FV, Aptecar E, Bach RG, Caracciolo EA, Donohue TJ, Rande JL, Geschwind HJ, Mechem CJ, Kane G, Teiger E, Wolford TL. Role of coronary artery lumen enlargement in improving coronary blood flow after balloon angioplasty and stenting: a combined intravascular ultrasound Doppler flow and imaging study. *J Am Coll Cardiol* 1997; 29:1520-1527.

46. Ge J, Erbel R, Zamorano J, Haude M, Kearney P, Gorge G, Meyer J. Improvement of coronary morphology and blood flow after stenting: assessment by intravascular ultrasound and intracoronary Doppler. *Int J Cardiac Imaging* 1995; 11:81-87.

47. Abizaid A, Mintz GS, Pichard A, Kent KM, Satler LF, Walsh CL, Popma JJ, Leon MB. Clinical, intravascular ultrasound and quantitative angiographic determinants of the coronary flow reserve before and after percutaneous transluminal coronary angioplasty. *Am J Cardiol* 1998; 82:423-428.

48. Carlier SG, Cespedes EI, Mastik F, Van Der Steen AF, Bom N, Serruys PW. Blood flow assessment with intravascular ultrasound catheters: the ideal tool for simultaneous assessment of coronary hemodynamics and

the vessel wall? *Semin Interv Cardiol* 1998; 3:21-29.

49. Lupotti FA, Cespedes EI, Steen AF. Decorrelation characteristics of trasverse blood flow along an intravascular array catheter: effects of aggregation of blood cells. *Ultrasound Med Biol* 2001; 27:409-417.

50. Pijls NH, De Bruyne B, Peels K, van der Voort PH, Bonnier HJ, Bartunek J, Koolen JJ. Measurement of fractional flow reserve to assess the functional severity of coronary-artery stenoses. *N Engl J Med* 1996; 334:1703-1708.

51. Takayama T, Hodgson JM. Prediction of the physiologic severity of coronary lesions using IVUS: validation by direct coronary pressure measurement. *Catheter Cardiovasc Interv* 2001; 53:48-55.

52. Briguori C, Anzuini A, Airoldi F, Gimelli G, Nishida T, Adamian M, Di Mario C, Colombo A. Intravascular ultrasound criteria for the assessment of the functional significance of intermediate coronary artery stenoses and correlation with fractional flow reserve. *Am J Cardiol* 2001; 87:136-141.

53. Brosh D, Higano ST, Slepian MJ, Miller HL, Kern MJ, Holmes DR, Lerman A. The effect of lesion length on the functional significance of coronary lesions. *J Am Coll Cardiol* 2002; 39:12A.

54. Albiero R, Rau T, Schluter M, et al. Comparison of immediate and intermediate-term results of intravascular ultrasound versus angiography-guided Palmaz-Schatz stent implantation in matched lesions. *Circulation* 1997; 96:2997-3005.

55. Hoffmann R, Mintz GS, Mehran R, et al. Intravascular ultrasound predictors of angiographic restenosis in lesions treated with Palmaz-Schatz stents. *J Am Coll Cardiol* 1998; 31:43-49.

56. Fitzgerald PJ, Oshima A, Hayase M, et al. Final results of the Can Routine Ultrasound Influence Stent Expansion (CRUISE) study. *Circulation* 2000; 102:523-530.

57. Katritsis DG, Ioannidis JP, Koroveis S, Giazitzoglou E, Parissis J, Webb-Peploe MM. Comparison of myocardial fractional flow reserve and intravascular ultrasound for the assessment of slotted-tube stents. *Cathet Cardiovasc Interv* 2001; 52:322-326.

58. Fearon WF, Luna J, Samady H, Powers ER, Feldman T, Dib N, Tuzcu M, Cleman MW, Chou TM, Cohen DJ, Ragosta M, Takagi A, Jeremias A, Fitzgerald PJ, Yeung AC, Kern MJ, Yock PG. Fractional flow reserve compared with intravascular ultrasound guidance for optimising stent deployment. *Circulation* 2001; 104:1917-1922.

59. Pijls NH, De Bruyne B, Bech GJ, Liistro F, Heyndrickx GR, Bonnier HJ, Koolen JJ. Coronary pressure measurements to assess the hemodynamic significance of serial stenosis within one coronary artery. Validation in humans. *Circulation* 2000; 102: 2371-2377.

60. Nishioka T, Amanullah AM, Luo H, Berglund MD, Kim CJ, Nagai T, Hakamata N, Katsushika S, Uehata A, Takase B, Isojima K, Berman DS, Siegel RJ. Clinical validation of intravascular ultrasound imaging for assessment of coronary stenosis severity. Comparison with stress myocardial perfusion imaging. *J Am Coll Cardiol* 1999; 33:1870-1878.

61. Abizaid AS, Mintz GS, Mehran R, Abizaid A, Lansky AJ, Pichard AD, Satler LF, Wu H, Pappas C, Kent KM, Leon MB. Long-term follow-up after percutaneous transluminal coronary angioplasty was not performed based on intravascular ultrasound findings. Importance of lumen dimensions. *Circulation* 1999; 100;256-261.

62. Kern MJ, Donohue TJ, Aguirre FV, Bach RG, Caracciolo EA, Wolford T, Mechem CJ, Flynn MS, Chaitman B. Clinical outcome of deferring angioplasty in patients with normal translesional pressure-flow velocity measurements. *J Am Coll Cardiol* 1995; 25:178-187.

63. Bech GJ, De Bruyne B, Bonnier HJ, Bartunek J, Wijns W, Peels K, Heyndrickx GR, Koolen JJ, Pijls NHJ. Long-term follow-up after deferral of percutaneous transluminal coronary angioplasty of intermediate stenosis on the basis of coronary pressure measurement. *J Am Coll Cardiol* 1998; 31:841-847.

64. Hermiller JB, Buller CE, Tenaglia AN, et al. Unrecognised left main coronary artery disease in patients undergoing interventional procedures. *Am J Cardiol* 1993; 71:173-176.

65. Nishimura RA, Higano ST, Holmes DR. Use of intracoronary ultrasound imaging for assessing left main coronary artery disease. *Mayo Clin Proc* 1993; 68:134-140.

66. Ger ber TC, Erbel R, Gorge G, Ge J, Rupprecht HJ, Meyer J. Extent of atherosclerosis and remodelling of the left main coronary artery determined by intravascular ultrasound. *Am J Cardiol* 1994; 73:666-671.

11

Value of Preintervention Imaging Before Interventions: Balloon Coronary Angioplasty

Fausto J. Pinto, MD

Lesion assessment before coronary ballon angioplasty. Predictors of restenosis. Imaging post-intervention (dissecions and other complications after intervention). Conclusion. References.

Intravascular ultrasound (IVUS) is a relatively new imaging technique with the unique ability to study vessel wall morphology *in vivo.*[1-5] *In vitro* and *in vivo* studies have demonstrated the accuracy and reproducibility of the method to measure vessel lumen dimensions and delineate wall morphology.[5-7] Intracoronary ultrasonic imaging is increasingly recognized for its ability to accurately display the details of vessel structure,[8] but quantitative angiography is still used as the gold standard to assess coronary artery disease. The coronary angiogram represents only a projectional image of the vessel lumen. Several comparative studies of angiography and pathology have demonstrated the shortcomings of angiography for the estimation of atheromatous plaques.[9-10] One of the major weaknesses of angiography is that selective contrast injections provide only longitudinal silhouette images of the vessel surface lining the lumen and provide no information about vascular wall architecture. Ultrasonic imaging can potentially provide information about tissue characteristics and atheroma area. This may be particularly relevant in the setting of coronary interventions, since the amount of wall «destruction» induced by different devices has been shown

on several pathology studies where the limitations of angiography to recognize these changes have been demonstrated.[11]

Several studies have shown the ability of intravascular imaging to assess vascular responses to pharmacological stimuli[12] and evaluate the acute success of mechanical interventions such as balloon angioplasty, stent placement, and atherectomy.[11, 13-16] IVUS detects measurable intimal proliferation and atheroma formation before angiographic evidence of coronary artery disease.[17] Therefore, it offers a unique potential to study atheromatous coronary artery disease at different stages, including following progression and regression of plaque atheroma.[18] IVUS has also been shown to be a safe and feasible imaging technique for the study of coronary artery disease, including during coronary interventions.[19, 20]

The use of IVUS during coronary interventions has been the subject of several recent publications, some with contradictory results, but altogether with enough data to allow us to draw some conclusions. Two important documents that were developed by the European Society of Cardiology and the American College of Cardiology have examined some of the issues implicated in the clinical use of IVUS.[21,22] In this chapter, we will discuss the use and advantages of IVUS before and during balloon angioplasty.

LESION ASSESSMENT BEFORE CORONARY BALLOON ANGIOPLASTY

IVUS has been shown to be useful in the identification of certain lesion characteristics that may be helpful in the selection of devices and in predicting intervention results. There are, however, some limitations to the pre-interventional use of IVUS, mostly related to the relation between luminal size and catheter size. In addition, the introduction of an imaging catheter inside a vessel with a tight lesion may result in flow occlusion and acute myocardial ischemia. Even if there is no flow occlusion, the catheter is usually stuffed inside the lesion (particularly in tight lesions), which is a limiting factor in luminal and plaque visualization and image interpretation. Alfonso et al.[23] showed that unsuccessful IVUS studies prior to intervention occur more frequently in vessels with proximal tortuosity or severe luminal narrowing, in calcified lesions, and when large imaging catheters are used. Despite these limitations, IVUS provides very important information about lesion composition, eccentricity, and length. This information may bring about modifications in treatment strategy in approximately 20 % of cases in some high-volume institutions.[24,25]

Sizing

The vessel can be sized at the lesion site and other simple measurements can be made by IVUS. All measurements should be performed under close to optimal conditions and, therefore, avoided if artifacts such as Non-Uniform Rotational Distortion (NURD) are present or if the IVUS catheter is not parallel to the vessel long axis. Area measure-

ments can also be added to calculate volumes.

Boundary identification

Measurements should be made at the leading edge of boundaries, never the trailing edge, as shown in Fig 11-1. With few exceptions, the location of the leading edge is accurate and reproducible, regardless of system settings or image-processing characteristics of different ultrasound scanners.[26] Measurements at the trailing edge are inconsistent and frequently yield erroneous results.

In muscular arteries such as the coronary arteries, there are frequently three layers.[7,27,28] The innermost layer consists of a complex of three elements: intima, atheroma (in diseased arteries), and internal elastic membrane. This innermost layer is relatively echogenic compared with the lumen and media. The trailing edge of the intima (which would correspond to the internal elastic membrane) cannot always be distinguished clearly. Moving outward from the lumen, the second layer is the media, which is usually less echogenic than the intima. In some cases, the media may appear artifactually thin because of blooming, an intense reflection from the intima or external elastic membrane (EEM). In other cases, the media can appear artifactually thick because of signal attenuation and the weak reflectivity of the internal elastic membrane. In elastic arteries such as the carotid artery, the media is more echoreflective because of the higher elastin content. The third and outer layer consists of the adventitia and periadventitial tissues

Lumen measurements

Lumen measurements are made using the interface between the lumen and the leading edge of the intima. In normal segments, the intimal leading edge is easily resolved be-

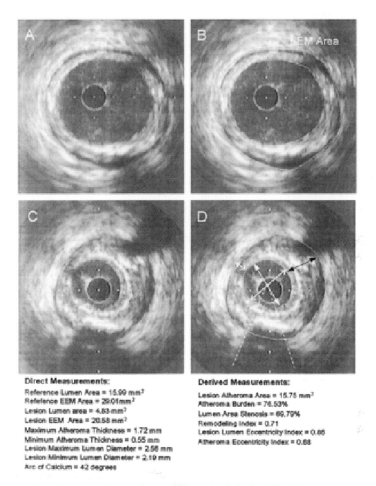

Direct Measurements:
Reference Lumen Area = 15.99 mm²
Reference EEM Area = 29.01mm²
Lesion Lumen area = 4.83 mm²
Lesion EEM Area = 20.58 mm²
Maximum Atheroma Thickness = 1.72 mm
Minimum Atheroma Thickness = 0.55 mm
Lesion Maximum Lumen Diameter = 2.56 mm
Lesion Minimum Lumen Diameter = 2.19 mm
Arc of Calcium = 42 degrees

Derived Measurements:
Lesion Atheroma Area = 15.75 mm²
Atheroma Burden = 76.53%
Lumen Area Stenosis = 69.79%
Remodeling Index = 0.71
Lesion Lumen Eccentricity Index = 0.86
Atheroma Eccentricity Index = 0.88

Figure 11-1. Example of commonly performed direct and derived IVUS measurements. Panels A and B illustrate the reference segment, whereas panels C and D represent the stenosis. In Panel B, the EEM and lumen areas are drawn. In panel D, the minimum and maximum lumen diameters are illustrated using a double-headed arrow (open and solid arrowheads, respectively). In panel D, minimum and maximum atheroma thickness are illustrated using double-headed arrows (white for minimum and black for maximum). Also in panel D, the EEM and lumen areas are drawn and the arc of calcification (dotted line) is shown. EEM = external elastic membrane (Reproduced from Ref 22).

cause the intima has thickened enough to be resolved as a separate layer and has an acoustic impedance that differs sufficiently from that of the lumen. Under such circumstances, the leading edge of the innermost echogenic layer should be used as the lumen boundary. Occasionally, particularly in younger normal subjects (e.g., post-transplantation), the vessel wall will have a single-layer appearance because the intima cannot be resolved as a discrete layer. In such cases, a thin, inner echolucent band corresponding to the intima and media is usually present and this is the boundary that should be measured. While lumen boundaries defined in this manner may include the intima, the thickness of this layer will be <160 μm and will add only a negligible error to the lumen measurement.

Once the lumen border has been determined, the following lumen measurements can be derived:

Lumen Cross Sectional Area (CSA): The area bound by the luminal border.

Minimum Lumen Diameter (MLD): The shortest diameter through the center point of the lumen.

Maximum Lumen Diameter: The longest diameter through the center point of the lumen.

Lumen Eccentricity: 1 ([Maximum Lumen Diameter minus Minimum Lumen Diameter] divided by Maximum Lumen Diameter).

Lumen area stenosis: (Reference Lumen CSA minus Minimum Lumen CSA)/Reference Lumen CSA. The reference segment used should be specified (proximal, distal, largest, or average) (see above).

Post-intervention (if dissection is present), it is important to state whether the lumen area is the true lumen or a combination of the true and false lumens.

EEM measurements

A discrete interface at the border between the media and the adventitia is almost invariably present in IVUS images and corresponds closely to the location of the EEM. The recommended term for this measurement is *EEM CSA*, rather than alternative terms such as vessel area or total vessel area.

External elastic membrane circumference and area cannot be measured reliably at sites where large side branches originate or in the setting of extensive calcification because of acoustic shadowing. If acoustic shadowing involves a relatively small arc (<90°), planimetry of the circumference can be performed by extrapolation from the closest identifiable EEM borders, although measurement accuracy and reproducibility will be reduced. If calcification is more extensive than 90° of arc, EEM measurements should not be

reported. In addition, some stent designs may obscure the EEM border and render measurements unreliable.

Disease-free coronary arteries are circular, but atherosclerotic arteries may remodel into a non-circular configuration. If maximum and minimum EEM diameters are reported, measurements should bisect the geometric center of the vessel rather than the center of the IVUS catheter.

Atheroma measurements

Because the leading edge of the media (the internal elastic membrane) is not well delineated, IVUS measurements cannot determine true histological atheroma area (the area bound by the internal elastic membrane).[26] Accordingly, IVUS studies use the EEM and lumen CSA measurements to calculate a surrogate for true atheroma area, the plaque plus media area. In practice, the inclusion of the media in the atheroma area does not constitute a major limitation of IVUS, because the media represents only a very small fraction of the atheroma CSA. The use of the term plaque plus media (or atheroma) has been suggested and the following measurements are made:

Plaque plus media (or atheroma) CSA: The EEM CSA minus the lumen CSA.

Maximum plaque plus media (or atheroma) thickness: The largest distance from the intimal leading edge to the EEM along any line passing through the center of the lumen.

Minimum plaque plus media (or atheroma) thickness: The shortest distance from intimal leading edge to the EEM along any line passing through the luminal center of mass.

Plaque plus media (or atheroma) eccentricity: (Maximum plaque plus media thickness minus minimum plaque plus media thickness) divided by maximum plaque plus media thickness.

Plaque (or atheroma) burden: Plaque plus media CSA divided by the EEM CSA. The atheroma burden is distinct from the luminal area stenosis. The former is the area within the EEM occupied by atheroma, regardless of lumen compromise. The latter is a measure of luminal compromise relative to a reference lumen analogous to the angiographic diameter stenosis.

Calcium detection

IVUS has a much higher sensitivity than coronary angiography for detection of calcifications.[29, 30] The presence, depth and circumferential distribution of calcifications are very important factors for selecting the type of interventional device and for estimating the risk of complications.[31, 32] For instance, the presence of an area of superficial calcium greater than 180 degrees is considered as an indication to use rotational atherectomy.[33] This will more easily create a smooth channel, which can be further enlarged by balloon angioplasty, directional atherectomy, or stent implantation with less risk than using directly any of these techniques instead of rotational atherectomy.[34] In addition, the presence of calcification is a major determinant of post-PTCA dissections, which are most likely to occur at the border between calcium and soft tissue.[35, 36]

Calcific deposits appear as bright echoes that obstruct the penetration of ultrasound, a phenomenon known as acoustic shadowing. Because high frequency ultrasound does not penetrate the calcium, IVUS can detect only the leading edge and cannot determine the thickness of the calcification. The calcification can also produce reverberations or multiple reflections that result from the oscillation of ultrasound between transducer and calcium and cause concentric arcs in the image at reproducible distances. Calcium deposits should be described qualitatively according to their location (e.g., lesion vs. reference) and distribution:

Superficial: The leading edge of the acoustic shadowing appears in the shallowest 50 % of the plaque plus media thickness.

Deep: The leading edge of the acoustic shadowing appears within the deepest 50 % of the plaque plus media thickness.

The arc of calcification can be measured (in degrees) by using an electronic protractor centered on the lumen. Because of beam-spread variability at given depths within the transmitted beam, this measurement is usually valid only to ±15°. Semi-quantitative grading has also been described, which classifies calcium as absent or subtending 1, 2, 3, or 4 quadrants. The length of the calcium deposit can be measured using motorized transducer pullback.

Plaque thickness and eccentricity

These are other elements of great importance in guiding interventions where IVUS has shown to be more sensitive than angiography. The presence of highly eccentric plaques, without significant sub endothelial calcification, may be an indication to use directional atherectomy. The origin of side branches from the diseased part of the vessel wall with an eccentric plaque is a predictor of occlusion after PTCA or stent deployment. IVUS can also clarify unusual lesion morphologies, such as aneurysm versus pseudoaneurysm. The ability to assess longitudinal vessel involvement and the degree of diffuse disease is particularly important in saphenous vein grafts, where IVUS can help in defining the extension and characteristics of wall morphology[37] and guide the type of intervention.[38] It is notable that only 9 % of the stents are optimally expanded when angiography is used to match the reference cross-sectional area in vein grafts.[39]

The ability to serially assess lesions that have been intervened and, therefore, to determine the mechanism of vessel remodeling (restenosis) is an important advantage of

IVUS.[40] It can basically distinguish between the two main types of vessel remodeling: negative remodeling, where expansion of total vessel area using a stent to avoid chronic vessel recoil may be the best therapeutic strategy, or positive remodeling, with plaque accumulation and a large plaque burden, where plaque debulking with adjunctive balloon angioplasty or stent implantation may be the best option. Dangas et al.[41] have shown in a total of 777 lesions in 715 patients treated with non-stent techniques that positive lesion-site remodeling is associated with a higher long term target lesion revascularization (TLR). In their study, lesions with positive remodeling had more revascularization events (31.2 % vs. 20.2 % for the negative/intermediate-remodeling group, p = 0.0001), despite a larger final IVUS lumen CSA after the interventional procedure. This adds to the evidence that long-term clinical outcome appears to be determined in part by preintervention lesion characteristics. These findings also suggest that positive-remodeling lesions should be targeted for treatment with interventions that have been shown to reduce restenosis, such as stents. Conversely, negative-remodeling lesions may be suitable for a provisional stent-implantation strategy.

IVUS during balloon angioplasty

IVUS has helped to understand the mechanism of balloon angioplasty.[11-13] It can detect plaque fractures or dissections at risk, which require immediate further treatment. In the setting of acute coronary syndromes it has shown that plaque area reduction is the major cause of luminal gain, suggesting that compression, redistribution, or dislodgment of a mural thrombus occurs in these syndromes.[42, 43]

The use of stents has increased dramatically over the last few years. Interestingly, stent availability has also improved the efficacy of stand-alone balloon angioplasty. With stents as a safety net, the operators can be more aggressive, optimizing the results of balloon angioplasty. IVUS guided balloon angioplasty has gained a new breath with the results from the CLOUT study.[44] In its pilot phase it reported that IVUS reference segment midwall dimensions could be used to safely upsize PTCA balloons.[44] In CLOUT, PTCA was first performed using conventional angiographic balloon sizing; then PTCA was repeated using IVUS balloon sizing. This study showed that on the basis of vessel size and extent of plaque burden in the reference segment evaluated with IVUS, 73 % of the lesions required larger balloons, even after achieving an optimal angiographic result [Nominal balloon size/artery ratios increased from 1.12 ± 0.15 to 1.30 ± 0.17 (p < 0.0001); and Quantitative Coronary Angiography (QCA) measured balloon/artery ratios increased from 1.00 ± 0.12 to 1.12 ± 0.13 (p < 0.0001)]. The success rate of IVUS-guided PTCA was 99.0 %. These IVUS guided balloon angioplasties (angiographically oversized) resulted in a greater final minimal lumen diameter (2.21 ± 0.47 mm) and a QCA DS decrease from 28 ± 15 % to 18 ± 14 %, without increased rates of dissection or ischemic complications.

The Washington group has published a study that extended the findings of CLOUT in three important areas: balloon sizing, acute endpoint determination, and long-term follow-up.[45] In CLOUT, the mid-wall dimensions of the proximal and distal reference segments were measured after angiographic-guided PTCA, and the smaller of the proximal and distal reference segment mid-wall dimensions was used for balloon sizing. The distal vessel is often small and underperfused pre-intervention, especially when the IVUS catheter is placed across the lesion. In their report, the pre-intervention lesion site EEM diameter was used to select the PTCA balloon size. They enrolled 284 consecutive patients with 438 native coronary artery stenosis in a study of IVUS-guided provisional stenting. The axial center of the target lesion was identified. Maximum and minimum EEM diameters were measured; and the two were averaged to select the balloon size. For any semi-compliant, or non-compliant balloon used; the manufacturer-supplied «in-air» nominal inflated balloon diameter had to match the lesion site EEM diameter at the maximum inflated pressure during the PTCA. If necessary, quarter-sized balloons were used for more exact size matching. When the operator felt that the best angiographic result had been achieved, IVUS was repeated. Patients were crossed-over to stent implantation if angiography showed less than TIMI-3 flow, an NHLBI grade C or greater dissection, or if post-PTCA IVUS did not show an optimal result. An optimal IVUS result was defined as 1) a minimum lumen CSA of 65% of the average of the proximal and distal reference lumen areas, or a minimum lumen CSA 6.0 mm^2, and 2) no major dissection. A major dissection was defined as 1) a mobile flap, 2) a dissection involving >90% of the vessel circumference, or 3) a dissection causing a sub-optimal true lumen CSA (excluding the area subtended by the dissection plane) as defined above. When necessary, stents were implanted using conventional techniques, followed by high-pressure adjunct PTCA. The IVUS criteria for optimum stent implantation were a minimum stent CSA >80% of the average reference lumen CSA (or an absolute minimum stent CSA ± 7.5 mm^2) and complete stent-vessel wall apposition. Overall, 206 lesions in 134 patients were treated with PTCA alone. Conversely, 232 lesions in 150 patients crossed over to stent implantation; this included 2 lesions (2 patients) that developed out-of-laboratory abrupt closure post-PTCA. Reasons for crossover were angiographic or IVUS flow-limiting or lumen compromising dissections in 65 (27.9%) or a sub-optimal IVUS minimum lumen CSA (as defined above) in 167 (72.1%). Sixty-three lesions (27.2%) were treated with Gianturco-Roubin stents and 169 (72.8%) with Palmaz-Schatz stents with an average of 1.2 ± 0.6 stents/lesion. Long-term follow-up was available in 96% of patients. There were no

deaths and one MI. The 1-year TLR rate was 8.2% for the PTCA group and 15.5% for the stent crossover group (p = 0.016). Using multivariate logistic regression analysis, the only predictor of TLR was use of the Gianturco-Roubin stent (odds ratio = 4.7, 95% confidence interval of 2.1 to 10.5, p = 0.0103). The TLR rate was 32.2% in the Gianturco-Roubin stent group (p = 0.001 vs. both PTCA and Palmaz-Schatz stents) and 10.4% in the Palmaz-Schatz group (p = 0.37 vs. PTCA).

A similar study was made at Tubingen, Germany.[46] The authors reported 252 patients who had 271 lesions treated with IVUS-guided balloon angioplasty. IVUS was performed before and after the intervention to determine the EEM diameter at the lesion site. The balloon catheter was sized according to the EEM diameter measured by IVUS. The mean balloon diameter was 4.1 ± 0.5 mm and the dilation time was 130 ± 60 seconds at a balloon pressure of 7.0 ± 2.0 atm. Clinical acute and 1-year long-term follow-up were obtained for all patients and follow-up angiography in 71% of patients. Acute events occurred post-interventionally in 5 patients (2%). The cumulative event rate during long-term follow-up was 14%. The angiographic restenosis rate (DS > 50%) after 1 year was 19%.

Haase et al.,[47] using a similar approach to CLOUT, confirmed that a larger final minimal lumen diameter (2.23 ± 0.58 mm) could be reached without an increase in in-hospital complications. The incidence of clinical events was 12% and the restenosis rate at one year of follow-up was 21%. The extension of this approach to more complex lesions and to diffuse disease still has to be proven, but may well be a good strategy for further reducing clinical events and restenosis in some problematic lesions.

PREDICTORS OF RESTENOSIS

IVUS has also been used to define predictors of lesion restenosis. In the early

1990s, studies were initiated to determine whether intravascular imaging could predict clinical and angiographic outcome after intervention. The goal of these investigations was to determine whether some morphological features, such as the presence or extent of dissection, or morphometric features (e.g., lumen size or plaque burden) were related to restenosis. The first multicenter trial, Post-IntraCoronary Treatment Ultrasound Result Evaluation (PICTURE), showed no statistically significant predictors of outcome in a relatively small cohort (250 patients) using early generation equipment.[48] Single-center studies, however, identified residual plaque burden as an independent predictor of outcome in multivariable analysis.[50] To examine this issue more completely, phase II of the Guidance by Ultrasound Imaging for Decision Endpoints (GUIDE) trial enrolled 524 patients undergoing angioplasty and/or atherectomy. Among the angiographic and ultrasound variables, ultrasound-derived residual percent plaque burden was the most powerful predictor of clinical outcome, with a risk ratio of 1.7.[50, 51] However, the long-term clinical impact of differences in angiographic result has not been well established.

Despite some contradictory results there is currently evidence that residual plaque burden is an important predictor of restenosis. In the GUIDE II trial, in addition to residual plaque burden, minimal luminal diameter measured by IVUS was also a predictor of restenosis.[51] Other studies have confirmed these results not only in balloon angioplasty but also in atherectomy, such as OARS[51] and ABACAS,[52] although no correlation was found in PICTURE, a study that enrolled 200 patients.[48]

For the first 15 years of interventional cardiology, investigators believed that the predominant mechanism of restenosis after angioplasty and atherectomy was intimal proliferation. Ultrasound studies in the peripheral vessels by Pasterkamp and colleagues[54] presented the first indication that negative remodeling, or localized shrinkage of the vessel, was a major mechanism of late lumen loss. Mintz et al.[55] studied 212 native coronary arteries in patients undergoing repeat catheterization for recurrent symptoms or dictated by research protocols after coronary interventions. At follow-up, there was a decrease in EEM area and an increase in plaque area at the target lesion. Interestingly, >70% of lumen loss was attributable to the decrease in EEM area, whereas the neointimal area accounted for only 23% of the loss. Moreover, the change in lumen area correlated more strongly with the change in EEM area than with the change in plaque area. For lesions with an increase in EEM area at follow-up (47% of segments studied), there was no change or an actual gain in lumen area and a reduction in angiographic restenosis (26% versus 62%; $P < 0.0001$).[55]

These observations have provided a key insight into the reduction of restenosis observed with stenting. Unlike the restenotic response to angioplasty or atherectomy, which is a mixture of arterial remodeling and neointimal growth, stent restenosis is primarily due to neointimal proliferation. In serial ultrasound studies, late lumen loss correlated strongly with the degree of in-stent neointimal growth ($r = 0.98$).[55, 56] The amount of intimal proliferation has been shown to correlate with the pre-stent plaque burden.[58, 59] In a serial study using IVUS of stented coronary segments, no significant change occurred in the area bound by stent struts, indicating that stents can resist the arterial remodeling process.[56] This phenomenon, combined with the greater initial lumen expansion accomplished with stenting, results in a lower net restenosis rate than that with angioplasty or atherectomy.

IMAGING POST-INTERVENTION (DISSECTIONS AND OTHER COMPLICATIONS AFTER INTERVENTION)

Intravascular ultrasound is commonly employed to detect and direct the treatment of dissections and other complications after intervention.[1,60-63] Dissections can be classified into five categories:

Intimal: Limited to the intima or atheroma not extending to the media.

Medial: Extending into the media.

Adventitial: Extending through the EEM.

Intramural hematoma: An accumulation of blood within the medial space, displacing the internal elastic membrane inward and EEM outward. Entry and/or exit points may or may not be observed.

Intra-stent: Separation of neointimal hyperplasia from stent struts, usually seen only after treatment of in-stent restenosis.

The severity of a dissection can be quantified according to: 1) depth (into plaque-useful only in describing intimal dissections that do not reach the media), 2) circumferential extension (in degrees of arc) using a protractor centered on the lumen, 3) length using motorized transducer pullback, 4) size of residual lumen (CSA), and 5) CSA of the luminal dissection. Additional descriptors of a dissection may include the presence of a false lumen, identification of mobile flap(s), the presence of calcification at the dissection border, and dissections in close proximity to stent edges. In a minority of patients, the dissection may not be apparent by IVUS because of scaffolding by the imaging catheter or because the dissection is located underneath a calcification. Usually, ultrasound-occult dissections can be demonstrated by angiography.

CONCLUSION

Intracoronary ultrasound has evolved over the last few years from its infancy to its early adulthood with some potential developments and applications still to be developed. After its reproducibility and safety were demonstrated, it became fundamental for understanding of the mechanism of action of some interventional devices, as well as in restenosis mechanisms. New concepts were introduced, such as negative remodeling, as a mechanism of restenosis. It was also due to IVUS that the deployment of stents was optimized and the burden of anticoagulation was eliminated, improving results and reducing costs, the ultimate goal of any new technology. Several new developments in IVUS may be important, by increasing the usefulness of IVUS before and during balloon angioplasty. Finally, we can easily admit that IVUS, although not needed all the time, can help, particularly in certain unclear situations, thus confirming the view that coronary intervention can be done without IVUS, but it can be done better when IVUS is available.

REFERENCES

1. Yock PG, Johnson EL, David DT. Intravascular ultrasound: Development and clinical potential. *Am J Cardiac Imaging* 1988; 2:185-193.

2. Potkin BN, Bartorelli AL, Gessert JM et al. Coronary artery imaging with intravascular high-frequency ultrasound. *Circulation* 1990; 81:1575-1585.

3. Nissen SE, Grines CL, Gurley JC et al. Application of a new phased-array ultrasound imaging catheter in the assessment of vascular dimensions. In vivo comparison to cineangiography. *Circulation* 1990; 81:660-666.

4. Chenzbraun A, Pinto FJ, Alderman EL et al. Distribution and Morphologic Features of Coronary Artery Disease in Cardiac Allografts: An Intracoronary Ultrasound Study. *J Am Soc Echocardiography* 1995; 8:1-8.

5. St. Goar FG, Pinto FJ, Stadius ML, Fitzgerald PJ, Alderman EL, Popp RL. Intravascular ultrasound imaging of angiographically normal coronary arteries: an in vivo comparison with quantitative angiography. *J Am Coll Cardiol* 1991; 18: 952-958.

6. Nishimura RA, Edwards WD, Warnes CA et al. Intravascular ultrasound imaging : In vitro validation and pathologic correlation. *J Am Coll Cardiol* 1990; 16:145-154.

7. Gussenhoven WJ, Essed CE, Lancee C et al. Arterial wall characteristics determined by intravascular ultrasound imaging: An in vitro study. *J Am Coll Cardiol* 1989; 14:947-952.

8. Waller BF, Pinkerton CA, Slack JD. Intravascular ultrasound: a histological study of vessels during life. The new «gold standard» for vascular imaging. *Circulation* 1992; 85:2305-10.

9. Marcus ML, Skorton DJ, Johnson MR, Collins SM, Harrison DG, Kerber RE. Visual estimates of percent diameter coronary stenosis: «A battered gold standard.» *J Am Coll Cardiol* 1988; 11:882-885.

10. Johnson DE, Alderman EL, Schroeder JS et al. Transplant coronary artery disease: Histopathological correlations with angiographic morphology. *J Am Coll Cardiol* 1991; 17:449-457.

11. Honye J, Mahon DJ, Jain A et al. Morphological effects of coronary balloon angioplasty in vivo assessed by intravascular ultrasound imaging. *Circulation* 1992; 85:1012-1025.

12. Pinto FJ, St.Goar FG, Fischell TA et al. Nitroglycerine-induced coronary vasodilation in cardiac transplant recipients: Evaluation with in vivo intravascular ultrasound. *Circulation* 1992; 85:69-77.

13. Gerber TC, Erbel R, George G, Ge G, Rupprecht HJ, Meyer J. Classification of morphologic effects of percutaneous transluminal coronary angioplasty assessed by intravascular ultrasound. *Am J Cardiol* 1992; 70:1546-54.

14. Umans VA, Baptista J, Di Mario C *et al.* Angiographic, ultrasonic and angioscopic assessment of the coronary artery wall and lumen area configuration after directional atherectomy: the mechanism revisited. *Am Heart J* 1995; 130:217-227.

15. Nakamura S, Colombo A, Gaglione A *et al.* Intracoronary ultrasound observations during stent implantation. *Circulation* 1994; 89:2026-34.

16. Colombo A, Hall P, Nakamura S *et al* . Intracoronary stenting without anticoagulation accomplished with intravascular ultrasound guidance. *Circulation* 1995; 91:1676-88.

17. St. Goar FG, Pinto FJ, Alderman EL et al. Intracoronary ultrasound in cardiac transplant recipients; In vivo evidence of «angiographically silent» intimal thickening. *Circulation* 1992; 85:979-987.

18. Pinto FJ, Chenzbraun A, St.Goar FG et al. Feasibility of Serial Intracoronary Ultrasound Imaging for Assessment of Progression of Intimal Proliferation in Cardiac Transplant Recipients. *Circulation* 1994; 90:2348-2355.

19. Pinto FJ, St.Goar FG, Gao SZ et al. Immediate and one year safety of intracoronary ultrasound imaging: evaluation with serial quantitative angiography. *Circulation* 1993; 88 (part 1):1709-1714.

20. Hassmann D, Erbel R, Albelli-Chemarin MJ *et al.* The safety of intracoronary ultrasound. A Multicenter Survey of 2207 Patients. *Circulation* 1995; 91:623-630.

21. Mario CD, Gorge G, Peters R et al. Clinical application and image interpretation in intracoronary ultrasound. Study Group on Intracoronary Imaging of the Working Group of Coronary Circulation and of the Subgroup on Intravascular Ultrasound of the Working Group of Echocardiography of the European Society of Cardiology. *Eur Heart J* 1998 Feb; 19(2):207-229.

22. Mintz GS, Nissen, Anderson WD et al. ACC clinical expert consensus document on standards for acquisition, measurement and reporting of intravascular ultrasound studies. *J Am Coll Cardiol* 2001; 37:1478-92.

23. Alfonso F, Goncalves M, Goicolea J et al. Feasibility of intravascular ultrasound studies: predictors of imaging success before coronary interventions. *Clin Cardiol* 1997; 20:1010-1016.

24. Mintz GS, Pichard AD, Kovach JA *et al.* Impact of preintervention intravascular ultrasound imaging on transcatheter treatment strategies in coronary artery disease. *Am J Cardiol* 1994; 73:423-30.

25. Abizaid A, Mintz GS, Pichard AD et al. Is intravascular ultrasound clinically useful or is it just a research tool? *Heart* 1997; 78:27-30.

26. Wong M, Edelstein J, Wollman J, Bond MG Ultrasonic-pathological comparison of the human arterial wall. Verification of intima-media thickness. *Arterioscler Thromb* 1993; 13:482-486.

27. Fitzgerald PJ , St. Goar FG, Connolly AJ et al. Intravascular ultrasound imaging of cor-

onary arteries. Is three layers the norm? *Circulation* 1992; 86:154-158.

28. Metz JA, Yock PG, Fitzgerald PJ. Intravascular ultrasound: basic interpretation. *Cardiol Clin* 1997; 15:1-15.

29. Mintz GS, Popma JJ, Pichard AD et al. Patterns of calcification in coronary artery disease. A statistical analysis of intravascular ultrasound and coronary angiography in 1155 lesions. *Circulation* 1995; 91:1959-65.

30. Tuzcu E.M, Berkalp B, De Franco AC et al. The dilemma of diagnosing coronary calcification: angiography versus intravascular ultrasound. *J Am Coll Cardiol* 1996; 27:832-838.

31. Baptista J, Di Mario C, Osaki Y et al. Impact of plaque morphology and composition on the mechanisms of lumen enlargement using intracoronary ultrasound and quantitative angiography after balloon angioplasty. *Am J Cardiol* 1996; 77:115-21.

32. Tenaglia AN, Buller CE, Kisslo KB et al . Intracoronary ultrasound predictors of adverse outcome after coronary artery interventions. *J Am Coll Cardiol* 1992; 20:1385-90.

33. Mintz GS, Kovach J, Javier SP et al. Mechanisms of lumen enlargement after coronary excimer laser angioplasty. An intravascular ultrasound study. *Circulation* 1995; 92:3408-14.

34. Mintz JS, Pichard AD, Poppma JJ et al. Preliminary experience with adjunct directional coronary atherectomy in the treatment of calcific coronary artery disease. *Am J Cardiol* 1994; 73:423-30.

35. Botas J, Clark DA, Pinto FJ, Chenzbraun A, Fischell TA. Balloon angioplasty results in increased segmental coronary distensibility: a likely mechanism of percutaneous transluminal coronary angioplasty. *J Am Coll Cardiol* 1994; 23:1043-1052.

36. Fitzgerald PJ, Ports TA, Yock PG. Contribution of localized calcium deposits to dissection after angioplasty in vivo assessed by intravascular ultrasound imaging. *Circulation* 1992; 86:64-70.

37. Mendelshon FO, Foster GP, Palacios IF, Weyman AE, Weissman NJ. In vivo assessment of enlargement in saphenous vein bypass grafts. *Am J Cardiol* 1995; 76:1066-9.

38. Keren G, Douek P, Oblon C, Bonner RF, Pichard AD, Leon MB. Atherosclerotic saphenous vein bypass grafts treated with

different intervention procedures assessed with intracoronary ultrasound. *Am Heart J* 1992; 124:198-206.

39. Painter JA, Mintz GS, Wong SG et al. Intravascular ultrasound assessment of biliary stent implantation in saphenous vein bypass grafts. *Am J Cardiol* 1995; 75:731-4.

40. Mintz GS, Poppma JJ, Pichard AD et al. Arterial remodeling after coronary angioplasty: A serial intravascular ultrasound study. *Circulation* 1996; 93:924-31.

41. Dangas G, Mintz GS, Mehran R et al. Preintervention arterial remodeling as an independent predictor of target-lesion revascularization after nonstent coronary intervention. An analysis of 777 lesions with intravascular ultrasound imaging. *Circulation* 1999; 99:3149-3154.

42. Kearney P, Koch L, Ge J, George G, Erbel R. Differences in morphology of stable and unstable coronary lesions and their impact on the mechanism of angioplasty. An in vivo study with IVUS. *Eur Heart J* 1996; 17:721-30.

43. Boksh WG, Schartl M, Beckmann SH, Dreysse S, Paeprer H. Intravascular ultrasound imaging in patients with acute myocardial infarction: comparison with chronic stable angina pectoris. *Coron Art Dis* 1994; 5:727-35.

44. Stone GW, Hodgson JM, St. Goar FG et al. for the clinical outcomes with ultrasound trial (CLOUT) investigators. Improved procedural results of coronary angioplasty with intravascular ultrasound guided balloon sizing. *Circulation* 1997; 95:2044-52.

45. Abizaid A, Pichard AD, Mintz GS et al. Acute and long-term results of an IVUS-guided PTCA/provisional stent implantation strategy. *Am J Cardiol* 1999; 84:1381-4.

46. Schroeder S, Baumbach A, Haase KK et al. Reduction of restenosis by vessel size adapted percutaneous transluminal coronary angioplasty using intravascular ultrasound. *Am J Cardiol* 1999; 83:875-9.

47. Haase KK, Athanasiadis A, Mahrholdt H et al. Acute and one year follow-up results after vessel size adapted PTCA using intracoronary ultrasound. *Eur Heart J* 1998; 19:263-272.

48. Peters RJ, Kok WE, Di Mario C, et al. Prediction of restenosis after coronary balloon

angioplasty: Results of PICTURE (Post-In-traCoronary Treatment Ultrasound Result Evaluation), a prospective multicenter intracoronary ultrasound imaging study. *Circulation.* 1997; 95:2254-2261.

49. Mintz GS, Popma JJ, Pichard AD, et al. Intravascular ultrasound predictors of restenosis after percutaneous transcatheter coronary revascularization. *J Am Coll Cardiol.* 1996; 27:1678-1687.

50. Fitzgerald PJ, Yock PG. Mechanisms and outcomes of angioplasty and atherectomy assessed by intravascular ultrasound imaging. *J Clin Ultrasound.* 1993; 21:579-588.

51. The GUIDE Trial Investigators. IVUS-determined predictors of restenosis in PTCA and DCA: an interim report from the GUIDE Trial, Phase II *Circulation* 1994; 90:4; 2:I-23 (113).

52. Simonton CA, Leon MB, Kuntz RE et al. Acute and late clinical and angiographic results of directional atherectomy in the optimal atherectomy restenosis study (OARS). *Circulation* 1995; 92:I-545.

53. Sumitsuji, Susuki T, Katoh O et al. for the ABACAS investigators. Restenosis mechanism after aggressive directional coronary atherectomy assessed by intravascular ultrasound in adjunctive balloolen angiop

lasty following coronary atherectomy study (ABACAS). *J Am Coll Cardiol* 1997; 129A.

54. Pasterkamp G, Wensing PJ, Post MJ, et al. Paradoxical arterial wall shrinkage may contribute to luminal narrowing of human atherosclerotic femoral arteries. *Circulation.* 1995; 91:1444-1449.

55. Mintz GS, Kent KM, Pichard AD, et al. Contribution of inadequate arterial remodeling to the development of focal coronary artery stenoses: an intravascular ultrasound study. *Circulation.* 1997; 95:1791-1798.

56. Painter JA, Mintz GS, Wong SC, et al. Serial intravascular ultrasound studies fail to show evidence of chronic Palmaz-Schatz stent recoil. *Am J Cardiol.* 1995; 75:398-400.

57. Hoffmann R, Mintz GS, Dussaillant GR, et al. Patterns and mechanisms of in-stent restenosis: a serial intravascular ultrasound study. *Circulation.* 1996; 94:1247-1254.

58. Hoffmann R, Mintz GS, Mehran R, et al. Intravascular ultrasound predictors of angiographic restenosis in lesions treated with Palmaz-Schatz stents. *J Am Coll Cardiol.* 1998; 31:43-49.

59. Prati F, Di Mario C, Moussa I, et al. In-stent neointimal proliferation correlates with the amount of residual plaque burden outside the stent: an intravascular ultrasound study. *Circulation.* 1999; 99:1011-1014.

12

Intravascular Ultrasound and Coronary Atherectomy

Javier Botas, MD
Jaime Elizaga, MD
Javier Soriano, MD

All atherectomy techniques share the common characteristic of directly eliminating plaque by extraction, pulverization or vaporization. The intervention is aimed at the plaque of a⇒theroma, as in other interventional cardiology procedures, but in this case the procedure seeks to eliminate it at least partially. The rationale for using intracoronary ultrasound is therefore sound as it allows direct visualization of the atheroma plaque and not just the impact of the plaque on the lumen, as in angiography. IVUS allows us to more accurately assess plaque extension, length, and composition, which helps in selecting the most adequate device according to lesion characteristics. It also allows to assess the amount of residual plaque remaining after the first passes of the device, thus determining the need to carry out additional atherectomy passes. Although aggressive atherectomy is technically complex, various studies have concluded that the amount of residual plaque following the procedure is the most powerful predictor of the patient's outcome in the case of balloon angioplasty or directional atherectomy (DA), carrying more weight than angiographic variables.[1-3]

INTRACORONARY ULTRASOUND AND DIRECTIONAL ATHERECTOMY

Introduction

In 1985, John Simpson[4] introduced a new device for cardiac interventions designed to extract atheroma plaque. At that time, the standard procedure was plain balloon angioplasty and this device was developed as a means to eliminate plaque selectively and in a directional manner with the hope of reducing restenosis. The device has undergone a series of refinements and variations over the last decade, but its basic design has nonetheless remained unchanged. The atherotome consists of a hollow torque tube drive shaft, a metal housing with an affixed balloon, and a nose-cone collection chamber. The system is advanced co-axially into the vessel over a coronary angioplasty guidewire. An externally powered cutter that is located inside the housing rotates at 2,000 rpm and cuts into plaque, storing the material removed in the nosecone. Typically, multiple passes are made aiming the window of the atherotome with the presumed location of the atheroma plaque.

The usefulness of intracoronary ultrasound during atherectomy resides in the possibility it offers of better selecting the cases in which the technique might be useful, in improving the safety and efficacy of the procedure, and in more accurately assessing any inconclusive angiographic images obtained during the procedure.

Finally, ultrasound imaging, particularly three-dimensional reconstructions obtained on repeated examinations of the target segments, have shown that late lumen loss after atherectomy is basically due to reduction of the total vessel area (negative remodeling) rather than to neointimal proliferation.[5]

Lesion Assessment and Device Selection

Ultrasound scanning allows direct visualization of the target of intervention, the atheroma plaque, and detailed assessment of its characteristics. Pre-intervention imaging allows to characterize the morphology and length of the plaque, as well as the presence and location of calcifications much more precisely than with angiography. The presence of calcification is the most im-

portant factor determining the success of atherectomy.[6,7] Extensive calcification, particularly if it is superficial, deposited on the lumen-plaque interface, is associated with poor tissue removal during the procedure. If the superficial calcification affects more than two quadrants of the vessel circumference, then an alternative type of intervention should probably be considered. Deep calcification inside the atheroma plaque is not a contraindication, even if it is extensive, as it does not prevent the more superficial plaque tissue from being removed. It actually constitutes a safety barrier against perforation of the vessel (Fig. 12-1).

In addition, pre-intervention assessment is useful for evaluating the true vessel size and therefore helps in choosing the most appropriate device size. Positive vessel remodeling at the site of the lesion is common, so the plaque burden may clearly be larger than suggested by angiography (Fig. 12-2). Furthermore, reference segments are almost always diseased, once more leading to underestimation of the plaque burden and the true size of the vessel. In a study of 884 patients, only 6.8 % of the reference segments considered to be normal by angiography turned out to be truly normal by ultrasound. Plaque

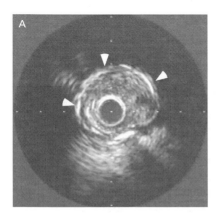 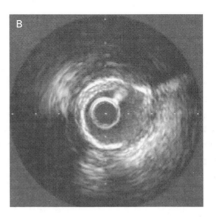

Figure 12-1. The IVUS baseline study (panel A) showed no residual lumen around the IVUS catheter, a large, soft, superficial plaque, and dense fibrosis/calcification deep inside the lesion (arrowheads). Post DCA (panel B), most of the soft plaque has been removed up to the level of the deep fibrosis/calcification.

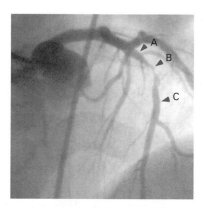

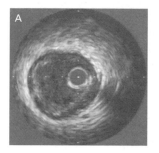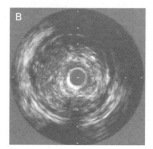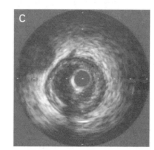

Figure 12-2. Severe stenosis of the anterior descending artery evaluated by IVUS at the lesion site (B), proximally (A), and distally (C). Although not noticeable by angiography, the vessel size (media to media) at the lesion site is much larger than distally and proximally. This is a typical example of positive remodeling, (outward vessel growth at the site of plaque accumulation).

occupied an average of 51% of the total cross-sectional area of these «normal» vessels.[8] All these factors must be taken into account when it comes to selecting the size of the device and inflation pressure. On the other hand, in some lesions negative remodeling is part of the stenosis mechanism, in other words there is vessel shrinkage at the lesion site. In these cases, the plaque burden is less than was initially estimated, meaning that the patient may not be such a good candidate for atherectomy, or extra care should be taken to avoid perforation.

Procedure Guidance

Because ultrasound is a tomographic technique, it allows the spatial distribution of the plaque in the vessel wall to be precisely located. With experience, the information supplied by angiography can be combined mentally with that obtained from ultrasound in order to direct the cutter selectively towards the area of interest. In practice, there are basically two techniques.

With the first technique, the operator considers the spatial relationship of the target plaque with respect to references that are easily identified by angiography. The reference points most often used are the take-offs of the secondary arterial branches, such as the diagonal and septal arteries from the anterior descending and the marginal arteries from the circumflex artery, or any other references that are easily recognizable with both techniques, such as an angiographically visible area of calcification. The relationship

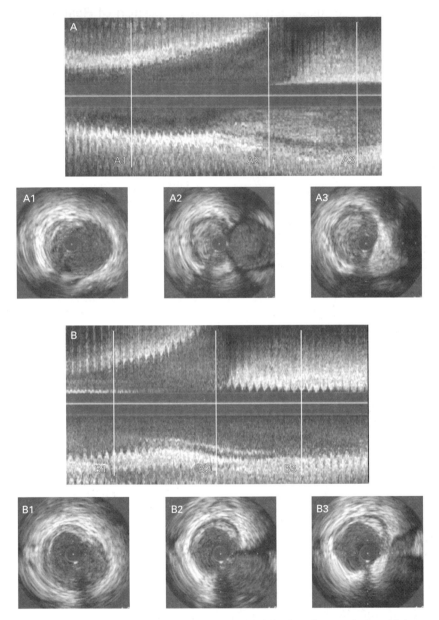

Figure 12-3. Panel A shows longitudinal reconstruction of the baseline study in which severe stenosis of the ostium of the anterior descending artery (LAD) was evaluated. The IVUS catheter is placed in the LAD and during automatic pullback interrogates the LAD (A3), the LAD ostium at the take off of the circumflex (A2), and the left main (A1). Note that the plaque extends into the left main (A), as it is usually the case in ostial LAD lesions. Also note that there is virtually no residual lumen around the catheter in the ostial (A2) and proximal LAD (A3). The plaque is eccentric and most of it is located just opposite the circumflex take-off (A2), so the device should be aimed in that direction to effectively remove the atheroma. Panel B shows the longitudinal reconstruction after standalone DCA. Most of the plaque has been successfully removed by aiming the device in the direction opposite to the circumflex take off (B, B1, B2, and B3).

between the plaque and these reference points, also visible by angiography, allows the cutter to be aimed at the area of interest. Furthermore, repeated ultrasound examinations during the procedure make it possible to precisely locate the residual plaque and target the area for subsequent cuts (Fig. 12-3). As discussed in previous chapters, in order to maintain a proper rotational orientation it is useful to remember that the diagonal branches take off are in the same direction as the circumflex artery and perpendicular to the take off of the septal branches.

The second technique, which is occasionally used, is to make a single initial cut with the atherotome in a direction that is easily recognizable by angiography and then to perform an ultrasound examination. The relationship between the initial cut and the residual plaque that we wish to tackle facilitates the integration of information from both techniques for subsequent cuts.

Optimization of Results

One of the most frequent surprises following atherectomy is to observe that there is still a large amount of residual plaque (Fig. 12-4) despite an angiographically satisfactory result.[7] The amount of residual plaque left after the procedure is one of the best predictors of restenosis.[1-3] Once more, direct visualization of the plaque clarifies the mechanism of residual stenosis and helps us to better assess the usefulness of additional atherectomy, adjunctive balloon angioplasty, or stent implantation (Fig. 12-5).

Ultrasound examination is particularly useful for the study of images that remain inconclusive after atherectomy, such as cuts that seem too deep by angiography, dissections, apparently over-dilated areas, or hazy images at the level of the treated segment. A better evaluation of these images is useful when it comes to deciding how to treat them. Not un-

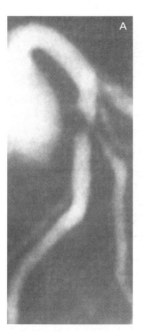 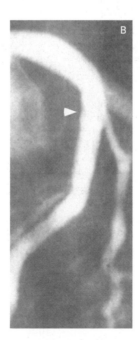 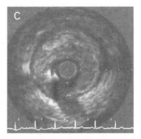

Figure 12-4. Panel A and B show the angiogram of a severe stenosis in the proximal anterior descending artery before and after DCA. Despite the excellent angiographic result, IVUS performed after DCA (C) showed that a substantial amount of plaque was not removed (note the take off of the diagonal at 6 o'clock at the lesion site).

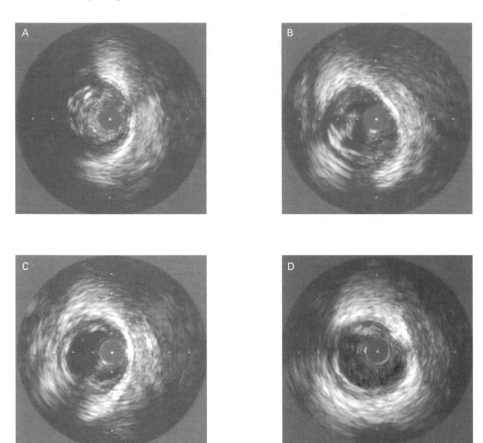

Figure 12-5. Panel A shows the baseline IVUS study of an eccentric lesion. After a few atherectomy passes (panel B), there is still substantial residual plaque, and a dissection at 9 o'clock. After successive passes of DCA aimed in that direction, the dissection was successfully removed and the lumen is now acceptable. Panel D shows the 6-month follow up study, in which there is negligible intimal proliferation and no vessel shrinkage.

commonly, dissections in the area at of the lesion have been treated with further atherectomy passes. If the dissection has occurred in the area of the plaque being treated, this is probably a reasonable approach (Fig. 12-6), although it may not be easy to perform. If the dissection is spiral or involves the untreated wall, further atherectomy passes are not the best option and stent implantation should be considered.

Optimal Atherectomy

The CAVEAT study[9] was undertaken in the early days of atherectomy and did not achieve the expected results. It revealed a tendency towards a lower rate of restenosis (50 % versus 57 %, p = 0.06), but at the expense of a larger number of complications. The main criticism of the CAVEAT study is that the atherectomies performed were conservative. The postprocedural angiographic percent diameter stenosis was 32 %, which could be translated into a residual plaque burden >70 %.[10] In this regard, a technique that allows direct plaque visualization and less conservative atherectomy might improve the results of this type of treatment. This hypothesis has been tested in various studies: OARS, ABACAS, BOAT and

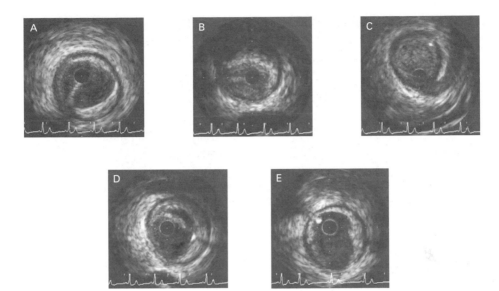

Figure 12-6. Panel A, B, and C show the baseline IVUS examination of the proximal reference, lesion, and distal reference. After several DCA passes, the angiographic image is good and there is a reasonable lumen (D), but a dissection clearly protrudes into the lumen on top of the IVUS catheter (from 12 to 3 o'clock). Additional cuts with the atherectomy catheter aimed at the dissection were able to resect it, resulting in a larger lumen (E).

START. In the OARS registry (Optimal Atherectomy Restenosis Study), the use of more aggressive atherectomy with ultrasound imaging yielded a restenosis rate of 28.9 % and a 6-months revascularization rate of 17.8 %.[11] Although the results were better than in previous reports, the study was criticized for not really being an ultrasound-guided study with clear targets to be achieved but rather a trial in which ultrasound was performed for purposes of observation. In fact, the post-procedural percent plaque burden of this study was 58 %.[10] The ABACAS trial (Adjunctive Balloon Angioplasty after Coronary Atherectomy Study) was designed to assess the effect of balloon angioplasty as a coadjuvant of atherectomy and the usefulness of ultrasound in achieving an optimal degree of atherectomy. The use of ultrasound as a guide for the procedure was associated with a lower residual plaque burden (42.6 % versus 45.6 % in the adjunctive balloon and stand-alone atherectomy groups,

respectively) and a lower restenosis rate (19.6 % versus 23.6 %, respectively, in the same groups).[12] These findings highlight the association between residual plaque burden and restenosis. In the BOAT study (Balloon versus Optimal Atherectomy Trial), the concept of optimal atherectomy was applied although ultrasound imaging was not used. A lower restenosis rate was obtained in patients who were treated with atherectomy than those randomized to balloon angioplasty (31.4 % versus 39.8 %, p = 0.016).[13] Finally, the START study (Stent versus Directional Coronary Atherectomy Randomized Trial) randomized 122 patients to study the hypothesis that rigorous atherectomy guided by ultrasound in order to leave as little residual plaque as possible might be equivalent or even superior to stent implantation. In this study,[14] atherectomy performed with ultrasound guidance significantly reduced restenosis when compared to stent implantation (16 % versus 33 %, p < 0.05).

Debulking
Prior to Stenting

Another potential use of atherectomy is the partial elimination of plaque prior to stent placement. The potential advantage is two-fold: to improve stent expansion and, perhaps, to reduce intimal proliferation (Fig. 12-7).

It is well known, and a consistent finding in all of the databases on coronary ultrasound imaging, that about one-third of the stents are under-expanded, despite the routine use of high implantation pressures. Even when ultrasound imaging is used to assess stent expansion, around 20 % of stents cannot be optimally expanded despite the choice of an appropriately sized balloon and the use of high pressure. The main force opposing stent expansion is the hoop resistance of the atheroma plaque.[15] It therefore seems logical to think that if the atheroma plaque were partially eliminated, it would be possible to increase the acute gain achieved with stenting without also increasing wall distension, thus reducing restenosis. The SOLD registry (Stenting after Optimal Lesion Debulking) was a pioneering study that tested this hypothesis. The restenosis rate and the need for revascularization in the 71 patients recruited for the trial were 11 % and 7 %, respectively.[16] A multicenter trial coordinated by our laboratory[17] underlined, albeit also in a small number of patients (n = 70), that the most important predictive factor of procedural acute gain and subsequent restenosis was the initial gain achieved by atherectomy, regardless of the use of stents. In addition, the results suggested that guiding the procedure by ultrasound imaging might reduce the restenosis rate (12.5 % versus 24 % in lesions with and without ultrasound guidance), but did not reach statistical significance (p = ns). The true clinical usefulness of atherectomy prior to stenting will have to await the definitive results of the randomized AMIGO trial, which has reported promising initial results,[18] as well as the long-term results of drug-eluting stents.

The second potential benefit of debulking prior to stenting derives from the more than likely link between the amount of residual plaque left outside the stent and subsequent intimal proliferation. This phenomenon has been reasonably well studied in the last few years with intracoronary ultrasound, particularly in the field of stenting. In a pioneering study with intravascular ultrasound in 50 patients, Prati et al.[19] showed that neointimal proliferation within the stent was directly influenced by the amount of residual atheroma outside the stent. These data, subsequently

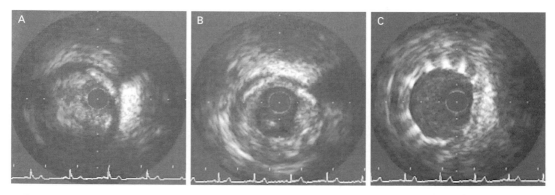

Figure 12-7.   Tight stenosis with a large plaque burden (A), treated with DCA (B) yielding a reasonable lumen (3 × 2 mm), which was further enlarged by subsequent stent implantation (C). Plaque removal with DCA allowed excellent stent expansion by removing some of the hoop resistance caused by the large plaque burden.

reproduced by other investigators,[20] confirm the potential value of debulking in reducing the restenosis rate.

INTRACORONARY ULTRASOUND AND ROTATIONAL ATHERECTOMY

Introduction

Rotational atherectomy (RA) uses a diamond-coated burr (rotablator) spinning at 100,000 to 200,000 rpm for ablation of the atheroma plaque. The burr is mounted on a flexible drive shaft, which is advanced into the coronary artery over a 0.009-inch guidewire. Coronary burr sizes range from 1.25-2.5 mm. The principle on which its action is based is called differential cutting,[21] meaning that it removes the more rigid fibrous-calcified tissue from the atheroma plaque while preserving the more elastic tissue that makes up the normal vessel wall. During ablation,

small particles (5-10 μ in diameter) that are generated embolize distally and are captured by the reticuloendothelial system. More than one burr is typically used, followed by a balloon or stent to optimize the result.

Mechanism of Action Assessed by Ultrasound Scan

The typical image seen after RA is one of selective plaque ablation, particularly calcified plaque (Fig. 12-8). The residual lumen is smooth, polished, and rounded. As with DCA, the large amount of residual post-procedural plaque is frequently striking, even when the angiographic result is good. Dissections are much less frequent than with balloon angioplasty, where they are practically the norm, and no distension of the vessel is observed, only tissue ablation,[22] which also contrasts with balloon angioplasty. The lumen obtained is usually 0.8 to 1.4 times the size of the burr used.[22] It may

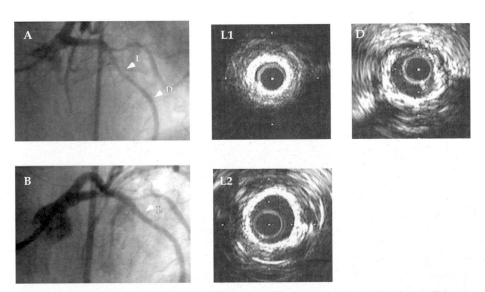

Figure 12-8. A long, significant lesion of the middle segment of the anterior descending artery (A). Baseline VUS examination showed 360° of superficial calcification at the lesion site (*L1*), with mild fibrocalcific disease at the distal reference (D). After standalone rotational atherectomy with a 2.0-mm burr, there is a nice smooth angiographic lumen (B) and a typical post-rotational atherectomy image, with a smooth, dissection-free lumen (*L2*).

be more than 1 in certain cases, basically due to a lack of co-axial alignment between the cutting burr and lumen, typically at bifurcations. If the plaque is severely calcified, the assessment is normally limited to quantifying the lumen, as the rest of the wall structures cannot be visualized unless the entire thickness of the calcified plaque is cut away, which is quite exceptional. There is a tendency to obtain a larger lumen in calcified plaques than in soft plaques, probably due to greater efficiency of the burr and/or lesser early loss due to elastic recoil.

Usefulness of Ultrasound Scanning in Rotational Atherectomy Procedures

Ultrasound is extremely sensitive when it comes to the detection of calcium in atheroma plaques. In the GUIDE I study and in numerous subsequent trials, ultrasound has been shown to be much more sensitive than angiography for the detection of calcifications.[2,23] The observation that a lesion is severely calcified is a good indication for considering the use of RA because the results of other techniques such as balloon angioplasty[24] or DCA[7] are frequently inadequate. Furthermore, the results obtained with stents in calcified lesions are worse than those obtained in non-calcified lesions or those treated with RA before stenting.[25] The location of the calcification, which can only be well assessed by ultrasound, also influences the decision as to when RA is more useful. Superficial calcification, close to the luminal interface, is the situation most often associated with poor results of other devices and the greatest benefit is obtained of RA. The thickness of the calcification cannot be assessed by ultrasound because of the existence of acoustic shadowing beyond the surface layer. It may also be difficult to evaluate the vessel size (media to media) if the calcification is extensive, although it is frequently possible to calculate it by extrapolation from

the immediately adjacent proximal and distal segments.

Procedure Guidance

The baseline ultrasound study allows the degree of calcification and size of the vessel to be assessed, unless the calcification is massive. The degree of calcification, measured in quadrants or in arc degrees, and its superficial or deep location are factors to be weighed when deciding if the lesion can benefit from RA. Occasionally, if the lesion is severe as well as calcified, or if there is marked proximal tortuosity, a baseline examination cannot be performed. It has, in fact, been suggested that failure to pass the ultrasound probe for the baseline study may in itself be an indication for carrying out RA. The minimal lumen diameter in the baseline examination determines the minimum burr size that must be used, which, logically, should be larger than the minimum lumen diameter. Furthermore, it must be remembered that the size of the burr must be smaller than the size of the distal reference in order to avoid perforation. This may be a problem if the lesion is located at a bifurcation and the vessel diameter tapers down abruptly. If the lesion is located on a curve, the maximum burr size should also be smaller. In this case, poor co-axial alignment between the vessel and the device may increase the intensity of ablation on one of the walls, thus increasing the risk of perforation. The length of the lesion is also significant when it comes to selecting the burr size. The amount of debris embolized depends on the plaque volume being treated, as well as plaque length, which is much more appropriately assessed by ultrasound imaging than by angiography. Generally speaking, in long lesions with a large plaque burden, it is appropriate to be less aggressive with the burr selection, particularly the final burr, in order to reduce the risk of no reflow.

Ultrasound assessment between the use of successive burrs helps to verify the degree of ablation achieved and the absence of complications, but it is not essential unless ambiguous angiography images must be clarified. A heated controversy exists regarding the best way to perform RA. For some, the ideal result is to achieve the maximum degree of atherectomy and obtain the greatest possible lumen dimension, whereas other operators only use small burrs to change the characteristics of the plaque and prepare the lesion for balloon angioplasty or stent placement. Lastly, the post-procedural assessment allows the presence of dissections or other complications to be evaluated. It must be remembered, however, that intravascular ultrasound is much more sensitive than angiography for the detection of dissections and that a small dissection with an adequate lumen is of no clinical consequence and does not require treatment. The assessment of the residual plaque, the lumen achieved, and its ratio to the reference lumen are all useful when deciding whether further atherectomy or adjunctive balloon angioplasty or stenting should be performed.

In-Stent Restenosis

In-stent restenosis is still a growing problem in cardiology. Focal restenosis is treated mainly with balloon angioplasty. In cases of diffuse restenosis, ablation techniques including RA and DCA have frequently been used in an attempt to reduce the tissue burden and improve the poor results obtained with balloon angioplasty. Intracoronary ultrasound imaging is a particularly useful tool in this setting.

First of all, if treatments other than balloon angioplasty are being considered, the ultrasound examination could be of great assistance because it allows detailed assessment of the mechanisms involved in restenosis. As has been mentioned, the studies made immediately after stent implantation have shown that around 25 % of stents are not optimally expanded. This lack of expansion is an important component of the residual stenosis at follow-up.[26] In cases in which this is the main mechanism, it seems logical to accept that the ideal treatment is re-expan-

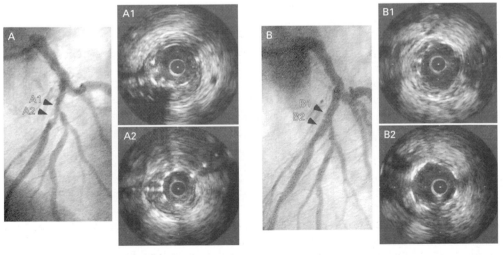

Figure 12-9.   In-stent restenosis of the proximal segment of the anterior descending artery (A). IVUS examination showed that, although there is some intimal tissue proliferation, most of the mechanism of the stenosis is due to inadequate stent expansion (A1 and A2). Although tissue ablation was initially planned, IVUS findings led to a change in strategy and only balloon dilation was performed. A 3.5-mm balloon at high pressures was used (B). A much larger lumen was achieved, mainly by improving stent expansion, as well as some tissue extrusion (B1 and B2).

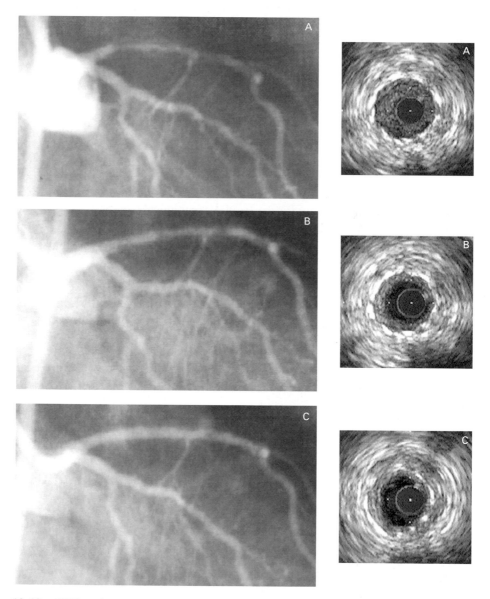

Figure 12-10. Diffuse in-stent restenosis of the anterior descending artery (A). IVUS showed that the stent lumen is filled up with intimal proliferation (A). Rotational atherectomy was performed with a 2.0 mm burr yielding a 2 × 2 mm lumen (B). Additional balloon dilation resulted in a larger lumen due to stent overexpansion (C).

sion of the stent using balloon angioplasty (Fig. 12-9). However, if stent restenosis is mainly due to intimal proliferation within the stent, an ablation technique might be useful, although it should be noted that there is very little evidence supporting this approach.

Ultrasound scans also allow operators to choose the maximum burr size that can pass between the struts without damaging them, thus permitting a maximal degree of atherectomy (Fig. 12-10). It must, however, be borne in mind that if the stent is on a curve, or the guidewire tends to position itself against one side of the stent, then it may not be possible to pass that particular burr size through the stent.

Few studies have assessed the use of atherectomy procedures for the treatment of in-stent restenosis and none has been designed to assess the role of ultrasound scanning in this context. Nonetheless, some data available suggest that ultrasound imaging may be really useful in this setting. In the ROSTER trial (Randomized Trial of PTCA versus Rotablator for Diffuse In-Stent Restenosis),[27] 200 patients with in-stent restenosis were randomly assigned to treatment with balloon angioplasty or RA. As part of the protocol, all patients considered for inclusion in the trial were assessed using intracoronary ultrasound. It is important to point out that one-third of the patients initially evaluated were not included because the presence of marked under-expansion of the stent played a key part in the stenosis mechanism. The study showed less need for revascularization in the RA group than in the group treated with balloon angioplasty (32 % versus 45 %, p = 0.04). Conversely, in the ARTIST study (Angioplasty versus Rotational Atherectomy for Treatment of Diffuse In-Stent Restenosis Trial)[28] performed on 298 patients, which had a similar design, the restenosis rate was higher in the RA group than in the plain balloon angioplasty group (65 % versus 51 %, p < 0.05). Although several factors may contribute to these markedly different results, one of the few clear differences between the two studies was the routine use of ultrasound guid-

ance in the ROSTER trial. Among other advantages, ultrasound allowed the exclusion of the patients in which stent under-expansion was an essential part of the restenosis mechanism. In fact, this factor is the most important limitation mentioned by the authors of the ARTIST study as an explanation for their results,[28] which underlines the potential usefulness of ultrasound in this type of procedure.

REFERENCES

1. Mintz GS, Popma JJ, Pichard AD, et al. Intravascular ultrasound predictors of restenosis after percutaneous transcatheter coronary revascularization. *J Am Coll Cardiol* 1996; 27:1678-87.

2. Fitzgerald PJ, Yock PG. Mechanisms and outcomes of angioplasty and atherectomy assessed by intravascular ultrasound imaging. *J Clin Ultrasound* 1993; 21:579-88.

3. The GUIDE trial investigators. IVUS-determined predictors of restenosis in PTCA and DCA: final report form the GUIDE trial (abstr.). *J Am Coll Cardiol* 1996; 27:156A.

4. Simpson JB, Johnson DE, Thapliyal HV, Marks DS, Braden LJ. Transluminal atherectomy: a new approach to the treatment of atherosclerotic vascular disease (abstr.). *Circulation* 1985; 72:III-146.

5. de Vrey EA, Mintz GS, von Birgelen C, et al. Serial volumetric (three-dimensional) intravascular ultrasound analysis of restenosis after directional coronary atherectomy. *J Am Coll Cardiol* 1998; 32:1874-80.

6. Popma JJ, Mintz GS, Satler LF, et al. Clinical and angiographic outcome after directional coronary atherectomy. A qualitative and quantitative analysis using coronary arteriography and intravascular ultrasound. *Am J Cardiol* 1993; 72:55E-64E.

7. Matar FA, Mintz GS, Pinnow E, et al. Multivariate predictors of intravascular ultrasound end points after directional coronary atherectomy. *J Am Coll Cardiol* 1995; 25:318-24.

8. Mintz GS, Painter JA, Pichard AD, et al. Atherosclerosis in angiographically «normal» coronary artery reference segments: an intravascular ultrasound study with clinical correlations. *J Am Coll Cardiol* 1995; 25:1479-85.

9. Topol EJ, Leya F, Pinkerton CA, et al. A comparison of directional atherectomy with coronary angioplasty in patients with coronary artery disease. The CAVEAT Study Group. *N Engl J Med* 1993; 329:221-7.

10. Honda Y, Yock PG, Fitzgerald PJ. Impact of residual plaque burden on clinical outcomes of coronary interventions. *Catheter Cardiovasc Interv* 1999; 46:265-76.

11. Simonton CA, Leon MB, Baim DS, et al. 'Optimal' directional coronary atherectomy: final results of the Optimal Atherectomy Restenosis Study (OARS). *Circulation* 1998; 97:332-9.

12. Suzuki T, Hosokawa H, Katoh O, et al. Effects of adjunctive balloon angioplasty after intravascular ultrasound-guided optimal directional coronary atherectomy: the result of Adjunctive Balloon Angioplasty After Coronary Atherectomy Study (ABACAS). *J Am Coll Cardiol* 1999; 34:1028-35.

13. Baim DS, Cutlip DE, Sharma SK, et al. Final results of the Balloon vs Optimal Atherectomy Trial (BOAT). *Circulation* 1998; 97:322-31.

14. Tsuchikane E, Sumitsuji S, Awata N, et al. Final results of the STent versus directional coronary Atherectomy Randomized Trial (START). *J Am Coll Cardiol* 1999; 34:1050-7.

15. Bermejo J, Botas J, Garcia E, et al. Mechanisms of residual lumen stenosis after high-pressure stent implantation: a quantitative coronary angiography and intravascular ultrasound study. *Circulation* 1998; 98:112-8.

16. Moussa I, Moses J, Di Mario C, et al. Stenting after optimal lesion debulking (SOLD) registry. Angiographic and clinical outcome. *Circulation* 1998; 98:1604-9.

17. Botas J, Peleato A, Angel J, Gomez Recio M, Garcia E, Anivarro I. Debulking Prior to Stenting: Insight Into the Best Technique of Use From a Prospective Study. *J Am Coll Cardiol* 2001; 37:648A.

18. Takagi T, Colombo A, Nishida T, et al. A randomized study of directional atherectomy prior to stenting versus stenting alone: a single site experience (abstr.). *Eur Heart J* 2001; 22:118.

19. Prati F, Di Mario C, Moussa I, et al. In-stent neointimal proliferation correlates with the amount of residual plaque burden outside the stent: an intravascular ultrasound study. *Circulation* 1999; 99:1011-4.

20. Okura H, Limpijankit T, Takagi A, et al. Extent of Neointima Predicts Subsequent Neointimal Proliferation in In-Stent Restenosis: A Volumetric Intravascular Ultrasound Study (abstr.). *J Am Coll Cardiol* 2000; 35:95A.

21. Kovach JA, Mintz GS, Pichard AD, et al. Sequential intravascular ultrasound characterization of the mechanisms of rotational atherectomy and adjunct balloon angioplasty. *J Am Coll Cardiol* 1993; 22:1024-1032.

22. Mintz GS, Potkin BN, Keren G, et al. Intravascular ultrasound evaluation of the effect of rotational atherectomy in obstructive atherosclerotic coronary artery disease. *Circulation* 1992; 86:1383-93.

23. Mintz GS, Douek P, Pichard AD, et al. Target lesion calcification in coronary artery disease: an intravascular ultrasound study. *J Am Coll Cardiol* 1992; 20:1149-55.

24. Fitzgerald PJ, Ports TA, Yock PG. Contribution of localized calcium deposits to dissection after angioplasty. An observational study using intravascular ultrasound. *Circulation* 1992; 86:64-70.

25. Hoffmann R, Mintz GS, Popma JJ, et al. Treatment of calcified coronary lesions with Palmaz-Schatz stents. An intravascular ultrasound study. *Eur Heart J* 1998; 19: 1224-31.

26. Dussaillant GR, Mintz GS, Pichard AD, et al. Small stent size and intimal hyperplasia contribute to restenosis: a volumetric intravascular ultrasound analysis. *J Am Coll Cardiol* 1995; 26:720-4.

27. Sharma SK, Kini AS, King T, et al. Multivariate predictors of target lesion revascularization in the Randomized Trial of PTCA versus Rotablator for Diffuse In-Stent Restenosis (ROSTER) (abstr.). *J Am Coll Cardiol* 2001; 37:648A.

28. vom Dahl J, Dietz U, Haager PK, et al. Rotational atherectomy does not reduce recurrent in-stent restenosis: results of the angioplasty versus rotational atherectomy for treatment of diffuse in-stent restenosis trial (ARTIST). *Circulation* 2002; 105:583-8.

13

Intravascular Ultrasound During Coronary Stenting. Criteria for Optimal Deployment

HARALD MUDRA, MD

Background. What is the Potential Impact of Intracoronary Ultrasound on Optimizing Stent Expansion? Ultrasound Criteria for Optimal Stent Deployment. Different Stents. Deployment Guidance and Optimization. Results of Randomized Studies. Practical Conclusion of Study Results. References.

BACKGROUND

Intracoronary stenting currently is the standard method of percutaneous catheter intervention. In Germany in 2001, stents were used in 79 % of 23,685 coronary angioplasties, as documented in the national ALKK-registry.[1] Intravascular ultrasound has obtained important insights into the anatomy of stented coronary segments that could not have been obtained with angiographic techniques alone. By depicting stent-expansion patterns in a cross-sectional view, intravascular ultrasound showed that many stents were underexpanded or did not have full vessel-wall apposition.[2,3] These insights led to a change in implantation techniques and the development of the so-called «high-pressure stent implantation» (A. Colombo). Due to the routine use of combined anti-platelet treatment with aspirin and ticlopidine or clopidogrel, paralleled by the use of this new implantation strategy, the rate of sub-acute stent thrombosis has fallen to less than 1 % in an average patient population.[4,5] However, despite these improvements, in-stent restenosis has emerged as a new disease that is difficult to treat and affects 10 % to 40 % of patients, depending on their risk profile.[6]

WHAT IS THE POTENTIAL IMPACT OF INTRACORONARY ULTRASOUND ON OPTIMIZING STENT EXPANSION?

Stent malapposition during the implantation procedure has decreased in frequency due to the change in procedural techniques mentioned above. However, when the acute results are examined systematically, the STRUT study has shown that 21 % of implanted stents are still not optimally apposed against the vessel wall.[7] In the POST registry of patients with documented stent thrombosis, this condition was present in 49 % of cases. Other qualitative and unique intravascular ultrasound aspects of a freshly implanted coronary stent refer also to the adjacent vessel segments with regard to plaque burden, persistent dissections, or intraluminal structures like fresh thrombi. Significant inflow/outflow disease (>40 plaque burden) was present in 30 %, edge dissection in 26 %, and in-stent thrombus in 23 % of cases, which was also a frequent prothrombotic factor in the POST registry in patients with stent thrombosis.[8] With the technical possibilities now available for longitudinal vessel reconstruction from a motorized catheter pull-back, documentation of optimal vessel wall apposition throughout the entire stent length is easy to obtain (Fig. 13-1).

The second controversial issue in relation to intravascular ultrasound in coronary stenting is the degree of stent expansion that must be reached in order to achieve what is called «optimal stent expansion.» This aspect was extremely important before the era of ticlopidine, clopidogrel, and glycoprotein IIb/IIIa antagonists, when it was thought that the achievement of laminar flow conditions throughout the stent was the major anatomical factor to be optimized in order to reduce the risk of thrombus formation.

The burning question of how to define «optimal stent expansion» addressed the problem of in-stent restenosis rates following different implantation strategies. In accordance with the idea that «the bigger the bet-ter,» which was introduced in relation to coronary interventions for different treatment modalities by Kuntz and colleagues in 1991,[9] the impact of optimal stent expansion on the rate of restenosis focused scientific interest and was supported by observational clinical studies.[10, 11] However, there is a correlation between the degree of vessel trauma in balloon angioplasty models and inflammation resulting from the activation of thrombocytes and several mitogenic factors, as well as exaggerated neointimal proliferation after excessive overdilatation.[12, 13] Consequently, intravascular ultrasound could achieve an optimal compromise between stent expansion relative to true coronary vessel dimensions, plaque volume, and plaque composition, on the one hand, and minimal vessel overstretching or trauma on the other hand.

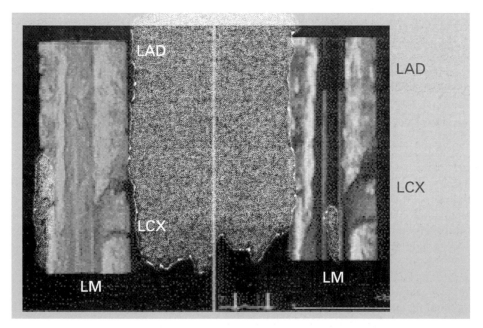

Figure 13-1. Longitudinal reconstruction of a motorized ECG-triggered catheter pull-back from the proximal left anterior descending (LAD) artery to the ostium of the left main stem (LM) after deployment of a slotted tube stent in the ostial left anterior descending artery. The left-hand panel depicts a three-dimensional reconstruction of the vessel segment in which the stent struts are partially visible. Note the adequate stent expansion with respect to the distal reference segment and the uncompromised take-off of the left circumflex artery (LCX).

ULTRASOUND CRITERIA FOR OPTIMAL STENT DEPLOYMENT

Qualitative criteria for optimal coronary stenting mainly follow the rationale of avoiding clinical complications like subacute stent thrombosis or vessel closure. The criteria listed in Table 13-1 have been identified empirically based on clinical case reports, personal communications, and retrospective clinical studies or registries.

There is still no consensus about the quantitative criteria that must be met for «optimal stent deployment.» Based on data showing that neointimal thickness is independent of stent size[14] and, therefore, is a minor problem in large stents, the absolute dimension of the minimal stent area dictates the resulting restenosis rate. It has been demonstrated in several series that a minimal in-stent lumen area of $\geqslant 9$ mm^2 incurs a low risk for restenosis. A result like this, however, can only be safely reached in larger coronary arteries since 9 mm^2 would mean 0 % residual stenosis in an artery with a diameter of 3.4 mm. The use of balloons larger than the true vessel size (within the external elastic membrane as the borderline to the adventitia) to maximize the in-stent lumen increases the risk of coronary rupture.[2]

For this reason, relative luminal criteria for «optimal stent expansion» were suggested, balancing a trade-off between lumen enlargement and vessel trauma. Relative luminal criteria, referring either to total vessel area within the EEM border or to the luminal dimensions proximal and distal to

Table 13-1. Qualitative Parameters of Optimal Stent Deployment

Adequate lesion coverage by the stent
Complete apposition against vessel wall
No intraluminal masses
Smoothly tapered inlet and outlet lumen dimensions adjacent to and within the stent
No persistent dissection

the stented segment, can be applied regardless of vessel size. One suggested criterion for optimal stent expansion, which derived from the observations of Glagov et al.[15] that suggested that plaque formation is compensated for by vessel enlargement up to a plaque burden of about 40 % of total vessel area, is that the minimal in-stent area be equivalent to 55 % or 60 % of total vessel area.[2, 16] This criterion is not easy to satisfy. Excessive plaque formation, present especially in the right coronary arteries, would result in an unphysiologically large lumen diameter when attempts are made to meet this criterion. In contrast, criteria that are based on hemodynamic considerations and attempt to create a smooth lumen channel in the stented segment in order to minimize turbulence are more widely accepted and easier to reach. However, they require more complex on-line measurements. Besides perfect vessel tapering, especially in longer stented lesions, to produce a gradual and continuous lumen decrease from the larger to the smaller reference segment, a minimal stent lumen area of 80 % to 90 % of the mean reference lumen area is established. In addition, a smooth stent inlet and outlet, with a stent mar-

Table 13-2. Quantitative Parameters of Optimal Stent Deployment

Intrastent MLCSA >9 mm^2
Intrastent MLCSA >55 or 60 % of vessel CSA (media to media)
Intrastent MLCSA >90 % of average reference lumen CSA
Intrastent MLCSA >80 % of average reference lumen CSA
Intrastent MLCSA >90 % of distal (or smaller) reference lumen CSA

MLCSA: Minimal lumen cross-sectional area.
CSA: Cross-sectional area.

ginal area of 90 % to 100 % of the corresponding reference site, have been proposed.[10]

All these criteria have been defined empirically instead of being evidence-based. Adherence to the guidelines of the American College of Cardiology Task Force on Clinical Expert Consensus Documents working group consensus report is recommended.[17] The most widely accepted, or at least the most widely used, criteria for «optimal stent expansion» in published studies are given in Table 13-2.

DIFFERENT STENTS

Most of the clinical studies that apply the proposed criteria for stent optimization are based on data obtained with the Palmaz-Schatz stent and its design successors. With a given balloon type, two major design-dependent features of different coronary stents dictate the resulting lumen dimension. These are radial force and lesion coverage as a result of relative metal surface coverage and the size of the areas between stent struts. For this reason, optimization of stent expansion usually correlates closely to lumen enlargement for all types of slotted-tube stents, the multicellular or corrugated-ring designs, as well as self-expanding mesh designs. However, with coil stents it might not be possible to fulfill the criteria of optimal stent expansion due to the limited radial force and tissue prolapse through the stent struts, which sometimes leads to the insertion of a second stent (stent in a stent).

DEPLOYMENT GUIDANCE AND OPTIMIZATION

Intravascular Ultrasound Before Stent Deployment

Whenever ultrasound guidance during stenting is planned, ultrasound imaging should be used before any other tool is introduced into the coronary artery to obtain the maximal gain in information in addition to angiography. In our opinion, the use of motorized pull-back, usually at a speed of 0.5 (sometimes 1.0) mm/s, is mandatory to ensure reproducible measurements without running any risk of losing information as a result of excessively fast manual catheter pullbacks. In some cases of significant involvement of the left main coronary that is not appreciated by angiography,[18] or of diffuse proximal plaque formation with less distal disease, the results of intravascular ultrasound may even induce a change in procedural strategy in favor of bypass surgery.[19]

Intravascular ultrasound allows for assessment of diffuse coronary atherosclerosis not visible by angiography and detailed quantification of stenosis severity with respect to the reference segment measurements based on both lumen and total vessel size. Moreover, it gives important information about plaque composition (soft, fibrous, or calcified) and its circumferential distribution (eccentric vs. concentric).[20] Based on these findings, we choose the proper length of stent and, if direct stenting does not seem to be feasible, the appropriate balloon size for predilatation. Appropriate balloon size is 1) the larger lumen diameter of the reference segments, 2) the average of the total vessel (EEM) and lumen diameters of both reference vessels or, in some cases, 3) the smaller EEM diameter, always taking into account the expected theoretical balloon diameter at a given inflation pressure. Thus, the ultrasound interrogation will result in a larger balloon size than a selection based on angiography alone. In some cases, alternative pretreatment modalities like a cutting balloon, or rotational or directional atherectomy are used before stent placement depending on the plaque type as assessed by intravascular ultrasound. Especially in tight ostial lesions and left main coronary procedures, we use these additional treatment options to ensure a maximal in-stent lumen gain in order to reduce restenosis.

Intracoronary Ultrasound Following Stent Placement

After stent placement, an intracoronary ultrasound evaluation is always indicated if the angiographic results are ambiguous. Such results include any unclear haziness within the stent that could be due to thrombus formation as well as non-uniform stent expansion due to focal lesion fibrosis or calcification. Sometimes, angiographically visible dissections at the stent margins are caused by a broken calcific shell, as assessed by ultrasound. If the lumen size is sufficient, no further stenting is needed. On the other hand, «pocket flaps» are usually an ultrasound indication for additional stent placement if there is luminal prolapse. Any plaque prolapse detected by ultrasound within the stent, which occurs predominantly in coil stents, is also an indication for further stent placement (stent in stent). If a balloon catheter cannot easily recross the stent, ultrasound occasionally reveals an unexpanded stent portion due to partial dislodgment of the stent by the balloon during insertion. Because the unexpanded part of the stent may be located in an angiographically undiseased segment, it may not be detected by angiography but can easily be corrected by a simple redilatation.

When stent deployment seems optimal as assessed by angiography, a standardized catheter pull-back is performed from a distance at least 15 mm distal to the stent to the ostium of the coronary artery, so that the distal reference segment is also properly assessed. The ultrasound catheter should be straightened in curved segments before the catheter is pulled back at the desired speed. The longitudinal reconstruction of this catheter pull-back is used to check the qualitative parameters (Table 13-1), including the integrity of the coronary vessel proximal to the stent. After calculation of the minimal in-stent lumen area, it is com-

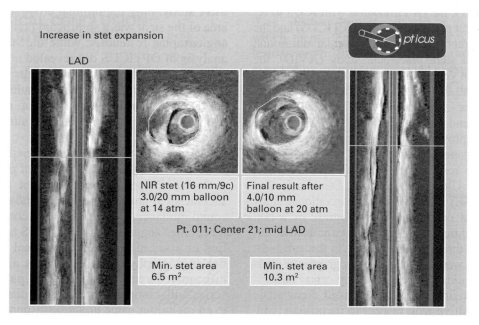

Figure 13-2. A stent placed in the left anterior descending artery (LAD) before (left) and after (right) ultrasound-guided optimization from an OPTICUS study case. Note the significant gain in stent expansion in both the longitudinal reconstruction and in the cross-sectional view of the tightest in-stent site. The lumen and adventitial borders are depicted.

14

In-Stent Restenosis

Jorge Luna, MD
Alan C. Yeung, MD

Overview. Predictors of Restenosis after Stent Placement. Intravascular Ultrasound During Repeated Intervention for in-Stent Restenosis. References.

OVERVIEW

Serial intravascular ultrasound studies have shown that restenosis after conventional balloon angioplasty represents a complex interplay between elastic recoil, smooth muscle proliferation, and vascular remodeling,[1,2] while restenosis after stent deployment is due almost entirely to smooth muscle hyperplasia and matrix proliferation.[3]

The role of intravascular ultrasound (IVUS) has gradually expanded, from the diagnostic merits, to the clinical application of stent implantation strategy for selected patient subsets. Several observational studies in selected patients have shown remarkably low restenosis rates after ultrasound-guided stent implantation; there is, however, still debate over whether or not routine IVUS guidance modifies the outcome of everyday coronary stenting interventions by reducing the rates of both restenosis and target vessel revascularization (TVR). Therefore, the current role for IVUS in the guidance of *de novo* coronary interventions in the stent era is probably limited to the assessment of complex lesions (i.e., bifurcation, ostial, long lesions) or to help in planning a bailout procedure when complications arise (i.e., peri-pro-cedural thrombus formation or coronary dissections). There is currently no class I indication for the use of IVUS in the year 2001 revision of the ACC/AHA Guidelines for Percutaneous Coronary Intervention. In the guidelines, its use is only recommended for evaluating results in high-risk procedures (i.e., patients with multiple stents, impaired TIMI grade flow or coronary flow reserve, and marginal angiographic appearance).[4] Thus, IVUS is not routinely used for stent optimization and there is no consensus regarding optimal procedural end-points.

A very important aspect of IVUS imaging is in the area of clinical research. Currently, this catheter-based imaging technology is widely accepted as being the new gold standard for follow-up studies of new treatment modalities for coronary artery disease, specifically those designed to prevent restenosis.

PREDICTORS OF RESTENOSIS AFTER STENT PLACEMENT

The beneficial effects of stent implantation on restenosis have been attributed to the larger acute lumen dimensions achieved compared with other interventions, as well as to the elimination of acute recoil after intervention.[5,6] Additionally, several studies have demonstrated that stents can withstand the remodeling forces that otherwise may have contributed to restenosis.[3] Thus, in addition to achieving larger post-procedural lumen dimensions and withstanding acute recoil, stents appear to reduce restenosis by resisting negative arterial remodeling.[7]

However, initial histological and angiographic studies have suggested that stents trigger the development of neointimal hyperplasia, whereas other studies have indicated that inadequate stent expansion and chronic stent recoil may also contribute to restenosis.[8] IVUS observations in humans, however, have confirmed that in-stent restenosis is primarily due to neointimal proliferation, thus leading to the major mechanism of late lumen loss after stent implantation. Also, serial IVUS studies have shown that late lumen loss correlates with neointimal tissue proliferation both overall, throughout the whole stent length by volumetric IVUS analysis, and at individual cross-sectional segments of the stent. Thus, the major limitation to stent implantation is the initiation of neointimal tissue proliferation within and adjacent to the stent.[3]

This phenomenon might respond to a stent-related exaggeration in neointimal tissue proliferation, since it has been shown to be independent of the acute results of stenting (i.e., larger acute lumen dimensions), and to the fact that stents appear to withstand negative arterial remodeling. Furthermore, early studies involving Palmaz-Schatz stents showed that the late neointimal formation was greater in the mid-portion of the stented segment. At first, it was thought that the presence of the central articulation in that particular stent design was the reason for this finding, but similar results were confirmed with non-articulated stent designs.[9]

In 1998, the MUSIC (Multicenter Ultrasound Stenting in Coronaries Study) investigators found that IVUS confirmation of optimal stent expansion was associated with low restenosis rates during follow-up (less than 10% at 6 months).[10] Also, the AVID (Angiography Vs. Intravascular ultrasound-Directed stent placement) study showed a dramatic decrease in the 12-month TVR, especially for vessels ≥ 2.5 mm (4.8% versus 10.6%, p = 0.02; relative reduction of 55%), vein grafts (5.4% versus 20.8%, relative reduction of 74%, p=0.04), and lesions with $\geq 70\%$ stenosis (3.5% versus 14.9%, relative reduction of 76 %, p = 0.003).[11]

In the era of «high pressure» stenting, several IVUS studies also showed that the degree of stent expansion correlates with TVR rate. In 1999, de Feyter et al.[12] showed an inverse relation between minimal stent area (MSA), as tracked by IVUS after angiographically successful deployment, and TVR. In a larger single-center study, Moussa et al. also showed an inverse relation between MSA and angiographic restenosis with 425 consecutive patients (496 lesions).[13] These findings were corroborated in a further single-center study by Hoffmann et al.,[14] who showed that IVUS after interventional stent dimensions was one of the most consistent predictors of angiographic in-stent restenosis. Also, in a large, single-center study, Kasaoka et al.[15] assessed angiographic and IVUS predictors of in-stent restenosis, and found by multivariate analysis that IVUS stent lumen CSA was a better independent predictor than the angiographic measurements. More recently, the CRUISE (Can Routine Ultrasound Influence Stent Expansion) study showed that IVUS-guided stent deployment resulted in significantly lower TVR rates at 9 months (8.5% versus 15.3%, p < 0.05; relative reduction of 44%), compared with angiographic-guided stenting. They also showed that these very low TVR rates could be achieved when a minimal in-stent area of more than 9 mm^2 was accomplished.[16]

On the other hand, the OPTICUS (OPTimization with ICUS to reduce stent restenosis) study investigators failed to show a beneficial effect of the routine use of ultrasound guidance for coronary stenting over angiography-guided optimization of tubular stents in a multicenter, randomized study in intravascular ultrasound-experienced centers.[17] They found no differences in angiographic restenosis, minimal lumen diameter, and percent diameter stenosis at 6 months. Also, the rates of major adverse cardiac events and repeat percutaneous interventions were not reduced in the ultrasound-guided group at 12 months of follow-up. Nevertheless, it is important to note that optimal stent placement (<10% diameter stenosis) was achieved in only 82.2% of patients of the ultrasound-guided group and that all 3 ultrasound MUSIC study criteria for optimal stent expansion were met by only 56.1% of patients in this group, leading to a mean stent area of 8.1 ± 2.3 mm^2 in the patients assigned to ultrasound guidance.

What is clear, however, is the lack of a standard guideline for the optimum post-stenting IVUS criteria to predict late outcomes, especially in vessels of smaller caliber. As a result, practitioners who use IVUS have to decide on the procedural end-point by a somewhat arbitrary assessment. Previous studies have indicated that MSA[13,14,18] and pre- or post-interventional plaque burden[14,19] may be important risk factors for in-stent restenosis. However, MSA has been the only independent predictor in the multivariate analyses that include other epidemiological, clinical and anatomical variables,[1] and thus represents the only parameter that can be manipulated by the operator at the time of stent deployment. Moreover, several studies used an MSA of 7.0 mm^2 as a reasonable cutoff value for the prediction of angiographic restenosis,[18,20] although little systematic evaluation has been made to determine the threshold in their methods in small vessels.

Several other criteria for optimal stent expansion have been used in IVUS-guided stent implantation trials, namely: MSA divided by mean reference lumen area (MSA/REFLA) ≥90% in the MUSIC[10] and

AVID trials,[11] and MSA/REFLA ≥80% in the RESIST (REStenosis after Ivus guided STenting) trial.[21] However, these criteria, based on MSA/REFLA, are considered to be less predictive for late outcomes, as proved by a recent investigation and a previous report.[20,22] In addition, an MSA divided by mean reference vessel area (MSA/REFVA) ≥55% might be another useful IVUS criterion to predict restenosis,[13] although the exact threshold is still controversial. In cases in which an MSA of 6.5 mm^2 may not be achieved, especially in smaller arteries, some weighted parameters such as MSA/REFVA, instead of an absolute MSA, may potentially be useful.[22]

Nevertheless, the main limitation of current investigations in this field is that all of them have been based on first-generation stent designs with uniformly aggressive stenting techniques. Although high-pressure dilation used in these trials is associated with the achievement of greater stent dimensions,[23] it might have also stimulated tissue proliferation within and surrounding the stents.[24] It is expected, therefore, that current non-articulated third-generation stent designs and lower-pressure techniques may result in better outcomes. As a matter of fact, in a recent IVUS study assessing the impact of different stent designs on intimal hyperplasia after implantation in atherosclerotic human coronary arteries, multivariate analysis proved that the tubular slotted stent type was the only independent predictor of intimal hyperplasia thickness at follow-up (P < 0.001).[25]

Thus, the role of IVUS guidance in further enhancing the results of current stent designs still needs to be established in future trials.

INTRAVASCULAR ULTRASOUND DURING REPEATED INTERVENTION FOR IN-STENT RESTENOSIS

Intracoronary ultrasound imaging has increased our understanding of the mechanisms of action of balloon angioplasty, coronary stenting ,and other interventions such as plaque-debulking techniques. In addition, the use of IVUS during follow-up studies of coronary stenting procedures has revealed many aspects and relevant pathophysiologic mechanisms of in-stent restenosis.[26]

IVUS offers several advantages over angiography in the assessment of in-stent restenosis. IVUS permits detailed, high-quality, cross-sectional imaging of the coronary arteries *in vivo*. Using this imaging technique, the normal coronary artery architecture, major components of the atherosclerotic plaque, and changes that occur in coronary arterial dimensions and anatomy with the atherosclerotic disease process, during transcatheter therapy, and on follow-up can be studied *in vivo* in a manner otherwise not possible. This includes the direct visualization of intensely echoreflective (but radiolucent) stainless steel stent struts, which can be difficult to visualize by angiography.[27-29] Stent borders are clearly demarcated and stent cross-sectional area can be accurately measured. Thus, by assessing the lumen and stent cross-sectional areas, the amount of neointimal tissue can be quantified.

Therefore, IVUS may prove to have clinical utility in the treatment of in-stent restenosis by helping to individualize device selection and sizing, and by more accurately assessing treatment results. Without doubt, it has been of great research value in the assessment of different treatment modalities for this problem. It is also still illustrating us about the long-term effect of neointimal inhibition by brachytherapy and, more recently, drug-eluting stents.[30-32]

REFERENCES

1. Mintz GS, Popma JJ, Pichard AD, et al. Intravascular ultrasound predictors of restenosis after percutaneous transcatheter coronary revascularization. *J Am Coll Cardiol* 1996; 27:1678-87.
2. Mintz GS, Popma JJ, Pichard AD, et al. Arterial remodeling after coronary angioplasty: a serial intravascular ultrasound study. *Circulation* 1996; 94:35-43.
3. Hoffmann R, Mintz GS, Dussaillant GR, et al. Patterns and mechanisms of in-stent restenosis. A serial intravascular ultrasound study. *Circulation* 1996; 94:1247-54.
4. Smith SC, Jr., Dove JT, Jacobs AK, et al. ACC/AHA guidelines of percutaneous coronary interventions (revision of the 1993 PTCA guidelines) —executive summary. A report of the American College of Cardiology/American Heart Association Task Force on Practice Guidelines (committee to revise the 1993 guidelines for percutaneous transluminal coronary angioplasty). *J Am Coll Cardiol* 2001; 37:2215-38.
5. Kuntz RE, Safian RD, Carrozza JP, Fishman RF, Mansour M, Baim DS. The importance of acute luminal diameter in determining restenosis after coronary atherectomy or stenting. *Circulation* 1992; 86:1827-35.
6. Kuntz RE, Gibson CM, Nobuyoshi M, Baim DS. Generalized model of restenosis after conventional balloon angioplasty, stenting and directional atherectomy. *J Am Coll Cardiol* 1993; 21:15-25.
7. Painter JA, Mintz GS, Wong SC, et al. Serial intravascular ultrasound studies fail to show evidence of chronic Palmaz-Schatz stent recoil. *Am J Cardiol* 1995; 75:398-400.
8. Gordon PC, Gibson CM, Cohen DJ, Carrozza JP, Kuntz RE, Baim DS. Mechanisms of restenosis and redilation within coronary stents —quantitative angiographic assessment. *J Am Coll Cardiol* 1993; 21:1166-74.
9. Mudra H, Regar E, Klauss V, et al. Serial follow-up after optimized ultrasound-guided deployment of Palmaz-Schatz stents. Instent neointimal proliferation without significant reference segment response. *Circulation* 1997; 95:363- 70.
10. de Jaegere P, Mudra H, Figulla H, et al. Intravascular ultrasound-guided optimized stent deployment. Immediate and 6 months clinical and angiographic results from the Multicenter Ultrasound Stenting in Coronaries Study (MUSIC Study). *Eur Heart J* 1998; 19:1214-23.
11. Russo RJ, Attubato MJ, Davidson CJ, et al. Angiography Versus Intravascular Ultrasound-Directed Stent Placement: Final Results from AVID. *Circulation* 1999; 100 (suppl I):I-234. Abstract.

12. de Feyter PJ, Kay P, Disco C, Serruys PW. Reference chart derived from post-stent-implantation intravascular ultrasound predictors of 6-month expected restenosis on quantitative coronary angiography. *Circulation* 1999; 100:1777-83.

13. Moussa I, Moses J, Di Mario C, et al. Does the specific intravascular ultrasound criterion used to optimize stent expansion have an impact on the probability of stent restenosis? *Am J Cardiol* 1999; 83:1012-7.

14. Hoffmann R, Mintz GS, Mehran R, et al. Intravascular ultrasound predictors of angiographic restenosis in lesions treated with Palmaz-Schatz stents. *J Am Coll Cardiol* 1998; 31:43-9.

15. Kasaoka S, Tobis JM, Akiyama T, et al. Angiographic and intravascular ultrasound predictors of in-stent restenosis. *J Am Coll Cardiol* 1998; 32:1630-5.

16. Fitzgerald PJ, Oshima A, Hayase M, et al. Final results of the Can Routine Ultrasound Influence Stent Expansion (CRUISE) study. *Circulation* 2000; 102:523-30.

17. Mudra H, di Mario C, de Jaegere P, et al. Randomized comparison of coronary stent implantation under ultrasound or angiographic guidance to reduce stent restenosis (OPTICUS Study). *Circulation* 2001; 104: 1343-9.

18. Hong MK, Park SW, Mintz GS, et al. Intravascular ultrasonic predictors of angiographic restenosis after long coronary stenting. *Am J Cardiol* 2000; 85:441-5.

19. Prati F, Di Mario C, Moussa I, et al. In-stent neointimal proliferation correlates with the amount of residual plaque burden outside the stent: an intravascular ultrasound study. *Circulation* 1999; 99:1011-4.

20. Schiele F, Seronde MF, Gupta S, et al. Optimal intravascular ultrasound criteria for stent deployment: comparison of different ultrasound criteria on the 6 months restenosis rate (abstr). *J Am Coll Cardiol* 1999; 33:101A.

21. Schiele F, Meneveau N, Vuillemenot A, et al. Impact of intravascular ultrasound guidance in stent deployment on 6-month restenosis rate: a multicenter, randomized study comparing two strategies-with and without intravascular ultrasound guidance. RESIST Study Group. REStenosis after Ivus guided STenting. *J Am Coll Cardiol* 1998; 32:320-8.

22. Morino Y, Honda Y, Okura H, et al. An optimal diagnostic threshold for minimal stent area to predict target lesion revascularization following stent implantation in native coronary lesions. *Am J Cardiol* 2001; 88:301-3.

23. Stone GW, St Goar FG, Hodgson JM, et al. Analysis of the relation between stent implantation pressure and expansion. Optimal Stent Implantation (OSTI) Investigators. *Am J Cardiol* 1999; 83:1397-400, A8.

24. Hoffmann R, Mintz GS, Mehran R, et al. Tissue proliferation within and surrounding Palmaz-Schatz stents is dependent on the aggressiveness of stent implantation technique. *Am J Cardiol* 1999; 83:1170-4.

25. Hoffmann R, Jansen C, Konig A, et al. Stent design-related neointimal tissue proliferation in human coronary arteries; an intravascular ultrasound study. *Eur Heart J* 2001; 22:2007-14.

26. Dussaillant GR, Mintz GS, Pichard AD, et al. Small stent size and intimal hyperplasia contribute to restenosis: a volumetric intravascular ultrasound analysis. *J Am Coll Cardiol* 1995; 26:720-4.

27. Goldberg SL, Colombo A, Nakamura S, Almagor Y, Maiello L, Tobis JM. Benefit of intracoronary ultrasound in the deployment of Palmaz-Schatz stents. *J Am Coll Cardiol* 1994; 24:996-1003.

28. Nakamura S, Colombo A, Gaglione A, et al. Intracoronary ultrasound observations during stent implantation. *Circulation* 1994; 89:2026-34.

29. Colombo A, Hall P, Nakamura S, et al. Intracoronary stenting without anticoagulation accomplished with intravascular ultrasound guidance. *Circulation* 1995; 91:1676-88.

30. Meerkin D, Tardif JC, Crocker IR, et al. Effects of intracoronary beta-radiation therapy after coronary angioplasty: an intravascular ultrasound study. *Circulation* 1999; 99: 1660-5.

31. Morino Y, Bonneau HN, Fitzgerald PJ. Vascular brachytherapy: what have we learned from intravascular ultrasound? *J Invasive Cardiol* 2001; 13:409-16.

32. Sousa JE, Costa MA, Abizaid AC, et al. Sustained suppression of neointimal proliferation by sirolimus-eluting stents: one-year angiographic and intravascular ultrasound follow-up. *Circulation* 2001; 104:2007-11.

15

Intravascular Ultrasound During Coronary Brachytherapy

MANEL SABATÉ, MD
GELA PIMENTEL, MD

Introduction. IVUS and the Mechanism of Action of Intracoronary Brachytherapy to Prevent Restenosis. IVUS and Limitations of Intracoronary Brachytherapy. IVUS and Radiation Dose Calculation. Conclusions. References.

INTRODUCTION

Percutaneous transluminal coronary angioplasty (PTCA) is an accepted treatment for coronary artery disease. However, angiographic restenosis is reported in 40 % to 60 % of patients after successful PTCA.[1,2] Mechanisms involved in the restenosis process are elastic recoil of the artery, local thrombus formation, vascular remodeling with vessel shrinkage, and an overactive healing process with neointimal hyperplasia.[2-5] Neointimal hyperplasia develops by the migration and proliferation of smooth muscle cells and myofibroblasts after balloon-induced trauma of the arterial wall, and by deposition of an extracellular matrix by the smooth muscle cells.[5-7] The introduction of the stent in the arsenal of the interventional cardiologist has reduced the restenosis rate to 15 % to 20 %,[8,9] by preventing elastic recoil and negative remodeling.[10] However, the occurrence of restenosis after stent implantation remains unresolved, especially in small vessels and long lesions, where it may exceed 30 % of cases.[11] It is primarily caused by neointimal hyperplasia, which occurs due to trauma of the arterial wall caused by stent struts. The treatment of in-stent restenosis with conventional techniques (balloon angioplasty or debulking) is rather disappointing, with restenosis rates of 27 % to 63 %, which increases with the number of re-interventions.[12-14] Because radiotherapy had proved to be effective in treating the exuberant fibroblastic activity of keloid scar formation and other nonmalignant processes such as ocular pterygium,[15,16] it was assumed that this adjunctive therapy would also prevent coronary restenosis.

The first experimental study in this field was carried out in 1964 by Friedman et al.,[17] who used iridium-192 (^{192}Ir) in cholesterol-fed rabbits. In 1992, Liermann et al.[18] performed brachytherapy in the first four cases, patients who had undergone a femoral percutaneous angioplasty. A second wave of experimental work was carried out in the United States by Wiedermann et al.[19] in New York, Waksman et al.[20] in Atlanta, and Mazur et al.[21] in Houston. At the same time, Verin et al.[22] of Geneva conducted experimental studies with the pure β-emitter yttrium-90 (^{90}Y) in carotid and iliac arteries of rabbits.

Radiation therapy can be delivered to the coronary arteries by external radiation or by brachytherapy methods, either using catheter-based systems or radioactive stents.[23] Catheter-based systems can handle either β —or γ-emitters, which can deliver the prescribed dose in either high or low-dose rate, manually or automatically. Radioactive stents use mainly pure β-emitters at a very low-dose rate.

The first clinical experience in coronary arteries in humans was carried out by Condado et al.,[24] using a ^{192}Ir wire hand-delivered using a non-centered, closed end-lumen catheter, and by Verin et al.,[25] using a β-source and a centered device. Both studies demonstrated that the delivery of radiation to the coronary artery is feasible and safe. Later, several randomized trials of γ-radiation reported positive results for the treatment of restenotic lesions after stent implantation,[26, 27, 28] which were confirmed with the use of β-radiation therapy.[29, 30, 31] The use of intracoronary brachytherapy has been further explored in patients with *de novo* lesions treated with plain balloon angioplasty.[32] In the higher prescribed dose group (18 Gy at 1 mm from the balloon surface), the restenosis rate dropped to a single-digit value (4 %). However, these results were not corroborated when a stent was implanted during brachytherapy in the only multicenter trial reported so far in this subset of patients.[33] Finally, the use of radioactive stents has been abandoned due to the occurrence of the so-called candy wrapper effect.[34]

In vivo intravascular ultrasound (IVUS) imaging studies have been helpful in determining the morphologic effect of brachytherapy on the vessel wall, as well as the nature of the complications and limitations of this technique. Further, a more accurate way to calculate the radiation dose delivered to a certain point of the vessel wall has been possible from IVUS analysis. This chapter will review the role of intravascular ultrasound in the development and understanding of this new therapy.

IVUS AND THE MECHANISM OF ACTION OF INTRACORONARY BRACHYTHERAPY TO PREVENT RESTENOSIS

Enhancement of positive remodeling. The effect of intracoronary radiation therapy on vascular remodeling has been clinically demonstrated in the BERT (Beta Energy Restenosis Trial) study. In this trial, only *de novo* lesions were treated and radiotherapy was delivered using a non-centered device (Beta-Cath system; Novoste Corp., Norcross, GA), which uses the pure β-emitter ^{90}Sr/Y. The dose was prescribed at 2 mm from the source and was randomly assigned to 12, 14, or 16 Gy.[35] In a careful volumetric analysis of the irradiated coronary segment following successful balloon angioplasty, vessel size (i.e., the volume encompassed by the external elastic membrane) appeared to increase significantly during the 6-month follow-up. This vessel enlargement (positive remodeling) accommodated a parallel increase in plaque volume. As a result, luminal volume remained unchanged at follow-up.[36] This morphologic evolution was not blunted by the implantation of a conventional stent at the site of the radiation therapy, as observed in a cohort of patients treated by means of a centered system (Guidant system; Guidant Corp., Santa Clara, CA), which uses the pure β-emitter phosphorus-32 (^{32}P).[37] Similarly, we have observed the same phenomenon in patients treated because of diffuse in-stent restenosis. During the 6-month follow-up, irradiated segments showed luminal enlargement on angiography (Fig. 15-1). Further IVUS analysis confirmed that the increase in total vessel volume at the irradiated site encompassed a lesser degree of plaque volume increase, leading to an increase in luminal volume (Figs. 15-2 and 15-3).

A distinct pattern was observed after radioactive stent implantation.[38] Both in low- (0.75 to 1.5 μCi) and high-activity (6 to 12 μCi) radioactive isostents, vessel remodeling was abolished outside the boundaries of the

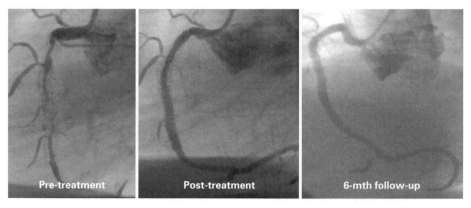

Figure 15-1. Angiographic image of a diffuse in-stent restenosis in the right coronary artery (left panel). Immediate result after balloon angioplasty and intracoronary brachytherapy (mid panel). Six-month angiographic follow-up (right panel). An increase in lumen dimensions is clearly visible on angiography.

stent, and neointimal hyperplasia was also inhibited in a dose-dependent manner[34, 38] (Fig. 15-4). Differences in activity and dose rate (catheter-based system: high-activity-high-dose rate; radioactive stent: low-activity-low-dose rate) may account for this dis-tinct morphologic change in vessel structures between both systems.

Inhibition of neointimal hyperplasia. The efficacy of gamma radiation therapy to prevent recurrence of in-stent restenotic lesions was serially assessed by IVUS. Data derived

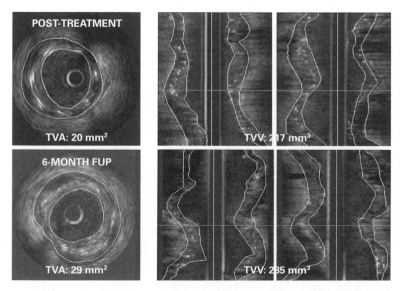

Figure 15-2. Cross-sectional and longitudinal IVUS images of the phenomenon depicted in Figure 15-1 on two perpendicular axes . Total vessel area and volume increased from post-treatment to 6 months of follow-up, resulting in an increase in luminal area and volume. TVA indicates total vessel area. TVV indicates total vessel volume.

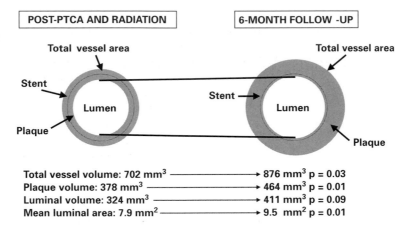

Figure 15-3. Average volumetric changes in our cohort of patients with in-stent restenosis treated with angioplasty and brachytherapy. A significant increase in total vessel volume is observed during the followup period, which can accommodate a significant increase in plaque volume, resulting in a significant increase in mean luminal area and a trend to larger luminal volume.

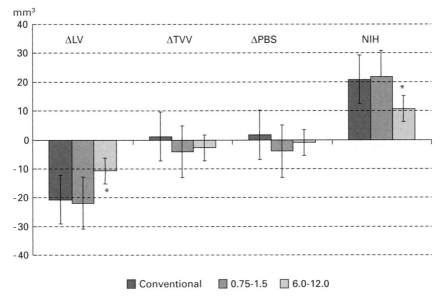

Figure 15-4. Morphologic changes within the stent margins (conventional stent versus 0.75 to 1.5-μCi adioactive stent versus 6 to 12-μCi radioactive stent). Lack of positive remodeling is demonstrated in the 3 groups of patients, which impeded plaque growth accommodation, resulting in a reduction in lumen dimensions. LV indicates lumen volume, TVV total vessel volume, PBS plaque behind stent, and NIH neointimal hyperplasia. *$P < 0.05$ between high-activity versus low-activity radioactive stent and conventional stents. (Adapted from reference 38.)

from IVUS analysis of various randomized trials[26, 39, 40] demonstrated that irradiated coronary arteries had significantly less increase in in-stent neointimal hyperplasia during follow-up than placebo.

IVUS AND LIMITATIONS OF INTRACORONARY BRACHYTHERAPY

Aneurysm Formation

Theoretically, the early beneficial effect of intravascular brachytherapy on arterial remodeling could lead to undesired aneurysm formation. The incidence of coronary aneurysm after balloon angioplasty or stent, defined as a coronary dilation that exceeded

the diameter of normal adjacent segments by 1.5 times, ranges between 3.4% and 5.4% and has not been associated with angiographic restenosis or unfavorable clinical outcome.[41] The incidence of aneurysm formation after radiation therapy is unknown.

Condado et al.[24] reported four cases (20%) within 2 months after γ-radiation. In two of them, a further increase in size was observed at 6 and 8 months, respectively, and remained unchanged at 2, 3, and 5 years (Condado, personal communication). This undesirable phenomenon was probably related to the high dose delivered to these coronary segments. Because the prescribed dose was 20 to 25 Gy to 1.5-mm depth, the actual dose calculated *a posteriori* ranged between 19 and 55 Gy.[24] In a cohort of patients included in the Rotterdam arm of the BERT-1.5 trial,

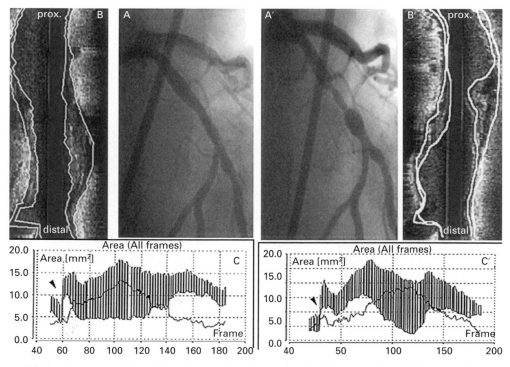

Figure 15-5. Aneurysm formation observed at 6 months of follow-up after balloon angioplasty intracoronary brachytherapy. Focal restenosis was evidenced proximal to the dilated area. A and A': angiographic image post-treatment and at 6 months of follow-up; B and B': IVUS longitudinal reconstruction post-treatment and at 6 months of follow-up; C and C': Chart showing volumetric data post-treatment and at 6 months of follow-up. (From reference 36 with permission.)

one case of aneurysm formation was observed in the irradiated segment. Interestingly, it was accompanied by a focal increase in the plaque burden proximal to the coronary dilatation, which led to restenosis[36] (Fig. 15-5). Besides, IVUS helped us to determine the actual dose delivered in both regions to the irradiated segment. By subsegmental analysis, a clear inhomogeneity in dose distribution to both regions was demonstrated: the segment that became restenotic received a rather low dose at the level of the adventitia as compared with that received by the region that was excessively dilated (4.6 vs 8.6 Gy, respectively). The presence of a coronary dissection, visible on IVUS, at the treated site might have precipitated the development

of such a coronary aneurysm in the context of a relatively high dose.[42] Recently, we have observed another case of aneurysm formation in an irradiated segment 6 months after stent implantation for a *de novo* lesion. In both cases, IVUS analysis confirmed the presence of the 3 layers of the coronary wall; thus, the diagnosis of true aneurysm was established.

Edge Effect (the «Candy Wrapper» Effect)

A potential limitation of intracoronary brachytherapy is the development of a new stenotic lesion at both edges of the irradiated

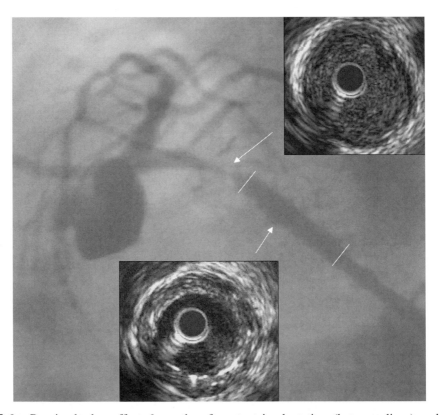

Figure 15-6. Proximal-edge effect 6-months after stent implantation (between lines) and catheter-based brachytherapy. IVUS images demonstrated minimal tissue growth within irradiated stent (bottom panel) and severe neointimal proliferation at the site of the proximal edge of the radiation source (upper right panel).

segments. This so-called edge effect, or «candy wrapper» effect, was originally described after high-activity (>3 μCi) radioactive stent implantation.[34] However, this phenomenon is not exclusive to radioactive stents, but may also affect coronary segments treated using a catheter-based system (Fig. 15-6).[36] Vessel wall injury[43] concomitantly to low-dose radiation at the edge of the irradiated segment[44] may be involved in the pathophysiology of this phenomenon. To integrate both components, a new concept in interventional cardiology was proposed: «the geographic miss.»[45] This concept is translated from a term in radio-oncology that defines a type of treatment failure due to low dose. In such cases, a small part of the treatment zone has either escaped irradiation or been inadequately irradiated because the total volume of the tumor was not appreciated, hence an insufficient margin was taken.[46] Typically, this phenomenon occurs by injuring the edges of the irradiated segment where, by definition, the dose received is rather low. Conceptually, after radioactive stent implantation, the incidence of geographic miss is 100%, because the length of the balloon used to deliver the stent is always longer than the radioactive stent. Thus, both edges are always injured and receive low-dose radiation. This would explain why the incidence of restenosis is high in the Milan dose-response study (52% in the low-activity group, 41% in the mid-activity group, and 50% in the high-activity group), but mostly at the expense of edge restenosis (31% in low-activity, 38% in mid-activity, and 39% in high-activity groups, respectively).[34] In addition, the authors identified the final balloon-to-artery ratio as an associated factor for the development of edge restenosis.[34]

Volumetric intravascular ultrasound studies demonstrated that the absence of positive remodeling, together with plaque increase, contributed to lumen shrinkage at both edges of the irradiated segment after catheter-based brachytherapy[36] (Fig. 15-7).

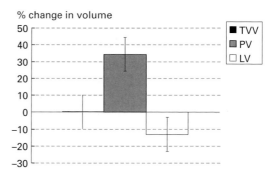

% change in volume

Figure 15-7. IVUS-derived volumetric changes occurring at the edges of the catheter-based radiation source: lack of positive vessel remodeling parallel to plaque increase leading to a decrease in luminal volume (adapted from reference 36). TVV indicates total vessel volume; PV indicates plaque volume; LV indicates luminal volume.

This phenomenon was later corroborated in the American series of patients treated with gamma-radiation for in-stent restenosis.[47]

To demonstrate that both low-dose radiation and injury have to coexist to induce the development of the «edge effect», Kozuma et al.[48] comparatively studied the geometric changes in the uninjured edges of irradiated and placebo segments using three-dimensional IVUS and volumetric analysis. Both groups showed similar degrees of plaque volume increase, total vessel volume changes, and luminal volume decrease during the follow-up period. Thus, the outcome of edges without macroscopic signs of injury was not negatively influenced by the low-dose radiation received during brachytherapy. This IVUS analysis confirmed previous angiographic evidence of the development of a higher-than-expected restenosis rate at injured edges compared to both irradiated segments and uninjured edges.[45] To minimize this harmful edge effect, the use of longer sources to allow enough margin to fully cover the injured segment has been advocated when catheter-based brachytherapy is applied.[49]

This «candy-wrapper» effect has been the Achilles heel of radioactive stents[34, 38].

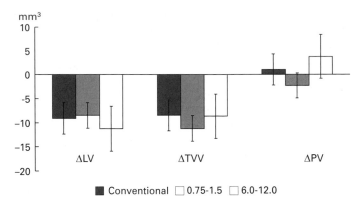

Figure 15-8. IVUS-derived volumetric changes occurring at the edges of the radioactive stent: in accordance with conventional stent edges, 0.75-1.5 radioactive stent edges, and 6.0-12.0 radioactive stent edges presented a decrease in total vessel volume at follow-up together with plaque volume increase. As a result, all groups showed a decrease in luminal volume at stent edges (adapted from reference 38). TVV indicates total vessel volume; PV indicates plaque volume; LV indicates luminal volume.

Again, IVUS analysis demonstrates that at the stent edge negative remodeling and plaque growth contributed to luminal narrowing (Fig. 15-8). Further attempts to either negate the impact of negative remodeling at the edges of the stent with «cold-end» radioactive stents, or reduce plaque growth with «hot-end» radioactive stents have not prevented occurrence of the problem. Cold-end stents caused a shift in the location of the IVUS-assessed neointimal hyperplasia toward the transition between the active and inactive parts of the stent.[50] Hot-end stents caused excess tissue growth, mainly at the proximal hot edge.[51] Finally, the use of a square-shouldered balloon to deliver the radioactive stent and, thus, to minimize edge injury, was also unsuccessful.[52] As a result, this device is no longer used for clinical purposes.

Late Thrombosis: Stent Malapposition/Persistent Dissection

The occurrence of coronary thrombosis beyond 1 month after angioplasty or stenting under a regimen of aspirin and ticlopidine or clopidogrel (for 15 days to 1 month) is anecdotal.[53] However, this undesirable phenomenon became apparent in the first series of patients treated with brachytherapy worldwide.[54, 55] In the first 92 patients treated with intracoronary brachytherapy in Rotterdam, a higher-than-expected incidence (6.6%) of thrombotic clinical events was observed 2 to 15 months after treatment.[54] This finding was confirmed in the American series of patients treated with γ-radiation. Data pooled from the WRIST (Washington Radiation for In-Stent Restenosis Trial), Long-WRIST, SVG-WRIST, Gamma-1, and BETA-WRIST trials demonstrated an incidence of late thrombotic occlusion of 9.1% as compared with 1.2% in the placebo groups 5.4 ± 3 months after the procedure.[55] The implantation of a conventional stent within the irradiated segment has been considered one of the contributors to this phenomenon. In this regard, the rate of late thrombosis, considering only the cohort of stented patients, reached 8.8% in the Rotterdam series and 14.6% in the American series.

The delay in stent re-endothelization has been considered a trigger mechanism of this event.[56] In addition, the possibility that brachytherapy may induce late stent malapposition by not being able to follow the vessel enlargement promoted by radiotherapy has been advocated in this process.[57, 58] Stent malapposition can be easily recognized on IVUS and has to be suspected when an obvious vessel enlargement is angiographically visible at the site of the original stent implantation (Fig. 15-9). In patients treated only with balloon angioplasty followed by intracoronary brachytherapy, the presence of unhealed dissections at 6 months of follow-up is a common phenomenon[59, 60] (Fig. 15-10). It remains to be seen whether persistent dissections are related to late thrombosis in non-stented patients.

To overcome this drawback, the long-term use (>6 months) of double antiplatelet therapy (aspirin and ticlopidine or clopidogrel) is clearly advocated when intracoronary radiation therapy is performed.

Black Hole

This term stands for an echolucent area in the lumen of the coronary artery that is only visualized with IVUS.[61] By definition, this type of lesion should have a homogeneous black appearance without backscatter (Fig. 15-11). This characteristic makes it possible to distinguish it from images with ring-down or other causes of relative echolucency, such as contrast, thrombus, or a lipid lake. This

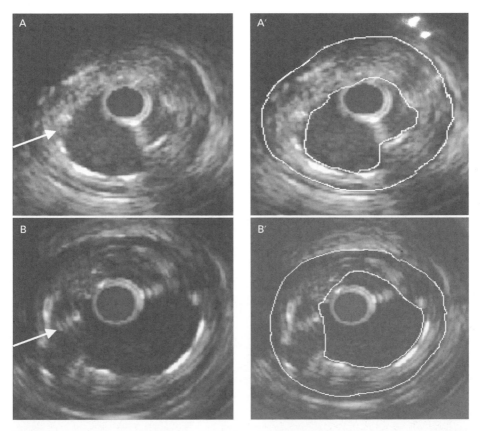

Figure 15-9. Late stent malapposition at 6 months of follow-up after intracoronary brachytherapy. A and A': IVUS cross-sectional image of the stent immediately after its implantation. B and B': Same cross-sectional IVUS image at 6 months of follow-up. Enlargement of the vessel size leading to stent strut malapposition is visible at 9 (arrow).

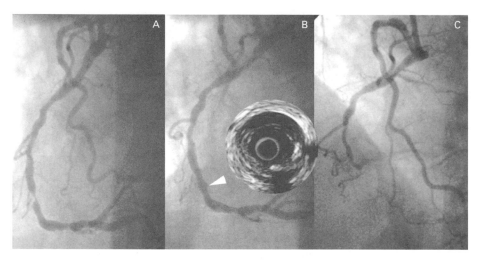

Figure 15-10.   Late thrombosis after balloon angioplasty and catheter-based brachytherapy. A. Target lesion on distal right coronary artery. B. IVUS imaging demonstrated a persistent submedial dissection at 6 months angiography. C. Thrombotic occlusion of the vessel at 8 months of follow-up.

phenomenon is genuinely associated with intracoronary radiation and more commonly with radioactive stent implantation (>6 μCi) in areas adjacent to the stent struts with radiation fall-off. In this subset of patients, the black hole was a dominant cause of restenosis, contributing to approximately 50% of the restenotic burden associated with neointimal hyperplasia seen at 6 month follow-up.[61] This relationship is less clear in patients treated with catheter-based radiation. Some atherectomy samples extracted from individuals with black holes after radiation therapy demonstrated the presence of myxoid, proteoglycan-rich matrix (mainly biglycan). It has been suggested that biglycan may contribute to the pathogenesis of atherosclerosis by trapping lipoproteins in the artery wall.[62] The long-term influence of this kind of lesions on the outcome of patients receiving

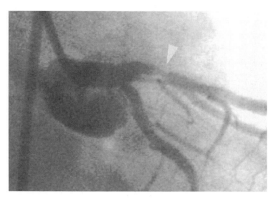 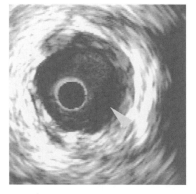

Figure 15-11.   Left panel: proximal edge restenosis after radioactive stent implantation (arrowhead). Right panel: IVUS appearance of a black hole (arrowhead) leading to restenosis at the proximal stent margin.

intracoronary radiation remains to be elucidated.

IVUS AND RADIATION DOSE CALCULATION

During intracoronary brachytherapy procedures, there may be a degree of dose non-homogeneity, which can have clinical implications. This phenomenon is inherent to the presence of a variable degree of vessel curvature, tortuosity, tapering, remodeling, and plaque extent and distribution. Further, the position of the radiation source in the lumen of a coronary segment is not fixed during the cardiac cycle and may vary in either axial or perpendicular direction during the dwell time. Finally, both the isotope (β- or γ-emitter) and the system used to deliver the radiation (centered or non-centered device, radioactive stent) may influence the dose distribution.

The dose delivered to the vessel wall may be calculated using the so-called dose-volume histograms.[63] This method condenses into a plot the information of the dose distribution data derived from IVUS analysis. In brief, radial distances (24 pie-slices, 15° for instance) from the center of the lumen (for centered systems) or from the IVUS probe (for non-centered system) to the lumen-intima and media-adventitia boundaries may be obtained from several equidistant cross-sectional areas within the irradiated coronary segment (every 0.2 mm, for instance). Given the prescribed dose, the type of isotope used and its activity at the time of the procedure, the dose received in those boundaries can be calculated and depicted as cumulative dose distribution over a specific volume. From this curve, the minimum dose received by 90 % of the adventitia or 90 % of the lumen can be also obtained (Fig. 15-12). Using dose-volume histograms, Carlier et al.[64] demonstrated in 23 patients enrolled in the BERT-1.5 trial that 90 % of the adventitial volume received only 37 % of the prescribed dose. By simulating a centering of the source and the use of a γ-emitter, this percentage of the dose received by the adventitia would increase to 49 % and 67 % of the prescribed dose, respectively. Further, in a subsegmental analysis of irradiated coronary segments by means of a non-centered device and the β-emitter ^{90}Sr/Y, the dose delivered to the

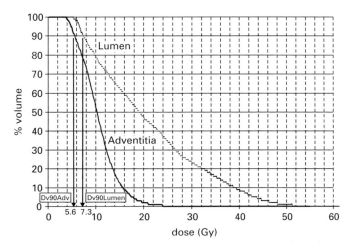

Figure 15-12. Dose-volume histogram of the cumulative dose received by the adventitia and lumen. From this histogram, the minimum dose received by 90 % of the adventitial (Dv90 adv) and luminal volumes (Dv90 lum) can be calculated.

adventitia appeared to vary considerably between subsegments, ranging from less than 2 Gy to 12 Gy. The delivered dose appeared to be an independent predictor of plaque volume at follow-up. This finding led to the conclusion that a minimum dose of 6 Gy had to be delivered to 90 % of the adventitia to be effective at 6 months of follow-up.[65] Another interesting finding derived from this accurate IVUS analysis was the fact that the type of plaque and amount of residual plaque burden were independent predictors of the plaque volume at follow-up in the irradiated segments. In brief, hard atherosclerotic plaques showed significantly less proliferation during the follow-up than soft plaques or segments with only intimal thickening at the time of the procedure.[65] The impact of vessel geometry on the response to radiation was further examined in the American series of patients treated with gamma radiation for in-stent restenosis.[66] In accordance with our previous findings,[65] maximum source-to-target distances (intravascular ultrasound catheter to external elastic membrane maximum distance), an elemental approach to dose measurement, significantly correlated with the change in minimum lumen area and the change in maximum intimal hyperplasia area.[66]

CONCLUSIONS

IVUS has been of the utmost importance in helping us to understand the pathophysiology of this new therapy and demonstrating its efficacy. Further, IVUS appears to be the gold standard for identifying the complications and limitations of intracoronary radiation therapy, as well as to accurately measure the dose delivered to the target site. Future development of new devices in the field of interventional cardiology has to take advantage of the knowledge emanated from IVUS in intracoronary brachytherapy in order to avoid repeating the same errors and to recognize or describe the new problems that these new techniques may originate.

REFERENCES

1. Holmes DR Jr, Vlietstra RE, Smith HC, et al. Restenosis after percutaneous transluminal coronary angioplasty (PTCA): a report from the PTCA Registry of the National Heart, Lung, and Blood Institute. *Am J Cardiol* 1984; 53:77C-81C.

2. Serruys PW, Luijten HE, Beatt KJ, et al. Incidence of restenosis after successful coronary angioplasty: a time-related phenomenon. A quantitative angiographic study in 342 consecutive patients at 1, 2, 3, and 4 months. *Circulation.* 1988; 77:361-371.

3. Schwartz RS, Holmes DR, Topol EJ. The restenosis paradigm revisited: an alternative proposal for cellular mechanisms. *J Am Coll Cardiol* 1992; 20:1284-1293.

4. Nobuyoshi M, Kimura T, Ohishi H, et al. Restenosis after percutaneous transluminal coronary angioplasty: pathologic observations in 20 patients. *J Am Coll Cardiol* 1991; 17:433-439.

5. Mintz GS, Popma JJ, Pichard AD, et al. Arterial remodeling after coronary angioplasty: a serial intravascular ultrasound study. *Circulation* 1996; 94:35-43.

6. MacLeod DC, Strauss BH, de Jong M, et al. Proliferation and extracellular matrix synthesis of smooth muscle cells cultured from human coronary atherosclerotic and restenotic lesions. *J Am Coll Cardiol* 1994; 23:59-65.

7. Guarda E, Katwa LC, Campbell SE, et al. Extracellular matrix collagen synthesis and degradation following coronary balloon angioplasty. *J Mol Cell Cardiol* 1996; 28:699-706.

8. Serruys PW, de Jaegere P, Kiemeneij F, et al. A comparison of balloon-expandable-stent implantation with balloon angioplasty in patients with coronary artery disease. Benestent Study Group. *N Engl J Med* 1994; 331:489-495.

9. Fischman DL, Leon MB, Baim DS, et al. A randomized comparison of coronary-stent placement and balloon angioplasty in the treatment of coronary artery disease. Stent Restenosis Study Investigators. *N Engl J Med* 1994; 331:496-501.

10. Haude M, Erbel R, Issa H, Meyer J. Quantitative analysis of elastic recoil after balloon

angioplasty and after intracoronary implantation of balloon-expandable Palmaz-Schatz stents. *J Am Coll Cardiol* 1993; 21:26-34.

11. Dussaillant GR, Mintz GS, Pichard AD, et al. Small stent size and intimal hyperplasia contribute to restenosis: a volumetric intravascular ultrasound analysis. *J Am Coll Cardiol* 1995; 26:720-724.

12. Sharma SK, Duvvuri S, Dangas G, et al. Rotational atherectomy for in-stent restenosis: acute and long-term results of the first 100 cases. *J Am Coll Cardiol* 1998; 32:1358-1365.

13. Eltchaninoff H, Koning R, Tron C, et al. Balloon angioplasty for the treatment of coronary in-stent restenosis: immediate results and 6-month angiographic recurrent restenosis rate. *J Am Coll Cardiol* 1998; 32:980-984.

14. Bauters C, Banos JL, Van Belle E, et al. Six-month angiographic outcome after successful repeat percutaneous intervention for in-stent restenosis. *Circulation* 1998; 97:318-321.

15. Kovalic JJ, Perez CA. Radiation therapy following keloidectomy: a 20-year experience. *Int J Radiat Oncol Biol Phys* 1989; 17:77-80.

16. Walter WL. Another look at pterygium surgery with postoperative beta radiation. *Ophthal Plast Reconstr Surg* 1994; 10:247-252.

17. Friedman M, Felton L, Byers S. The anti-atherogenic effect of iridium192 upon the cholesterol-fed rabbit. *J Clin Invest* 1964; 43:185-192.

18. Liermann D, Bottcher HD, Kollath J, et al. Prophylactic endovascular radiotherapy to prevent intimal hyperplasia after stent implantation in femoropopliteal arteries. *Cardiovasc Intervent Radiol* 1994; 17:12-16.

19. Wiedermann JG, Marboe C, Amols H, et al.: Intracoronary irradiation markedly reduces neointimal proliferation after balloon angioplasty in swine: persistent benefit at 6-month follow-up. *J Am Coll Cardiol* 1995; 25:1451-1456.

20. Waksman R, Robinson KA, Crocker IR, et al.: Intracoronary low-dose beta-irradiation inhibits neointima formation after coronary artery balloon injury in the swine restenosis model. *Circulation* 1995; 92:3025-3031.

21. Mazur W, Ali MN, Khan MM, et al. High dose rate intracoronary radiation for inhibition of neointimal formation in the stented and balloon-injured porcine models of restenosis: angiographic, morphometric, and histopathologic analyses. *Int J Radiat Oncol Biol Phys* 1996; 36:777-788.

22. Verin V, Popowski Y, Urban P, et al. Intraarterial beta-irradiation prevents neointimal hyperplasia in a hypercholesterolemic rabbit restenosis model. *Circulation* 1995; 92:2284-2290.

23. Waksman R. *Vascular Brachytherapy, 2nd ed.* Armonk, New York: Futura Publishing Co.; 1999.

24. Condado JA, Waksman R, Gurdiel O, et al. Long-term angiographic and clinical outcome after percutaneous transluminal coronary angioplasty and intracoronary radiation therapy in humans. *Circulation* 1997; 96:727-732.

25. Verin V, Urban P, Popowski Y, et al. Feasibility of intracoronary beta-irradiation to reduce restenosis after balloon angioplasty. A clinical pilot study. *Circulation* 1997; 95:1138-1144.

26. Teirstein PS, Massullo V, Jani S, et al.: Catheter-based radiotherapy to inhibit restenosis after coronary stenting. *N Engl J Med* 1997; 336:1697-1703.

27. Waksman R, White L, Chan R, et al. Intracoronary radiation therapy after angioplasty inhibits recurrence in patients with in-stent restenosis. *Circulation* 2000; 101:2165-2171.

28. Leon MB, Teirstein PS, Moses JW, et al. Localized intracoronary gamma-radiation therapy to inhibit the recurrence of restenosis after stenting. *N Engl J Med* 2001; 344:250-256.

29. Waksman R, Bhargava B, White LR, et al. Intracoronary beta-radiation therapy inhibits recurrence of in-stent restenosis. *Circulation* 2000; 101:1895-1898.

30. Popma JJ, Sumtharalingam M, Lansky AJ, et al. Randomized trial of ^{90}Sr/^{90}Y β-radiation versus placebo control for treatment of in-stent restenosis. *Circulation* 2002; 106:1090-1096.

31. Waksman R, Raizmer AL, Yeung AC, Lansky AJ, Vandortriel L. Use of localised intracoronary β-radiation in treatment of in-stent restenosis: the INHIBIT randomised controlled trial. *Lancet* 2002; 359:551-557.

32. Verin V, Popowski Y, de Bruyne B, et al. Endoluminal beta-radiation therapy for the prevention of coronary restenosis after balloon angioplasty. *N Engl J Med* 2001; 344: 243-249.

33. Kuntz RE. Clinical and angiographic outcomes after use of Sr-90 beta-radiation for the treatment of de novo and restenotic coronary lesions: Results from the Betacath study. *J Am Coll Cardiol* 2001; (abstract).

34. Albiero R, Adamian M, Kobayashi N, et al. Short- and intermediate-term results of 32P radioactive beta-emitting stent implantation in patients with coronary artery disease. The Milan dose-response study. *Circulation* 2000; 101:18-26.

35. King SB III, Williams DO, Chogule P, et al. Endovascular beta-radiation to reduce restenosis after coronary balloon angioplasty. Results of the Beta Energy Restenosis Trial (BERT). *Circulation* 1998; 97:2025-2030.

36. Sabaté M, Serruys PW, van der Giessen WJ, et al. Geometric vascular remodeling after balloon angioplasty and betaradiation therapy: a three-dimensional intravascular ultrasound study. *Circulation* 1999; 100:1182-1188.

37. Costa M, Sabaté M, Serrano P, et al. The effect of 32P beta-radiotherapy on both vessel remodeling and neointimal hyperplasia after coronary balloon angioplasty and stenting. A three-dimensional intravascular ultrasound investigation. *J Invasive Cardiol* 2000; 12:113-120.

38. Kay IP, Sabaté M, Costa M, et al.: Positive geometric vascular remodeling is seen after catheter-based radiation followed by conventional stent implantation, but not after radioactive stent implantation. *Circulation* 2000; 102:1434-1439.

39. Ahmed JM, Mintz GS, Waksman R, et al. Serial intravascular ultrasound assessment of the efficacy of intracoronary gamma-radiation therapy for preventing recurrence in very long, diffuse, in-stent restenosis lesions. *Circulation* 2001; 104:856-xxx.

40. Mintz GS, Weissman NJ, Teirstein PS et al. Effect of intracoronary gamma radiation therapy on in-stent restenosis: an intravascular ultrasound analysis from the Gamma-1 Study. *Circulation* 2000; 102:2915-2918.

41. Bal ET, Plokker T, van den Berg EMJ, et al. Predictability and prognosis of PTCA-induced coronary aneurysms. *Cathet Cardiovasc Diagn* 1991; 22:85-88.

42. Sabaté M, Serruys PW, van der Giessen WJ, et al. Coronary aneurysm after endovascular brachytherapy: true or false? *Circulation* 2000; 102:e121 (letter to the editor).

43. Schwartz RS, Huber KC, Murphy JG, et al. Restenosis and proportional neointimal response to coronary artery injury: results in a porcine model. *J Am Coll Cardiol* 1992; 19:267-274.

44. Weinberger J, Amols H, Ennis RD, et al. Intracoronary irradiation: dose response for prevention of restenosis in swine. *Int J Rad Oncol Biol Phys* 1996; 36:767-775.

45. Sabaté M, Costa MA, Kozuma K, et al. Geographic miss: a cause of treatment failure in radio-oncology applied to intracoronary radiation therapy. *Circulation* 2000; 101:2467-2471.

46. Paterson R: *The Treatment of Malignant Disease by Radiotherapy.* London, UK: Edward Arnold Publishers; 1963.

47. Ahmed JM, Mintz GM, Waksman R, et al. Serial intravascular ultrasound analysis of edge recurrence after intracoronary gamma radiation treatment of native artery in-stent restenosis lesions. *Am J Cardiol* 2001; 87:1145- 1149.

48. Kozuma K, Costa MA, Sabaté M, et al. Three-dimensional ultrasound assessment of non-injured edges of betairradiated coronary segments. *Circulation* 2000; 102: 1484-1489.

49. Pötter R, van Limbergen E, Dries W, et al. Recommendations of the EVA GEC ESTRO Working Group: prescribing, recording, and reporting in endovascular brachytherapy. Quality assurance, equipment, personnel and education. *Radiother Oncol* 2001; 59:339-360.

50. Albiero R, Nishida T, Wardeh AJ et al. Final results of the hot ends 32P radioactive beta-emitting stent implantation in patients with CAD. The Milan and Rotterdam experience (abstract): *J Am Coll Cardiol* 2001; 37:1A-648A.

51. Wardeh AJ, Albiero R, Kay IP, et al. Angiographic follow-up after 32P beta-emitting radioactive cold ends isostent implantation. Results from Aalst, Milan and Rotterdam.

52. Wardeh AJ, Knook AHM, Regar E, et al. Square shouldered balloons. The final op-

tion to prevent edge restenosis after radioactive stent implantation (abstract). *J Am Coll Cardiol* 2001; 37:1A-648A.

53. Colombo A, Hall P, Nakamura S, et al.: Intracoronary stenting without anticoagulation accomplished with intravascular ultrasound guidance. *Circulation* 1995; 91:1676-1688.

54. Costa M, Sabaté M, van der Giessen WJ, et al.: Late coronary occlusion after intracoronary brachytherapy. *Circulation* 1999; 100:789-792.

55. Waksman R, Bhargava B, Mintz GS, et al. Late total occlusion after intracoronary brachytherapy for patients with in-stent restenosis. *J Am Coll Cardiol* 2000; 36:65-68.

56. Farb A, Tang A, Virmani R: The neointima is reduced but endothelialization is incomplete 3 months after 32P beta-emitting stent placement [abstract]. *Circulation* 1998; 98(suppl I):I-770.

57. Sabaté M, van der Giessen WJ, Deshpande NV, et al. Late thrombotic occlusion of a malapposed stent 10 months after intracoronary brachytherapy. *Int J Cardiovasc Interv* 1999; 2:55-59.

58. Kozuma K, Costa MA, Sabaté M, et al. Late stent malapposition occurring after intracoronary beta-irradiation detected by intravascular ultrasound. *J Invas Cardiol* 1999; 11:651-655.

59. Kay IP, Sabaté M, van Langenhove G: The outcome from balloon-induced coronary artery dissection after intracoronary beta-radiation. *Heart* 2000; 83:332-337.

60. Meerkin D, Tardif JC, Bertrand OF, et al. The effects of intracoronary brachytherapy on the natural history of postangioplasty dissections. *J Am Coll Cardiol* 2000; 36:59-64.

61. Kay IP, Ligthart JMR, Virmani R, et al. The black-hole: echo-lucent tissue observed following intracoronary radiation. *Eur Heart J* 2002; (in press).

62. O'Brien KD, Olin KL, Alpers CE, et al. Comparison of apolipoprotein and proteoglycan deposits in human coronary atherosclerotic plaques. Colocalization of biglycan with apolipoproteins. *Circulation* 1998; 98:519-527.

63. Drzymala RE, Mohan R, Brewster L, et al. Dose-volume histograms. *Int J Radiat Oncol Biol Phys* 1991; 21:71-78.

64. Carlier SG, Marijnissen JPA, Coen VLMA, et al. Comparison of brachytherapy strategies based on dose-volume histograms derived from quantitative intravascular ultrasound. *Cardiovasc Radiat Med* 1999; 1:115-124.

65. Sabaté M, Marijnissen JPA, Carlier SG, et al. Residual plaque burden, delivered dose and tissue composition predict the 6-month outcome after balloon angioplasty and beta-radiation therapy. *Circulation* 2000; 101:2472-2477.

66. Ahmed JM, Mintz GS, Waksman R, et al. Serial intravascular analysis of the impact of lesion length on the efficacy of intracoronary gamma-irradiation for preventing recurrent in-stent restenosis. *Circulation* 2001; 103:188-191.

16

Diagnostic and Therapeutic Ultrasound Application for Interventional Cardiology: From Current Practice to Future Potential

Peter J. Fitzgerald, MD

Introduction. Diagnostic application of intravascular ultrasound. Stent optimization. Drug eluting stent. Detection of vulnerable plaque. Therapeutic application of intravascular ultrasound. Intravascular sonotheraphy. Application of intravascular ultrasound for chronic total occlusion. Therapeutic application of extravascular ultrasound. Augmentation of pharmacolofical trombolysis. Application of ultrasound for vascular closure device. References

INTRODUCTION

Over the past decade, ultrasound technology has been broadly applied to the practical setting in interventional cardiology, mainly as an intravascular diagnostic tool. With its ability to visualize the details of coronary atherosclerosis, intravascular ultrasound (IVUS) is currently well accepted as a diagnostic tool for the evaluation of coronary artery disease and often plays a critical role in optimizing the acute results of coronary interventions. Furthermore, recent advancements in ultrasound technology have further broadened ultrasound applications into the therapeutic domain, offering another treatment modality to the field of interventional cardiology.

DIAGNOSTIC APPLICATION OF INTRAVASCULAR ULTRASOUND

Stent Optimization

As the concept of «bigger is better» regarding luminal dimension has gained ac-

ceptance to reduce in-stent restenosis after bare metal stent deployment, IVUS-guided stenting, which enables precise examination inside the treated vessel, has become a more accepted practice to optimize stent deployment. With IVUS, valuable information regarding inadequate stent deployment can be obtained during the stent procedure.[1,2] Figure 16-1 illustrates potential observations of inadequate stent deployment that are better visualized with IVUS than angiography. Incomplete stent expansion occurs when some portions of the stented segment are not adequately expanded compared to the proximal and distal reference segments. Since final minimal lumen area (or minimal stent area) immediately after bare metal stenting is the most powerful predictor of subsequent instent restenosis,[3,4] the diagnosis of incomplete stent expansion is critical for optimizing stent deployment and determining additional stent expansion with larger balloon(s) or higher inflation pressures. Incomplete stent apposition refers to the situation in which more than one stent strut is clearly separated from the vessel wall, with evidence of blood speckles behind the stent at the site

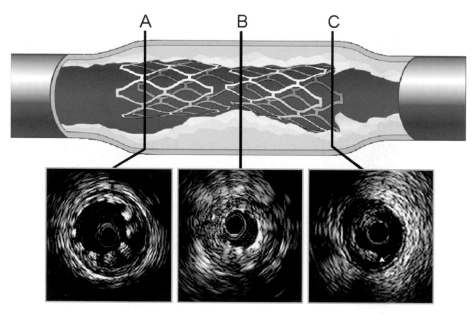

Figure 16-1. IVUS-detected problems with stent deployment. A: Incomplete apposition. B: Incomplete expansion. C: Edge dissection (indicated by white arrow). (Adapted from Honda, et al. Topol textbook of interventional cardiology 4th edition. 893-917.)

without side branch involvement. Immediately after stenting, this condition may be seen with incomplete stent expansion or inadequate stent size selection. IVUS can also detect edge dissection or the magnitude of the reference disease, both of which may impact the subsequent development of adverse cardiac event(s) and restenosis after stenting.[1] Preinterventional IVUS may also determine the range that needs to be covered by the stent and stent size selection, thereby minimizing vessel injury.

Drug Eluting Stent

Current results of European and U.S. clinical trials regarding drug-eluting stent enthusiastically support the potential of this new device as the most effective approach to preventing in-stent restenosis.[5-8] As shown in Figure 16-2, since the main cause of in-stent restenosis, intimal hyperplasia, is

better visualized with IVUS than with angiography, IVUS has played a major role examining the effects of various drugs on neointimal suppression by providing information for calculating both volumetric and cross-sectional intimal and lumen parameters. Also, several reports regarding IVUS follow-up of drug-eluting stents have suggested the late development of incomplete apposition, characterized by the vessel wall moving away from the stent struts, accompanied by vessel expansion during the follow-up period.[9] Although the exact clinical impact of late incomplete apposition is still not clear, it may be important to regularly evaluate vessel dimensions as well as neointimal growth over a longer follow-up period. In addition, IVUS should also be useful to optimize drug-eluting stent deployment. For instance, despite the dramatic reduction of restenosis inside the stented segment, the development of persistent edge stenosis still remains to be solved. Although

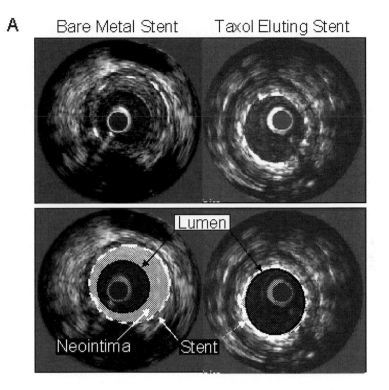

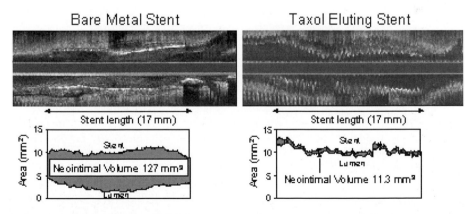

Figure 16-2.   Representative cases of bare-metal and drug-eluting stents. A: Cross-sectional IVUS images at 6 months of follow-up demonstrate abundant neointimal hyperplasia in bare metal stent versus minimal neointimal hyperplasia in a 7-hexanoyltaxol-eluting stent. B: Longitudinal reconstruction of IVUS images at 6 months of follow-up. Exaggerated neointimal hyperplasia is observed in bare metal stent, whereas the 7-hexanoyltaxol-eluting stent shows distinct inhibition of neointimal growth along the entire stented segment. (Adapted with modifications from Kataoka, et al. Circulation. 2002; 106: 1788-1793).

the exact mechanism involved is unclear, stent edge injury or residual persistent disease may be related to persistent edge stenosis after drug-eluting stent implantation. In this regard, using IVUS to precisely evaluate vessel size and lesion length prior to drug-eluting stent selection and implantation may minimize these potential causes of edge stenosis. Furthermore, complete stent strut apposition to the vessel wall is critical for adequate drug delivery to the vessel wall. Thus, the evaluation of stent strut apposition after stent deployment may be useful in maximizing the effect of this device.

Detection of Vulnerable Plaque

Vulnerable plaque, which consists of an atheromatous plaque core covered by a thin fibrous cap with ongoing inflammation, is now generally considered as a major cause of acute coronary syndrome. As this type of plaque may develop without luminal narrowing, it is possible that arterial segments that appear relatively undiseased by angiography are more prone to the development of vulnerable plaque.[10] The detection of vulnerable plaque by IVUS involves contrasting between two heterogeneous tissue types. Although conventional IVUS is an effective technique for producing structural component images of the arterial wall, the disadvantages of limited resolution ($110 \ \mu m$)[11] or acoustic shadowing caused by superficial calcification[12] may limit the characterization of the vessel wall composition. Accordingly, alternative approaches to using ultrasound, such as radiofrequency intravascular ultrasound (IVUS-RF) or IVUS elastography, are

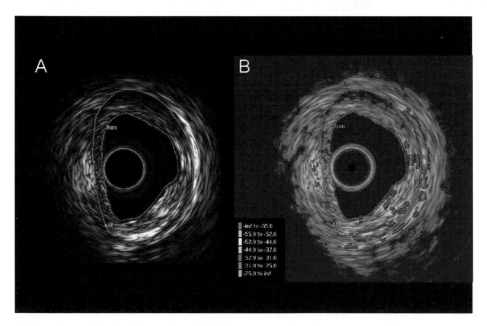

Figure 16-3. Example of a conventional IVUS image (A) and a parametric image based on radiofrequency IVUS (IVUS-RF) data (B). A superimposed color-mapping scheme in the parametric image can be used to display any of several quantitative parameters, calculated in small regions of interest throughout the entire image. In the example shown, the color of each pixel reflects the backscatter intensity (BI) of a small region surrounding the pixel relative to the BI detected from a reflection off a steel plate. The backscatter intensity is calculated in the frequency domain. Low-intensity regions, which may reflect increased lipid content, are assigned dark red colors, while high-intensity regions, which represent fibrous tissue and/or calcium, are presented as bright blue colors.

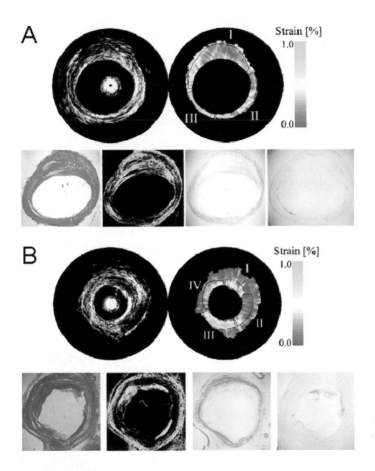

Figure 16-4. Examples of cases of IVUS elastography. IVUS image (top left) and elastogram (top right) of diseased human femoral artery with corresponding histology: (bottom row, left to right) picro-Sirius red, picro-Sirius red with polarized light microscopy, anti-actin, and anti-CD-68 antibody. A: Original image reveals eccentric plaque (region I). Elastogram reveals low strain in plaque (0.24 %), similar strain in undiseased vessel wall between 3 and 7 o'clock positions (0.32 %), and high strain in vessel wall between 7 and 9 o'clock positions (0.96 %). Histology reveals fibrous composition of plaque (bottom row, first 2 panels on left). Region with high strain contains fatty foam cells at lumen-vessel wall boundary and increased macrophage activity (bottom row, far right). B: Echogram shows concentric plaque with different echogenicities for regions. Elastogram reveals 2 soft regions (region I and region III) and 2 harder regions (region II and region IV). Histology shows that 2 soft regions contain fatty material and 2 harder regions contain mainly fibrous material. The macrophage concentration is also increased in soft regions. (Adapted with modification from de Korte CL, et al. *Circulation.* 2000;102:617-623.

currently under development to further identify lipid, collagen, and cellular infiltrates within plaques.

Radiofrequency Intravascular Ultrasound (IVUS-RF): IVUS-RF has advantages over conventional IVUS in the identification of vulnerable plaque components. Conventional IVUS supplies grayscale imaging that is sometimes unable to accurately distinguish plaque components such as a lipid core and fibro-fatty atheroma. On the other hand, IVUS-RF grossly discriminates between early lesions and advanced lesions with high sensitivity and specificity (Figure 16-3).[13] Since RF data use a raw digitized ultrasound signal, frequency-based analyses rely less on subjective interpretation than conventional IVUS. The normalized signal power provides objective indices over the entire frequency bandwidth to better predict the likely presence of a vulnerable plaque.[14]

Attenuation of the ultrasound signal occurs as a factor of the distance of the region of interest (ROI) from the catheter. Furthermore, artery wall tissue between the lumen and ROI can attenuate the signal. Despite some signal losses, however, IVUS-RF provides relatively clear discrimination between plaque components.[14]

IVUS Elastography: Since IVUS displays less sensitivity and selectivity for detecting a lipid core, it benefits from complementary technology to characterize plaque components. Intravascular elastography uses an IVUS echogram system and a pressure differential to distinguish between hard and soft tissue under the premise that soft material displays more radial strain than harder material under a given force. Furthermore, marked differences in average strain exist among fibrous tissue, fibro-fatty tissue, and fatty tissue, with strain values increasing for each respective group as marked by histology (Figure 16-4).[15] Such subtle differences are not discriminated in independent IVUS echogram images. Thus, since it is possible to discriminate between lipid-rich and fibrous tissue according to strain values, vulnerable plaques may be identified by elastography. Finally, a thin fibrous cap and collagen destruction by macrophages may be identified by increased strain on the elastogram (Figure 16-4).[16]

One of the greatest advantages of IVUS elastography is that the instruments are currently available for clinical application. For an IVUS elastogram, two IVUS echograms are needed at two intraluminal pressures. Therefore, an IVUS elastogram requires only an IVUS catheter and a pressure sensor.[15] Furthermore, in contrast with the IVUS echogram apparatus, no additional processing is necessary. Hence, IVUS elastography may serve as a useful complementary tool to conventional IVUS to mechanically discriminate plaque components.

THERAPEUTIC APPLICATION OF INTRAVASCULAR ULTRASOUND

Intravascular Sonotherapy

Previous studies using cell cultures have shown that high-energy ultrasound has a direct physiologic impact on cell viability, migration, and adhesion, thereby leading to a reduction of cellular proliferation.[17, 18] Based upon these results, the concept of intravascular sonotherapy (IST) to inhibit vascular smooth muscle cell proliferation was introduced.

One IST system (URX, PharmaSonics Inc., Sunnyvale, CA) has recently been developed and introduced into clinical evaluation. Presently, two types of IST catheters are available for the treatment of peripheral and coronary lesions. The catheters incorporate single or multiple cylindrical ultrasonic transducers operating in a pulsed mode at a center frequency of 700 KHz (8 Fr peripheral) or 1 MHz (5 Fr coronary). In the preliminary animal studies using a swine femoral and coronary artery stent model, IST demonstrated feasible neointimal reduction as compared to a control group.[19, 20] Furthermore, one animal study using IST for a coronary stent model showed no evidence of thrombi as well as complete endothelialization on the surface of implanted stents at 180 days.

On the basis of these favorable preclinical data, several human trials have been initiated in the United States and Europe. However, despite favorable preclinical results, the results of the SILENT and EuroSPAH trials recently reported failed to demonstrate the superiority of IST over the control group in terms of clinical outcome.

Application of Intravascular Ultrasound for Chronic Total Occlusion

The ability to deliver high-frequency mechanical energy to the tip of an endovascular catheter has demonstrated initial feasibility in the recanalization of vascular occlusions.[21] One method of generating mechanical energy is to use an external ultrasound transducer to create, amplify, and transmit energy through an internal wire in a specially designed catheter (Figure 16-5). The energy is propagated to the tip of the catheter through a compression wave and vibrates the tip of the catheter at the frequency range of 20-40 kHz. These vibrations created at the catheter tip have notable effects on vascular obstructions. Methods of action include the creation of tiny microbubbles, commonly referred to as cavitation, and mechanical impact. When applied to the occlusion, the forces created by these effects cause a change in occlusion compliance, thus facilitating the passage of obstructive material (usually comprised of organized fibrotic tissue impregnated with

calcium) using standard guidewire techniques.

Recent improvements in catheter design have led to the development of more flexible catheters capable of withstanding a wide range of energies without whipping, material stress, and fatigue. Catheter optimization has allowed the use of two energy modes with a single catheter design. Two modes thought to be beneficial in the recanalization of vascular occlusions are pulsed mode (50% duty cycle) and continuous mode. Pulsed-mode provides more displacement of the catheter tip and allows more energy to be applied through the catheter without increasing stress on the catheter structure. Continuous mode results in a more frequent, but lower, mechanical displacement. The continuous mode is thought to be more useful in fibrotic occlusions, whereas pulsed mode has demonstrated superior ablating efficiency in calcified occlusions.

THERAPEUTIC APPLICATION OF EXTRAVASCULAR ULTRASOUND

Augmentation of Pharmacological Thrombolysis

Early initiation of coronary thrombolysis has been proved to reduce mortality and pre-

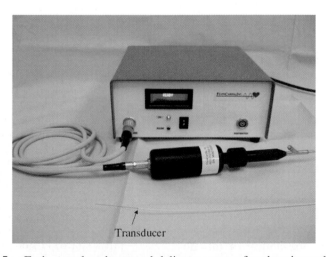

Figure 16-5. Endovascular ultrasound delivery system for chronic total occlusion.

serve ventricular function in myocardial infarction. However, the effect of this treatment is limited by the frequency of success and bleeding complications. Low-frequency ultrasound has been suggested to facilitate clot lysis in the absence of heat production with a minimal mechanical effect on the clot, both *in vitro* and *in vivo*, using animal peripheral arteries.[22-24] Accordingly, a noninvasive transthoracic ultrasound device is currently being developed to augment the effect of pharmacological coronary arterial thrombolysis. This device, with low-frequency ultrasound (27 kHz), can be applied to the anterior chest wall while an intravenous thrombolytic drug is administered simultaneously. In fact, one animal study of a canine coronary thrombotic occlusion demonstrated the potential benefit of this device for augmentation of pharmacological thombolysis.[25] Based on these favorable pre-clinical results, clinical trials are currently underway.

Application of Ultrasound for Vascular Closure Device

Another application of externally applied ultrasound is wound closure. This technology has matured into a defense application for the external application of ultrasound for acoustic hemostasis. Thus, this technology may be directly applied for the closure of femoral arteries in the catheterization laboratory. One device currently under development enables external ultrasound to be precisely focused on the targeted pinhole component at the puncture sight. Furthermore, by allowing the interaction between the sheath and vascular puncture sight to be visualized, this device allows one to precisely target the ultrasound energy. A few seconds of ultrasound application generates enough heat to cause vessel and adventitial bonding, thus producing a quick and efficient vascular closure. Unlike other mechanical or sealing technologies, the ability of this device to visualize the femoral puncture site

and its potential as a second application further broaden the use of this technology either in the holding room or on the patient ward. Although the equipment capital is somewhat dependent on a miniaturized ultrasound system, this technology has also seen significant digital miniaturization over the past few years. Combining the precise visualization of the puncture site, the use of focused ultrasound for vessel closure may be effective in the catheterization laboratory for quick and proper wound sealing at the puncture site. This device also should be welcome in our day-to-day practice, specifically in settings involving aggressive antiplatelet therapy.

REFERENCES

1. Honda Y, Fitzgerald PJ, Yock PG. Intravascular Ultrasound. *Topol Textbook of Interventional Cardiology 4th edition* 2002:893-917.

2. Takahashi T, Honda Y, Russo RJ, Fitzgerald PJ. Intravascular ultrasound and quantitative coronary angiography. *Catheter Cardiovasc Interv* 2002; 55:118-128.

3. Hoffmann R, Mintz GS, Mehran R, Pichard AD, Kent KM, Satler LF, Popma JJ, Wu H, Leon MB. Intravascular ultrasound predictors of angiographic restenosis in lesions treated with Palmaz-Schatz stents. *J Am Coll Cardiol* 1998; 31:43-49.

4. Kasaoka S, Tobis JM, Akiyama T, Reimers B, Di Mario C, Wong ND, Colombo A. Angiographic and intravascular ultrasound predictors of in-stent restenosis. *J Am Coll Cardiol* 1998; 32:1630-1635.

5. Leon MB, Moses JW, Popma JJ, Fishell T, Wong SC, Midei M, Douglas J, Lambert C, Mooney M, Teirstein P, Kuntz R. A Multicenter Randomized Clinical Study of the Sirolimus-Eluting Stent in Native Coronary Lesions: Angiographic Results (abstract). *Circulation* 2002; 106(Suppl II):II-392.

6. Kataoka T, Grube E, Honda Y, Morino Y, Hur SH, Bonneau HN, Colombo A, Di Mario C, Guagliumi G, Hauptmann KE, Pitney MR, Lansky AJ, Stertzer SH, Yock PG, Fitzgerald PJ. 7-hexanoyltaxol-eluting stent for prevention of neointimal growth: an in-

travascular ultrasound analysis from the Study to COmpare REstenosis rate between QueST and QuaDS-QP2 (SCORE). *Circulation* 2002; 106:1788-1793.

7. Regar E, Serruys PW, Bode C, Holubarsch C, Guermonprez JL, Wijns W, Bartorelli A, Constantini C, Degertekin M, Tanabe K, Disco C, Wuelfert E, Morice MC. Angiographic findings of the multicenter Randomized Study With the Sirolimus-Eluting Bx Velocity Balloon-Expandable Stent (RAVEL): sirolimus-eluting stents inhibit restenosis irrespective of the vessel size. *Circulation* 2002; 106:1949-1956.

8. Degertekin M, Serruys PW, Foley DP, Tanabe K, Regar E, Vos J, Smits PC, van der Giessen WJ, van den Brand M, de Feyter P, Popma JJ. Persistent inhibition of neointimal hyperplasia after sirolimus-eluting stent implantation: long-term (up to 2 years) clinical, angiographic, and intravascular ultrasound follow-up. *Circulation* 2002; 106:1610-1613.

9. Serruys PW, Degertekin M, Tanabe K, Abizaid A, Sousa JE, Colombo A, Guagliumi G, Wijns W, Lindeboom WK, Ligthart J, de Feyter PJ, Morice MC. Intravascular ultrasound findings in the multicenter, randomized, double-blind RAVEL (RAndomized study with the sirolimus-eluting VElocity balloon-expandable stent in the treatment of patients with de novo native coronary artery Lesions) trial. *Circulation* 2002; 106:798-803.

10. Kinlay S. What has intravascular ultrasound taught us about plaque biology? *Curr Atheroscler Rep* 2001; 3:260-266.

11. Patwari P, Weissman NJ, Boppart SA, Jesser C, Stamper D, Fujimoto JG, Brezinski ME. Assessment of coronary plaque with optical coherence tomography and high-frequency ultrasound. *Am J Cardiol* 2000; 85:641-644.

12. Jang IK, Bouma BE, Kang DH, Park SJ, Park SW, Seung KB, Choi KB, Shishkov M, Schlendorf K, Pomerantsev E, Houser SL, Aretz HT, Tearney GJ. Visualization of coronary atherosclerotic plaques in patients using optical coherence tomography: comparison with intravascular ultrasound. *J Am Coll Cardiol* 2002; 39:604-609.

13. Komiyama N, Berry GJ, Kolz ML, Oshima A, Metz JA, Preuss P, Brisken AF, Pauliina Moore M, Yock PG, Fitzgerald PJ. Tissue characterization of atherosclerotic plaques by intravascular ultrasound radiofrequency signal analysis: an in vitro study of human coronary arteries. *Am Heart J* 2000; 140:565-574.

14. Stahr PM, Hofflinghaus T, Voigtlander T, Courtney BK, Victor A, Otto M, Yock PG, Brennecke R, Fitzgerald PJ. Discrimination of early/intermediate and advanced/complicated coronary plaque types by radiofrequency intravascular ultrasound analysis. *Am J Cardiol* 2002; 90:19-23.

15. de Korte CL, Pasterkamp G, van der Steen AF, Woutman HA, Bom N. Characterization of plaque components with intravascular ultrasound elastography in human femoral and coronary arteries in vitro. *Circulation* 2000; 102:617-623.

16. de Korte CL, Sierevogel MJ, Mastik F, Strijder C, Schaar JA, Velema E, Pasterkamp G, Serruys PW, van der Steen AF. Identification of atherosclerotic plaque components with intravascular ultrasound elastography in vivo: a Yucatan pig study. *Circulation* 2002; 105:1627-1630.

17. Lejbkowicz F, Zwiran M, Salzberg S. The response of normal and malignant cells to ultrasound in vitro. *Ultrasound Med Biol* 1993; 19:75-82.

18. Alter A, Rozenszajn LA, Miller HI, Rosenschein U. Ultrasound inhibits the adhesion and migration of smooth muscle cells in vitro. *Ultrasound Med Biol* 1998; 24:711-721.

19. Fitzgerald PJ, Takagi A, Moore MP, Hayase M, Kolodgie FD, Corl D, Nassi M, Virmani R, Yock PG. Intravascular sonotherapy decreases neointimal hyperplasia after stent implantation in swine. *Circulation* 2001; 103:1828-1831.

20. Post MJ, Moore P, Menahem N, Bao J, Virmani R, Kolodgi FD, Corl D, Kuntz RE. Intravascular sonotherapy prevents intimal hyperplasia in a coronary stent pig model without long term adverse effects (abstract). *Circulation* 2000; 102(Suppl II):II-733.

21. Cannon LA, John J, LaLonde J. Therapeutic ultrasound for chronic total coronary artery occlusions. *Echocardiography* 2001; 18:219-223.

22. Suchkova V, Siddiqi FN, Carstensen EL,

Dalecki D, Child S, Francis CW. Enhancement of fibrinolysis with 40-kHz ultrasound. *Circulation* 1998; 98:1030-1035.

23. Riggs PN, Francis CW, Bartos SR, Penney DP. Ultrasound enhancement of rabbit femoral artery thrombolysis. *Cardiovasc Surg* 1997; 5:201-207.

24. Birnbaum Y, Luo H, Nagai T, Fishbein MC, Peterson TM, Li S, Kricsfeld D, Porter TR, Siegel RJ. Noninvasive in vivo clot dissolution without a thrombolytic drug: recanalization of thrombosed iliofemoral arteries by transcutaneous ultrasound combined with intravenous infusion of microbubbles. *Circulation* 1998; 97:130-134.

25. Siegel RJ, Atar S, Fishbein MC, Brasch AV, Peterson TM, Nagai T, Pal D, Nishioka T, Chae JS, Birnbaum Y, Zanelli C, Luo H. Noninvasive, transthoracic, low-frequency ultrasound augments thrombolysis in a canine model of acute myocardial infarction. *Circulation* 2000; 101:2026-2029.

SECTION III

Intracardiac and Great Vessels Ultrasound

fitted at the proximal end of the catheter and provides a 360° field of view, perpendicular to the axis around which it turns, with a radius of about 4 cm. The main disadvantage of catheters with mechanical transducers is that they need to be purged with distilled water injected through the tip of the catheter. The entry orifice produced by the needle facilitates the entry of blood into the transducer chamber, particularly if the catheter has to be purged more than once, which may affect image quality. In addition, if the catheter curves in excess, the image may be lost when the rotor stops. Even so, most of the work in ICE has been carried out with these catheters.

The second system uses a 10 F catheter (Acuson Corporation; Mountain View, California) with a «phased array» technology comprising 64 elements with electronically controlled frequencies ranging from 5.5 to 10 MHz. It can be aligned in four directions and two planes to offer 90° sections with a penetration of up to 15 cm.[10-12]

Both catheters are usually inserted into the right femoral vein using a pre-formed sheath and are connected to a console (either a conventional or a dedicated ICE console) to provide real-time two-dimensional images of the cardiac structures and any other devices or catheters located inside the heart. Comparatively, catheters with «phased array» technology allow greater depth of field and may be used to obtain Doppler images (in color, continuous, pulsed, and tissue imaging), whereas mechanical technology has a better resolution.

Thanks to post-processing of the images, investigators have recently begun to study the three-dimensional echocardiographic reconstruction of the different chambers of the heart.

CLINICAL APPLICATIONS OF INTRACARDIAC ECHOCARDIOGRAPHY

ICE requires insertion of the catheter, generally into a vein. This is why it is per-formed in interventional cardiology laboratories, where its usefulness has been demonstrated.

Intracardiac Echocardiography in Congenital Heart Disease

One of the most frequent congenital heart diseases is atrial septal defect. Over the last few years various devices have been designed to close these defects without surgery. These devices are also used to close patent foramen ovale in patients with cerebrovascular accidents in which the suspected cause could be a paradoxical embolism. ICE has been shown to be a very effective technique for viewing the defect, analyzing its characteristics, and studying its relationship with neighboring cardiac structures.[13-15] This information helps to ensure the correct insertion of the percutaneous closure device and to optimize its position.

Usefulness of Intracardiac Echocardiography in Electrophysiology

In the last 10 years, therapeutic electrophysiology has succeeded in treating most cardiac arrhythmias, thanks to ablation using a radiofrequency catheter. The ablation sites are located using the radiological position of the catheters and local electrograms as reference points. ICE is useful in reducing fluoroscopy times. Although new mapping methods have been introduced to eliminate the need for fluoroscopy, the X-ray exposure time during ablation procedures is still very long.[16] The images obtained by ICE make it possible to view the position of the catheters in relation to fluoroscopically invisible anatomical structures (such as the crista terminalis or fossa ovalis), and the point of contact between the ablation electrode and underlying cardiac tissue[16-27] (Fig. 17-1). In addition, certain complications, such as pericardial effusion secondary to cardiac perforation or the formation of intracavitary thrombi, can be detected immediately.[23] In these circumstances, early diagnosis is a key to preventing further complications.

Generally speaking, catheters can be viewed with ICE, although the technique still cannot differentiate between various catheters placed inside a cardiac chamber. The ablation catheter can be distinguished because it has a distal electrode that is generally larger than the other mapping electrodes. An ultrasound beam emitted toward the ablation catheter produces a characteristic triangular echogenic shadow that indicates the exact position of the distal electrode (Fig. 17-1). This allows the point of contact between the ablation catheter and target tissue to be analyzed. Surprisingly, the ablation

catheter is unstable in up to one-third of radiofrequency applications, despite fluoroscopic evidence of stability.[24,25] This is an important finding as the conventional stability markers used during radiofrequency applications are the fluoroscopic image, local electrogram recordings (which often are unclear during application), and the impedance of the ablation electrode. ICE has shown that electrode impedance may not be reliable, as the formation of thrombi and microbubbles (signs of poor contact) have been observed in the absence of significant changes in impedance.[24]

Another advantage of ICE is its precision in locating anatomical structures. Chu et al.[16] studied this property in the right atrium of anesthetized dogs. Guided only by ICE, they attempted to produce lesions at three points of the right atrium: the junction between the

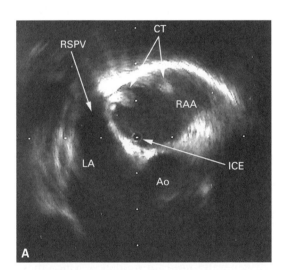 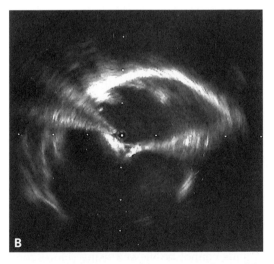

Figure 17-1. A) The right atrial appendage (RAA) can be seen, in this case with two extensions of the crista terminalis (CT). The echocardiography catheter lies in the area of the right atrium close to the aortic valve (Ao). Immediately behind it, the left atrium (LA) and outflow of the right superior pulmonary vein (RSPV) are visible.

B) An ablation catheter has been placed in contact with the atrial wall at the same level as the ICE catheter. The distal catheter electrode produces a typical acoustic shadow. Electrical activity can be mapped as the ablation catheter slips over the surface of the atrium until it reaches the CT prolongations. This makes it possible to determine whether the earliest electrical activity during atrial tachycardia originates in the CT. If the earliest electrical activity is observed in the area adjacent to the pulmonary vein, the atrial tachycardia probably originates from this vein and a left-side approach will be required for to cure the ablation.

lateral wall and superior vena cava (upper crista terminalis), the junction with the inferior vena cava at the base of the atrial appendage on the fossa ovalis, and the ostium of the coronary sinus. Subsequent histopathological studies showed that in 87 % of cases the lesions were within 2 mm of the target. A good correlation between the size of the echocardiographic image visible after radiofrequency applications and the size of the lesion created has also been shown.[25, 26] Things are not so simple with a beating heart in clinical practice and currently available methods cannot always assess the magnitude of the lesion created, although it can be recognized.

Inappropriate Sinus Tachycardia

Inappropriate sinus tachycardia is a rare disease characterized by an abnormally high heart rate both at rest and with minimal effort. Its etiology is still unknown, but potential causes that have been proposed involve an abnormal influence of the autonomic nervous system or an increase in the intrinsic automaticity of the sinus node. Regardless of its cause, in clearly symptomatic patients who do not respond to negative chronotropic drugs, good results have been reported with sinus node ablation.[28-31] This procedure requires the ablation of an area of atrial tissue starting at the superolateral part of the crista terminalis and ending at the lateral part of this anatomical landmark. The crista terminalis cannot be viewed using fluoroscopy and it is difficult to stabilize an ablation catheter on it, so ICE is useful.[28-31] The procedure is safe and effective when performed with ICE. The echocardiographic characteristics of the lesions that have been found to correlate with a reduction of approximately 30 % in intrinsic heart rate are hypodense or echo-free linear lesions from the endocardium to the epicardium in the area corresponding to the sinus node.[30]

Atrial Tachycardias

When the heart is structurally normal, atrial tachycardias usually have a focal origin, such as the crista terminalis, coronary sinus ostium, atrial appendages around the pulmonary veins, or the mitral annulus. However, when structural heart disease is present, tachycardias are generally not focal and are usually due to macroreentry favored by scars or anatomical obstacles. A typical example can be seen in the tachycardias that originate around the scars left by surgical correction of certain congenital malformations. ICE allows the study of the anatomical structures that originate or contribute to arrhythmogenesis[32] and it may be decisive in doubtful cases, such as tachycardia whose electrical origin is in the upper right atrium.[20] In these cases, it is necessary to differentiate between tachycardia arising from the upper crista terminalis, which requires a right atrial therapeutic approach, or from the right upper pulmonary vein, which requires a left atrial approach, generally with transseptal puncture.

Transseptal Puncture

The transseptal approach is used for the ablation of arrhythmias with a left atrial substrate, unless there is a patent foramen ovale. To perform transseptal catheterization, the catheter must be passed through the interatrial septum in the area of the fossa ovalis with the aid of a Brockenbrough needle. Anatomical references, like the aortic valve, are generally used for guidance. Since these anatomical structures are not visible fluoroscopically, they are located by visualizing the position of the catheter in contact with them.

ICE allows the needle to be exactly positioned at the fossa ovalis.[33-37] As the needle presses against the fossa, a characteristic tent-shaped deformation of the membrane appears, then disappears as the membrane recovers its normal position when the needle pierces it (Fig. 17-2).

Transseptal catheterization is increasingly performed in electrophysiology laboratories by operators with no prior experience of this technique. This is because certain patients require ablation treatment of accessory pathways for atrial tachycardia or atrial fibrillation. Positioning an ultrasound catheter in the right atrium makes it easier to learn the transseptal puncture procedure. It also makes the procedure more effective and safer for the patient since it allows the cardiac anatomy to be recognized reliably, particularly the location and size of the fossa ovalis. This is as important in pathological hearts with dilation of the chambers or aortic root, and in small hearts, where failure to pass the interatrial septum at the proper site may lead to perforation and cardiac tamponade.[37]

Atrioventricular Nodal Reentrant Tachycardia

The substrate of A-V nodal reentrant tachycardia is located close to the A-V node. Ablation of the region of Koch's triangle, next to the ostium of the coronary sinus, is effective in almost 100 % of cases, with an incidence of A-V block of less than 1 %. The site of application of radiofrequency is at the insertion of the septal leaflet of the tricuspid valve, in the muscular region of the atrioventricular septum. This area has been shown to contain the slow nodal pathway that is the target of ablation in patients with A-V nodal reentrant tachycardias. ICE has proved to be a reliable technique for its recognition.[38-40] Nonetheless, since the conventional ablation technique (guided by electrograms and fluoroscopy) is usually simple, ICE is reserved for selected cases with a particularly difficult fluoroscopic anatomy. It is also used in cases in which the situation of the patient (for example pregnant women) makes it necessary to perform ablation without relying on ionizing radiation. The same rationale applies to the ablation of atrioventricular accessory pathways, which occasionally require a left transseptal approach.[41, 42]

Exceptionally, radiofrequency ablation is performed inside the coronary sinus and ICE is useful as it visualizes the area of the sinus where energy is being released. ICE also serves to monitor the appearance of pericardial effusion as a result of the application of radiofrequency (Fig. 17-3).

Atrial Flutter

Common atrial flutter is characterized by the presence of typical F waves in the surface electrocardiogram and is due to counterclockwise reentry of the activation front around the tricuspid annulus. Ablation is performed in this condition using a radiological anatomical guide to create a line of ablation in the cavotricuspid isthmus. ICE is generally not required for this technique, but it has made a special contribution to our knowledge of the electrical anatomy of this common arrhythmia. ICE has made it possible to correlate the direction of electrical activation with anatomical structures of the right atrium that are invisible to conventional fluoroscopy.[43] This technique has revealed how the crista terminalis and edge of the Eustachian valve constitute anatomical barriers that block the activation front and favor reentry around the tricuspid ring.

Atrial Fibrillation

Atrial fibrillation is the most frequent sustained arrhythmia and it has recently been discovered that it may have a focal origin in some patients. In these cases, the ectopic foci are located inside or close to the pulmonary veins. It is not unusual for patients to have several of these ectopic foci.[44, 45] In patients with this type of atrial fibrillation, various therapeutic alternatives have been proposed, including ablation of the focus, when possible, or electrical isolation of one or more pulmonary veins. Different methods, applied in conjunction with either electrical or ana-

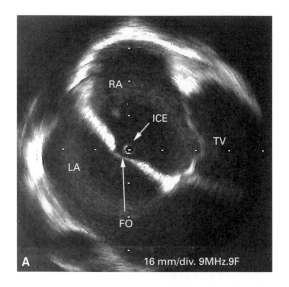

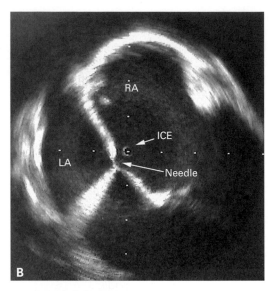

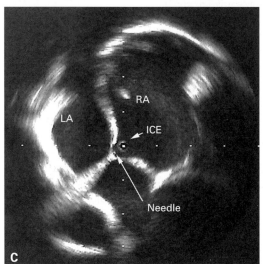

Figure 17-2. Usefulness of intracardiac echocardiography (ICE) for transseptal puncture. A) The ICE catheter is located in the right atrium near the fossa ovalis (FO).
B) The Brockenbrough needle is positioned exactly at the fossa ovalis, casting an echogenic shadow over the left atrium.
C) When the Brockenbrough needle is pressed against the fossa ovalis, it produces a tent-shaped deformation of the interatrial septum that disappears when the interatrial septum is pierced. See Figure 17-1 for abbreviations.

tomical guidance, may be used to isolate the pulmonary veins. The most frequent complications are stenosis of the pulmonary veins, pericardial effusion, and cerebral embolism.

Another treatment proposed for atrial fibrillation acts on the atrial substrate to reduce the spread of activation fronts. This is done by compartmentalizing the atria with ablation

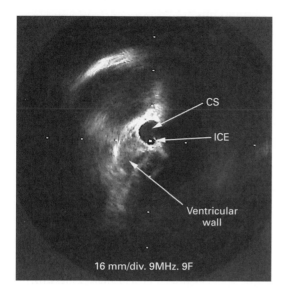

Figure 17-3. Intracardiac echocardiography (ICE) catheter inside the coronary sinus (CS). The lumen of the coronary sinus and wall of the left ventricle can be seen.

lines created by radiofrequency applications instead of surgery, as was previously used.

The use of ICE in radiofrequency ablation of atrial fibrillation is important from the very start of the procedure, as it facilitates transseptal puncture and monitoring for the onset of complications. In addition, ICE is used to examine the pulmonary veins and the alignment of the ablation electrode(s) with respect to the target tissue[46-48] (Figs. 17-4 and 17-5). Nonetheless, passage of the ultrasound catheter into the left atrium is still troublesome with mechanical ICE systems, as it requires the use of a special sheath that is larger than the sheaths used to insert mapping or ablation catheters. Strict anticoagulation is essential, as well as extreme care, if embolism is to be prevented because catheters often have to be exchanged one or more times inside the sheath before reaching the pulmonary vein or veins targeted.

Ventricular Tachycardia

The site of origin of some ventricular tachycardias makes ablation particularly dif-

ficult, due to the proximity of the tachycardia substrate to important structures that can be damaged by the application of radiofrequency. For instance, in ventricular left outflow tract tachycardias, the origin of the tachycardia may lie close to the aortic valve and coronary ostium. ICE facilitates the inspection of this area and ensures catheter stability during ablation.[49]

In our experience, ICE is useful in patients with ventricular tachycardias originating in the right ventricle, such as idiopathic ventricular right outflow tract tachycardia and tachycardia associated with arrhythmogenic right ventricular dysplasia. The images obtained with the ICE catheter placed in the right ventricle allow the ablation catheter to be stabilized in extremely trabecular areas, where it would otherwise be impossible to ensure stability during radiofrequency applications (Fig. 17-6).

OTHER APPLICATIONS

Researchers are currently studying the usefulness of ICE for locating and measuring

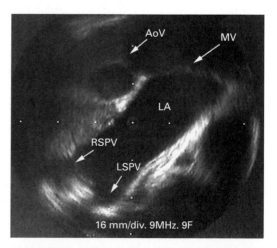

Figure 17-4. Intracardiac echographic (ICE) catheter inside the left atrium (LA) at the level of the aortic (AoV) and mitral (MV) valves. Tangential slices of the right superior pulmonary vein (RSPV) and left superior pulmonary vein (LSPV) are shown.

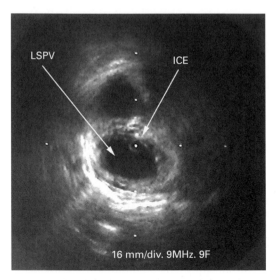

Figure 17-5. Intracardiac echocardiography (ICE) of the left superior pulmonary vein (LSPV) in a patient treated for a focal atrial fibrillation arising from that vein. The plane view is perpendicular to the longaxis of the vein.

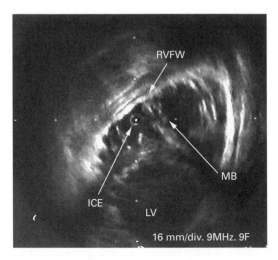

Figure 17-6. Intracardiac echocardiography (ICE) of the right ventricle in a patient with arrhythmogenic dysplasia. LV: left ventricle; MB: moderator band; RVFW: right ventricular free wall.

the magnitude of myocardial ischemia during percutaneous procedures.[50-54] Furthermore, the effect of radiofrequency on myocardial infarction scars is being studied to guide the ablation of ischemic ventricular tachycardias.[55] ICE has also been used as a guide in the biopsy of intracardiac masses, septostomy in patients with pulmonary hypertension, direct injection of genes into the myocardium, the analysis of aortic valve anatomy, and even for the monitoring of right and left ventricular performance.[56-60]

FUTURE

The future of ICE to depends on whether or not its current limitations can be overcome. Catheters must be thin and steerable to allow complete visualization of the heart and pulmonary veins from the right atrium or ventricle, preferably by three-dimensional imaging.[61] ICE catheters should have a Doppler sensor to assess blood flow and velocity. Ideally, it should be possible to integrate information about anatomical structures and local electrical activation on the same catheter, as well as deliver radiofrequency. This would make ICE indispensable in the interventional cardiology laboratory, where current technology already allows certain procedures to be conducted under the guidance of this technique alone, as well as for monitoring in the cardiac operating theatre or critical care unit.[62]

REFERENCES

1. Glassman E, Kronzon I. Transvenous intracardiac echocardiography. *Am J Cardiol* 1981; 47:1255-9.

2. Pandian NG. Intravascular and intracardiac ultrasound imaging. *Circulation* 1989; 80:1091-4.

3. Schwartz SL, Pandian N G, Kusay BS, et al. Real-time intracardiac two-dimensional echocardiography: An experimental study of in vivo feasibility, imaging planes, and echocardiographic anatomy. *Echocardiography* 1990; 7:443-S5.

4. Seward JB, Khandheria BK, McGregor CGA, Locke TJ, Tajik AJ. Transvascular and intracardiac two-dimensional echocardiography. *Echocardiography* I990; 7:457-64.

5. Belohlavek M, Foley DA, Gerber TC, Kinter TM, Greenleaf JF, Seward JB. Three- and four-dimensional cardiovascular ultrasound imaging: a new era for echocardiography. *Mayo Clin Proc* 1993; 68:221-40.

6. Tardif JC, Cao QL, Schwartz SL, Pandian NG. Intracardiac echocardiography with a steerable low-frequency linear-array probe for left-sided heart imaging from the right side: experimental studies. *J Am Soc Echocardiogr* 1995; 8:132-8

7. Seward JB, Packer DL, Chan RC, Curley M, Tajik AJ. Ultrasound cardioscopy: embarking on a new journey. *Mayo Clin Proc* 1996; 71:629-35.

8. Bruce CJ, Packer DL, Seward JB. Intracardiac Doppler Hemodynamics and flow: new vector phased array ultrasound tipped catheter *Am J Cardiol* 1999; 83:1509-12.

9. Belohlavek M, MacLellan-Tobert SG, Seward JB, Greenleaf JF. Toroidal geometry: novel three-dimensional intracardiac imaging with a phased-array transducer. *J Am Soc Echocardiogr* 1997; 10:493-8.

10. Caspari GH, Muller S, Bartel T, Koopmann J, Erbel R. Full performance of modern echocardiography within the heart: in vivo feasibility study with a new intracardiac, phased array ultrasound-tipped catheter. *Eur J Echocardiogr* 2001; 2: 100-7.

11. Bruce CJ, Nishimura RA, Rihal CS et al. Intracardiac echocardiography in the interventional catheterization laboratory: preliminary experience with a novel, phased array transducer. *Am J Cardiol* 2002; 89: 635-640.

12. Packer DL, Stevens CL, Curley MG, Bruce CJ, Miller FA, Khanderia BK, Oh JK, Sinak LJ, Seward JB. Intracardiac Phased-Array Imaging: Methods and Initial Clinical Experience with High Resolution, Under Blood Visualization. *J Am Coll Cardiol* 2002; 39: 509-516.

13. Hijazi Z, Wang Z, Cao Q, Koenig P, Waight D, Lang R. Transcatheter closure of atrial septal defects and patent foramen ovale under intracardiac echocardiographic guidance: feasibility and comparison with tran-

sesophageal echocardiography. *Catheter Cardiovasc Interv* 2001; 52:194-9.

14. Jan SL, Hwang B, Lee PC, Fu YC, Chiu PS, Chi CS. Intracardiac ultrasound assessment of atrial septal defect: comparison with transthoracic echocardiographic, angiocardiographic, and balloon-sizing measurements. *Cardiovasc Intervent Radiol* 2001; 24: 84-9.

15. Hijazi Z, Wang Z, Cao Q, Koenig P, Waight D, Lang R. Transcatheter closure of atrial septal defects and patent foramen ovale under intracardiac echocardiographic guidance: feasibility and comparison with transesophageal echocardiography. *Catheter Cardiovasc Interv* 2001; 52:194-9.

16. Chu E, Fitzpatrick AP, Chin MC, Sudhir K, Yock PG, Lesh MD. Radiofrequency catheter ablation guided by intracardiac echocardiography. *Circulation* 1994; 89:1301-8.

17. Stellbrink C, Siebels J, Hebe J, et al. Potential of intracardiac ultrasonography as an adjunct for mapping and ablation. *Am Heart J* 1994; 127:1095-101.

18. Tardif JC, Vannan MA, Miller DS, Schwartz SL, Pandian NG. Potential applications of intracardiac echocardiography in interventional electrophysiology. *Am Heart J* 1994; 127:1090-4.

19. Chu E, Kalman JM, Kwasman MA, et al. Intracardiac echocardiography during radiofrequency catheter ablation of cardiac arrhythmias in humans. *J Am Coll Cardiol* 1994; 24:1351-7.

20. Kalman JM, Olgin JE, Karch MR, Lesh MD. Use of intracardiac echocardiography in interventional electrophysiology. *Pacing Clin Electrophysiol* 1997; 20:2248-62.

21. Ban J, Schwartzman D, Callans D, Mareblioski FE, Gottlieb CD, Chaudhry FA. Imaging technique and clinical utility for electrophysiologic procedures of lower frequency (9 MHz) intracardiac echocardiography. *Am J Cardiol* 1998; 82:1557-60.

22. Marchlinski FE, Ren JF, Schwartzman D, Callans DJ, Gottlieb CD. Accuracy of fluoroscopic localization of the Crista terminalis documented by intracardiac echocardiography. *J Interv Card Electrophysiol* 2000; 4:415-21.

23. Clark CB, Davies LR, Kerber RE. Intracardiac echocardiography identifies pericardial

fluid and can monitor the success of pericardiocentesis: experimental studies. *J Am Soc Echocardiogr* 2001; 14:712-4.

24. Kalman JM, Fitzpatrick AP, Olgin JE, et al. Biophysical characteristics of radiofrequency lesion formation in vivo: dynamics of catheter tip-tissue contact evaluated by intracardiac echocardiography. *Am Heart J* 1997; 133:8-18.

25. Kalman JM, Jue J, Sudhir K, Fitzgerald P, Yock P, Lesh MD. In vitro quantification of radiofrequency ablation lesion size using intracardiac echocardiography in dogs. *Am J Cardiol* 1996; 77:217-9.

26. Ren JF, Callans DJ, Schwartzman D, Michele JJ, Marchlinski FE. Changes in local wall thickness correlate with pathologic lesion size following radiofrequency catheter ablation: an intracardiac echocardiographic imaging study. *Echocardiography* 2001; 18:503-7.

27. Epstein LM, Mitchell MA, Smith TW et al. Comparative study of fluoroscopy and intracardiac echocardiographic guidance for the creation of linear atrial lesions. *Circulation* 1998; 98:1796-1801.

28. Kalman JM, Lee RJ, Fisher WG, et al. Radiofrequency catheter modification of sinus pacemaker function guided by intracardiac echocardiography. *Circulation* 1995; 92:3070-81.

29. Lee RJ, Kalman JM, Fitzpatrick AP, et al. Radiofrequency catheter modification of the sinus node for «inappropriate» sinus tachycardia. *Circulation* 1995; 92:2919-28.

30. Ren JF, Marchlinski FE, Callans DJ, Zado ES. Echocardiographic lesion characteristics associated with successful ablation of inappropriate sinus tachycardia. *J Cardiovasc Electrophysiol* 2001; 12:814-8.

31. Callans DJ, Ren JF, Schwartzman D et al. Narrowing of the superior vena cava-right atrium junction during radiofrequency catheter ablation for inappropriate sinus tachycardia: analysis with intracardiac echocardiography. *J Am Coll Cardiol* 1999; 33:1667-1670.

32. Kalman JM, Olgin JE, Karch MR et al. Cristal tachycardias: origin of right atrial tachycardias from crista terminalis identified by intracardiac echocardiography. *J Am Coll Cardiol* 1998; 31:451-459.

33. Hung JS, Fu M, Yeh ICH, Chua S, Wu JJ, Chen YC. Usefulness of intracardiac echocardiography in transseptal puncture during percutaneous transvenous mitral commissurotomy. *Am J Cardiol* 1993; 72:853-4.

34. Hung JS, Fu M, Yek KH, Wu CJ, Wong P. Usefulness of intracardiac echocardiography in complex transseptal catheterization during percutaneous transvenous mitral commissurotomy. *Mayo Clin Proc* 1996; 71:134-40.

35. Epstein LM, Smith T, TenHoff H. Nonfluoroscopic transseptal catheterization: safety and efficacy of intracardiac echocardiographic guidance. *J Cardiovasc Electrophysiol* 1998; 9:625-630.

36. Szili-Torok T, Kimman G, Theuns D, Res J, Roelandt JR, Jordaens LJ. Transseptal left heart catheterization guided by intracardiac echocardiography. *Heart* 2001; 86:E11.

37. Cafri C, de la Guardia B, Barasch E, Brink J, Smalling RW. Transseptal puncture guided by intracardiac echocardiography during percutaneous transvenous mitral commissurotomy in patients with distorted anatomy of the fossa ovalis. *Catheter Cardiovasc Interv* 2000; 50:463-7.

38. Fisher WG, Pelini MA, Bacon ME. Adjunctive intracardiac echocardiography to guide slow pathway ablation in human atrioventricular nodal reentrant tachycardia. *Circulation* 1997; 96:3021-29.

39. Batra R, Nair M, Kumar M, et al. Intracardiac echocardiography guided radiofrequency catheter ablation of the slow pathway in atrioventricular nodal reentrant tachycardia. *J Interv Card Electrophysiol* 2002; 6:43-49.

40. DeLurgio DB, Frohwein SC, Walter PF, Langberg JJ. Anatomy of atrioventricular nodal re-entry investigated by intracardiac echocardiography. *Am J Cardiol* 1997; 80:231-4.

41. Ren JF, Schwartzman D, Callans DJ, Marchlinski FE, Zhang LP, Chaudhry FA. Intracardiac Echocardiographic Imaging in Guiding and Monitoring Radiofrequency Catheter Ablation at the Tricuspid Annulus. *Echocardiography* 1998; 15:661-664.

42. Szili-Torok T, Kimman GJ, Tuin J, Jordaens L. How to approach left-sided accessory pathway ablation using intracardiac echocardiography. *Europace* 2001; 3:28.

43. Olgin JE, Kalman JM, Fitzpatrick, Lesh MD. Role of right atrial endocardial struc-

tures as barriers to conduction during human type I atrial flutter: activation and entrainment mapping guided by intracardiac echocardiography. *Circulation* 1995; 92:1839-48.

44. Haissaguerre M, Jais P, Shah DC et al. Spontaneous initiation of atrial fibrillation by ectopic beats originating in the pulmonary veins. *N Engl J Med* 1998; 339:659-666.

45. Haissaguerre M, Jais P, Shah DC et al.: Electrophysiological end point for catheter ablation of atrial fibrillation initiated from multiple pulmonary venous foci. *Circulation* 2000; 101:1409-1417.

46. Cooper JM, Epstein LM. Use of intracardiac echocardiography to guide ablation of atrial fibrillation. *Circulation* 2001; 104:3010-3013.

47. Morton JB, Sanders P, Byrne MJ, Power J, Mow C, Edwards GA, Kalman JM. Phased-Array intracardiac echocardiography to guide radiofrequency ablation in the left atrium and at the pulmonary vein ostium. *J Cardiovasc Electrophysiol* 2001; 12:343-8.

48. Olgin JE, Kalman JM, Chin M et al.: Electrophysiological effects of long linear atrial lesions placed under intracardiac ultrasound guidance. *Circulation* 1997; 96:2715-2721.

49. Lamberti F, Calo L, Pandozi C, et al. Radiofrequency catheter ablation of idiopathic left ventricular outflow tract tachycardia: utility of intracardiac echocardiography. *J Cardiovasc Electrophysiol* 2001; 12:529-535.

50. Schwartz SL, Pandian NC, Hsu TL, Weintraub A, Cao QL. Intracardiac echocardiographic imaging of cardiac abnormalities, ischemic myocardial dysfunction, and myocardial perfusion: studies with a 10 MHz ultrasound catheter *J Am Soc Echocardiogr* 1993; 6:345-SS.

51. Spencer KT, MelCay CB, Kerber RE. Intracardiac ultrasound detection of right ventricular infarction in a canine model. *J Am Soc Echocardiogr* 1997; 10:352.

52. Ren JF, Callans DJ, Michele JJ, Dillon SM, Marchlinski FE. Intracardiac echocardiographic evaluation of ventricular mural swelling from radiofrequency ablation in chronic myocardial infarction: irrigated-tip versus standard catheter. *J Interv Card Electrophysiol* 2001; 5:27-32.

53. Bissing JW, Ryan AJ, Kerber RE. Coronary risk area measurement by intracardiac echocardiography and ultrasound contrast. *J Am Soc Echocardiogr* 2001; 14:706-11.

54. Pislaru C, Bruce CJ, Belohlavek M, Seward JB, Greenleaf JF. Intracardiac measurement of pre-ejection myocardial velocities estimates the transmural extent of viable myocardium early after reperfusion in acute myocardial infarction. *J Am Coll Cardiol* 2001; 38:1748-56.

55. Callans DJ, Ren JF, Narula N, Michele J, Marchlinski FE, Dillon SM. Effects of linear, irrigated-tip radiofrequency ablation in porcine healed anterior infarction. *J Cardiovasc Electrophysiol* 2001; 12:1037-42.

56. Jiang L, de Prada JA, Lee MY, et al. Quantitative assessment of stenotic aortic valve area by using intracardiac echocardiography: in vitro validation and initial in vivo illustration. *Am Heart J* 1996; 132:137-44.

57. Segar DS, Bourdillon PD, Elsner C, Kesler IC, Feigenbaum H. Intracardiac echocardiography-guided biopsy of intracardiac masses. *J Am Soc Echocardiogr* 1995; 8:927-9.

58. Jiang L, Weissman NJ, Guerrero JL, et al. Percutaneous trans-venous intracardiac ultrasound imaging in dogs: a new approach to monitor left ventricular function. *Heart* 1996; 76:442-8.

59. Park SW, Gwon HC, Jeong JO, Byun J, Kang HS, You JR, Cho SS, Lee MJ, Lee Y, Kim S, Kim DK. Intracardiac echocardiographic guidance and monitoring during percutaneous endomyocardial gene injection in porcine heart. *Hum Gene Ther* 2001; 12:893-903.

60. Moscucci M, Dairywala IT, Chetcuti S, Mathew B, Li P, Rubenfire M, Vannan MA. Balloon atrial septostomy in end-stage pulmonary hypertension guided by a novel intracardiac echocardiographic transducer. *Catheter Cardiovasc Interv* 2001; 52:530-4.

61. Dairywala IT, Li P, Liu Z, et al. Catheter based interventions guided solely by a new phased-array intracardiac imaging catheter: in vivo experimental studies. *J Am Soc Echocardiogr* 2002; 15:150-8.

62. Light ED, Idriss SF, Wolf PD, Smith SW. Real-time three-dimensional intracardiac echocardiography. *Ultrasound Med Biol* 2001; 27:1177-83.

18

Intravascular Ultrasound in the Diagnosis of Aortic and Pulmonary Diseases

RAIMUND ERBEL, MD, CLEMENS VON BIRGELEN, MD
JUNBO GE, MD, HOLGER EGGEBRECHT, MD
DIETRIC BAUMGART, MD

Introduction. Aorta and Great Vessels. Pulmonary Artery Imaging. References.

INTRODUCTION

Echocardiography has become the standard non-invasive method for the analysis of normal and abnormal cardiac morphology, global and regional ventricular function, congenital and acquired valvular heart disease, coronary artery disease, cardiomyopathy, hypertensive heart disease, and cardiac involvement in systemic diseases.[1]

Transesophageal echocardiography has opened a new window on the heart, improving decision-making for surgery with its high accuracy and resolution.[2,3] It has even become possible to image the coronary arteries.[4]

The use of intravascular ultrasound (IVUS) for the examination of the heart and great vessels was proposed when ultrasound first began to be used in medicine, as reported by Bom et al.[5] Due to technical limitations and the lack of clinical perspectives, the use of this technique was not pursued further. In the last ten years, however, new miniaturized electronic and mechanical scanners have been developed.[7,8] Steerable systems and even micromotor-based systems (Fig. 18-1) have become available.[9,10] However, the breakthrough of the introduction of a linear phased-array ultrasound catheter made possible IVUS with all imaging modalities of echocardiography and Doppler, combined with steerability.[12-14]

AORTA AND GREAT VESSELS

With a size of 6.2 F, IVUS was first used for imaging the great vessels and aorta.[15-18] *In vitro* studies demonstrated it was highly accurate in estimating the diameters of the aorta and other vessels.[19,20] In the great vessels, results were compared to digital subtraction angiography. The superiority of IVUS was demonstrated, particularly in evaluating the vessel wall.[21,22] Similarly, IVUS of the aorta showed a high resolution with cross-sectional imaging.[18,19,23] The mean difference between IVUS and aortography was only 0.3 ± 2.3 mm and for the area 9 ± 80 mm^2 (ns).[16]

A major limitation was the scan's depth of field, which was limited to 2 cm using 20-MHz transducers. Thus, only aortic diameters up to 4 cm could be visualized.[16] Recently, low-frequency mechanical and electronic scanners using 10 MHz transducers were introduced, which allows a scanning depth of 4 cm. Depending on the catheter position, even large aneurysms can be imaged,

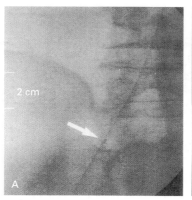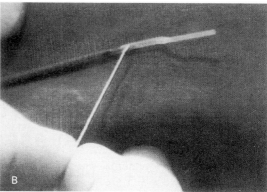

Figure 18-1. Fluoroscopy (A) and photography (B) of the catheter embedded micromotor used for the first time in 1997[10].

but they may be out of the scan field of an eccentrically positioned catheter.

Changes in aortic shape during the cardiac cycle can be recorded to obtain an estimate of aortic compliance, a major determinant of cardiac risk.[24, 25] This is further improved by making simultaneous pressure measurements and taking vessel hysteresis into account. The best way, however, is direct measurement as proposed by Toutouzas et al.[26]

Aortic sclerosis can be regarded as a degenerative disease that develops with aging of the aorta. Aortic sclerosis is related to risk factors like hypertension, smoking, and hypercholesterolemia, in addition to other risk factors. The disease is graded as follows:[27]

Grade I = minimal intimal thickening
Grade II = extensive intimal thickening
Grade III = sessile atheroma
Grade IV = protruding atheroma
Grade V = mobile atheroma

Similarly, traumatic damage to the aorta, mainly as a result of blunt chest trauma caused by traffic accidents, is graded:[27]

Grade I = intimal hemorrhage
Grade II = intimal hemorrhage with ulceration
Grade III = medial ulceration
Grade IV = complete ulceration
Grade V = false aneurysm formation

Recently, aortic disease leading to acute aortic syndromes that result in acute aortic dissection or rupture has been classified into five classes, in addition to the classic system of grading by location of the disease process.[27]

Stanford Classification

Type A dissection = ascending aorta and descending aorta.
Type B dissection = descending aorta.

De Bakey Classification

Type 1 dissection = ascending and descending aorta
Type 2 dissection = ascending aorta
Type 3 dissection = descending aorta

European Task Force Classification of Acute Aortic Syndromes According to Svenson et al.[33]

Class 1 = classic dissection with intimal flaps
Class 2 = intramural hematoma / hemorrhage
Class 3 = discrete / subtle dissection

Class 4 = plaque ulceration / rupture
Class 5 = traumatic/iatrogenic dissection

The diameter of the normal aorta tapers down from the ascending to the descending part. Normal values have been assessed by transthoracic and transesophageal echocardiography, as well as computed tomography and angiography.[27] Males have larger diameters than females. Depending on the body surface area, aortic diameter increases nonlinearly in a range between 0.5 and 2 m^2.[29] All methods agree on an upper normal limit of 4 mm for aortic wall thickness.[27]

During life, the diameter of the aorta increases by 1-2 mm every 10 years.[30, 31] This rate is enhanced during aneurysm formation. Expansions of 1.3 ± 1.2 mm/year and 3.1 ± 3.2 mm/year have been reported for the ascending and abdominal aorta, respectively. Arteriosclerosis is the main cause of aneurysm formation, other causes being inherited diseases, media necrosis, inflammatory, traumatic, and toxic diseases.[27]

Using IVUS, aortic sclerosis has been recognized at early stages. The diagnostic accuracy of IVUS compared to computed tomography and angiography has been demonstrated.[2, 16, 21, 22] Resolution has improved with the use of 10 MHz transducers.[33] From the beginning, there have been a wide variety of indications for IVUS, such as renal artery stenosis, tumor infiltration, and Budd Chiari syndrome.[16] IVUS is now a standard technique in the catheterization laboratory, providing deeper insights into vessel wall morphology when magnetic resonance imaging, computed tomography, and angiography prove inconclusive.

The most important indication has become aortic dissection (Fig. 18-2), particularly the confirmation, localization, classification, and description of the extension of disease.[17, 35-41]

IVUS complements ultrasound examination of the aorta because of the blind spot of the ascending aorta for transesophageal echocardiography (TEE). In addition, the abdominal aorta and iliac arteries can be imaged with high resolution, particularly the side branch involvement in aortic dissection.[37, 39] Visualization of the relation between the true and false lumen[36, 39] became important not only for class 1 but also for

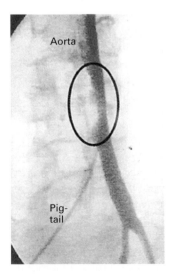 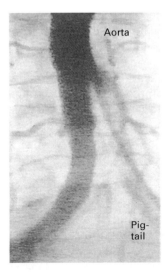 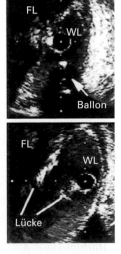

Figure 18-2. Aortography of the true lumen, false lumen (middle part) and IVUS images of the balloon fenestration of aortic dissection (right side). TL/FL = true/false lumen. Lücke = Tear[43].

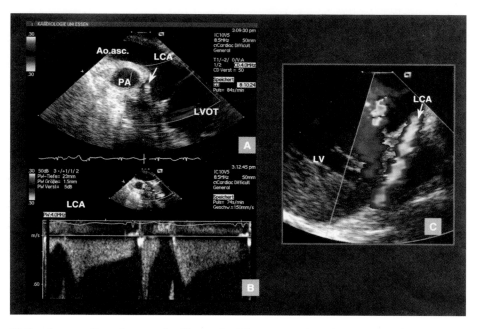

Figure 18-3. Intracardiac ultrasound with the AcuNev system, imaging ascending aorta (Ao asc), pulmonary artery (PA), left coronary artery (LCA), left ventricle and left ventricular outflow tract (LVOT).[13]

other types like class 2 dissection. IVUS was found to be of diagnostic value in patients in which other imaging techniques were inconclusive.[40]

Since IVUS provides complete imaging of the aorta, it was introduced for monitoring and guiding interventional techniques like aortic fenestration[42, 43] and aortic stent implantation.[44, 45] In particular, longitudinal scanning with 3-D reconstruction is helpful for evaluating the correct positioning of stent or graft stents.[44] The relief of ischemia of the bowel, kidney, or limb has been demonstrated.[43, 45] False lumen thrombosis is regarded as the best sign of successful stent deployment.[47, 48]

Furthermore, IVUS became an important scanning technique for the evaluation of aortic coarctation because it yields true cross-sectional images with a high resolution that allow exact angioplasty and stent selection.[46-48] Intimal flaps are nearly always visualized, which explains the importance of stenting in aortic coarctation.[49]

Currently, IVUS imaging is possible only before and after the intervention. In the future, an alternative may be to image from the right side, superior and inferior vena cava, or right ventricle because the whole aorta and its side branches can be visualized, including Doppler flow-imaging.[13, 14] The results of preliminary experiences (Figs. 18-3, 18-4) are promising. TEE has been used with IVUS to visualize the total aortic arch (Figs. 18-5, 18-6), a technique called «lighthouse TEE.»[50]

PULMONARY ARTERY IMAGING

Early on, IVUS was used to image the pulmonary artery because only the contour method, angiography, was available. However, cross-sectional imaging techniques were necessary to visualize vessel walls.[7, 8, 17, 51-54] IVUS has become an important tool for evaluating the cause of pulmonary hypertension. Thrombus formation (Fig. 18-7) can be detec-

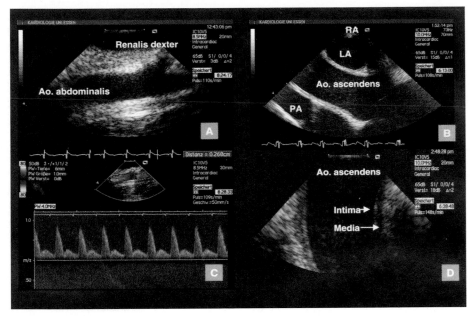

Figure 18-4. Intracardiac ultrasound with the AcuNev system (Acuson, Siemens, Erlangen, Germany) imaging the right/left atrium (RA/LA), pulmonary artery (PA), and aorta. High resolution during visualization of the aortic wall[13].

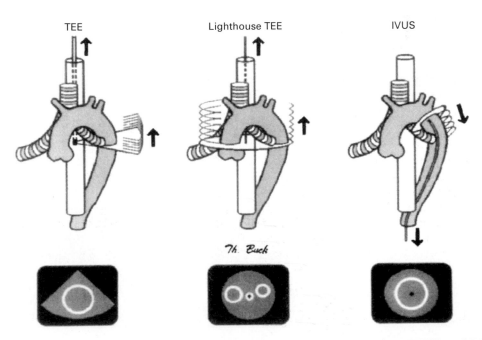

Figure 18-5. Transesophageal echocardiography (TEE), intravascular ultrasound (IVUS) and IVUS of the esophagus as lighthouse TEE[50].

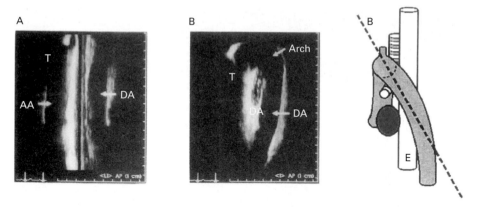

Figure 18-6.   Lighthouse TEE of the descending aorta (DA) and aortic arch as well as ascending aorta (AA).[50]

ted.[51-53] In order to increase diagnostic accuracy, IVUS has been combined with angioscopy to better visualize mural thrombus formation.[53-54]

In patients with precapillary pulmonary hypertension, surgery can be performed and may lead to full recovery of patients. The diagnosis is difficult.[55] By studying shape changes and recorded pressures, the compliance of the pulmonary artery can be assessed and the response to drug treatment evaluated.[56]

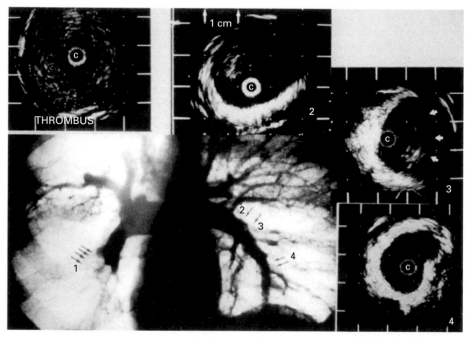

Figure 18-7.   Pulmonary angiogram of a patient with embolism. By IVUS thrombotic material is demonstrated in different locations (arrows).[65]

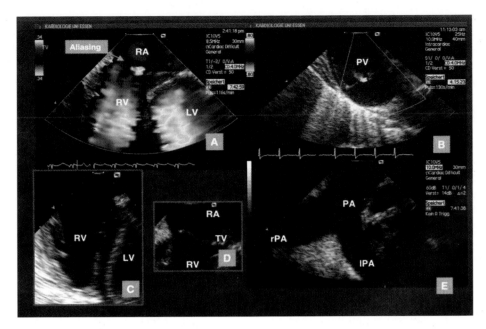

Figure 18-8. Pulmonary artery visualization from intracardiac catheters. Unique view of the main stem (PA), right and left (r/l) PA, right atrium and ventricle (RA/RV), left ventricle (LV), tricuspidal valve (TV).[13]

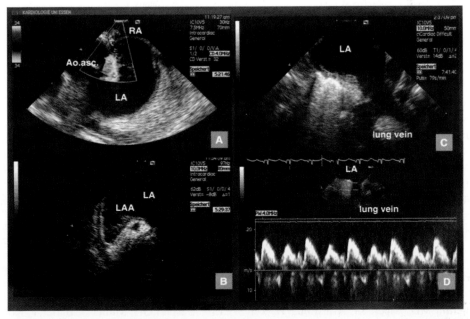

Figure 18-9. Intracardiac ultrasound images of the left atrium (LA) with imaging of the left atrium appendage and pulmonary (lung) veins.[13]

Arteriosclerosis of the vessel wall can be imaged.[57,58] A typical presentation is a three-layer appearance of the otherwise monolayer vessel wall in pulmonary hypertension.

After the first report describing the visualization of pulmonary thrombi by suprasternal scanning[59] and TEE,[60] we could also report the imaging of pulmonary thrombi by IVUS.[61] IVUS is superior to angiography in visualizing pulmonary thrombi, thus confirming the findings of early experimental studies.[62-64] The diameter of the pulmonary artery can be determined with the two techniques with a mean difference of only ± 1.5 mm. In pulmonary embolism, free-floating thrombi (type A thrombi) as well as mural thrombus formation (type B) are detected by IVUS in 87% and 13% of patients, respectively. IVUS revealed thrombi in 34% of angiographically normal pulmonary segments (with type A thrombi in 53% and type B thrombi in 47% of patients[65]). IVUS with TEE has also been proposed for follow-up studies during thrombolytic therapy.[66]

Currently, IVUS catheters are advanced into the pulmonary artery using guide catheters. Imaging is excellent on the periphery of the artery, but of lower quality in large pulmonary arteries when 20 to 30 MHz transducers are used.

Therefore, pulmonary artery imaging is best done with 10 MHz to detect changes in vessel wall morphology. Due to the position of the guidewires, only a limited number of pulmonary artery segments can be visualized. Hopefully, new steerable catheters will allow better imaging (Figs. 18-8, 18-9) of the pulmonary tree.[12-14] The full extent of involvement of major side branches needs to be evaluated, otherwise, the occlusion of small side branches may be overlooked.

REFERENCES

1. Cheitlin MD, Alpert JS, Armstrong WF, et al. ACC/AHA guidelines for the clinical application of echocardiography: executive summary. A report of the American College of Cardiology/American Heart Association Task Force on practice guidelines. *J Am Coll Cardiol* 1997; 29:862-79.

2. Erbel R, Khandheria BK, Brennecke R, Meyer J, Seward JB, Tajik AJ. Transesophageal echocardiography. Springer Verlag Berlin, Heidelberg, New York, London, Paris Tokyo Hong Kong 1989.

3. Erbel R, Engberding R, Daniel W, Roelandt J, Visser CM, Rennollet H. Echocardiography in diagnosis of aortic dissection. *Lancet* 1989; 1:457-61.

4. Erbel R. Transesophageal echocardiography. New window to coronary arteries and coronary blood flow. *Circulation* 1991; 83: 339-341.

5. Bom N. Lancee CT, van Egmond FC. An ultrasonic intracardiac scanner. *Ultrasonics* 1972; 10:72-76.

6. Bom N, Roelandt J (eds). Intravascular ultrasound. 1989 Kluwer Academic Publishers, Dordrecht, The Netherlands.

7. Pandian NG, Hsu, TL. Intravascular ultrasound and intracardiac echocardiography: concepts for the future. *Am J Cardiol* 1992; 69: 6H-17H.

8. Roelandt J, Serruys PW, Tuccillo B, Gussenhoven WJ. Clinical perspectives of intravascular ultrasound. *Echocardiography* 1990; 7:503-14.

9. Görge G, Ge J, Haude M, Baumgart D, Buck T, Erbel R. Initial experience with a steerable intravascular ultrasound catheter in the aorta and pulmonary artery. *Am J Card Imaging* 1995; 9:180-84.

10. Erbel R, Roth T, Koch L, Ge J, Görge G, Serruys PW, Bom N, Lancee CT, Roelandt J. IVUS of micromotors for cardiovascular imaging. *Min Invas Ther & Allied Technol* 1997; 6:195-198.

11. Bruce CJ, Packer DL, Seward JB. Intracardiac Doppler hemodynamics and flow: new vector, phased-array ultrasound-tipped catheter. *Am J Cardiol* 1999; 83:1509-1512.

12. Bruce CJ, Packer DL, Seward JB. Transvascular imaging: feasibility study using a vector phase array ultrasound catheter. *Echocardiography* 1999; 16:425-30.

13. Caspari GH, Müller S, Bartel T, Koopmann J, Erbel R. Full performance of modern echocardiography within the heart: *in vivo*

feasibility study with a new intracardiac, phased-array ultrasound-tipped catheter. *Eur J Echocardiography* 2001; 2:100-107.

14. Fu M, Hung JS, Lo PH, Wu CJ, Chang KC, Lau KW. Intracardiac echocardiography via the transvenous approach with use of 8F 10 MHz ultrasound catheter. *Mayo Clin Proc* 199; 74:777-83.

15. Pandian NG, Kreis A, Weintraub A, Motarjeme A, Desnoyers M, Isner JM, Konstam M, Salem DN, Millen V. Real-time intravascular ultrasound imaging in humans. *Am J Cardiol* 1990; 65:1392-96.

16. Düber C, Klose KJ, Erbel R, Schmiedt W, Thelen M. Intravaskuläre Sonographie: erste klinische Ergebnisse. *Fortschr Röntgenstr* 1991; 154:164-171.

17. Gerber T, Erbel R, Görge G, Ge J, Meyer J. Comparison of aortic diameter and area as determined by angiography and intravascular ultrasound. *Herz Kreisl* 1991; 23:403-8.

18. Nishimura RA, Kennedy KD, Warnes CA, Reeder GS, Holmes DR, Tajik AJ. Intravascular ultrasonography: image interpretation and limitations. *Echocardiography* 1990; 7: 469-473.

19. Pandian NG, Kreis A, Brockway B, Isner JM, Sacharoff A, Boleza E, Caro R, Müller D. Ultrasound angioscopy: real-time, two-dimensional, intraluminal ultrasound imaging of blood vessels. *Am J Cardiol* 1988; 62: 493-494.

20. Gussenhoven WJ, Essed CE, Frietman P, Mastik F, Lancée C, Slager C, Peterman H, Bom N. Intravascular echocardiographic assessment of vessel wall characteristics: a correlation with histology. *Int J Cardiac Imaging* 1989; 4:105-116.

21. Davidson CJ, Sheikh KH, Harrison JK, Himmelstein SI, Leithe ME, Kisslo KB, Bashore TM. Intravascular ultrasonography versus digital subtraction angiography: a human in vivo comparison of vessel size and morphology. *J Am Coll Cardiol* 1990; 16:633-636.

22. Nissen SE, Grines CL, Gurlex C, Sublett K, Haynie D, Diaz C, Booth DS, DeMaria AN. Application of a new phased-array ultrasound imaging catheter in the assessment of vascular dimensions: in vivo comparison to cineangiography. *Circulation* 1990; 81:660-663.

23. Yock PG, Johnson EL, Linker DT. Intravascular ultrasound: development and clinical potential. *Am J Cardiac Imaging* 1988; 2: 185-189.

24. Stefanidis C, Dernellis J, Tsiamis E, Stratos C, Diamantopoulos L, Michaelides A, Toutouzas P. Aortic stiffness as a risk factor for recurrent acute coronary events in patients with ischemic disease. *Eur Heart J* 2000; 21:390-396.

25. Madhavan S, Ooi WL, Chohen H, Alderman MH. Relation of pulse pressure and blood pressure reduction to the incidence of myocardial infarction. *Hypertension* 1994; 23: 395-401.

26. Stefanidis C, Stratos C, Vlachopoulos C, Marakas S, Boudoulas H, Kallikazaros I, Tsiamis E, Toutouzas K, Sioros L, Toutouzas P. Pressure-diameter relation of the human aorta: a new method of determination by the application of a special ultrasonic dimension catheter. *Circulation* 1995; 92:2210-2219.

27. Erbel R, Alfonso F, Boileau C, Dirsch O, Eber B, Haverich A, Rakowski H, Struyven J, Radegran K, Sechtem U, Taylor J, Zollikofer CH. Diagnosis and management of aortic dissection. Recommendations of the Task Force on Aortic Dissection, European Society of Cardiology. *Eur Heart J* 2001; 22:1642-1681.

28. Svensson LG, Labib SB, Eisenhauer AC, Butterly JR. Intimal tear without hematoma. *Circulation* 1999; 99:1331-6.

29. Roman MJ, Devereux RB, Kramer-Fox R, O'Loughlin J. Two-dimensional echocardiographic aortic root dimensions in normal children and adults. *Am J Cardiol* 1989; 64: 507-12.

30. Taylor KM. Diseases of the aorta. In: Julian DG, Camm AJ, Fox KM, Hall RJC, Poole-Wilson PA, eds. Diseases of the Heart, 1st Ed., London. *Baailliere Tindall* 1989; 1338- 62.

31. Mohr-Kahaly S, Erbel R. Advantages of biplane and multiplane transesophageal echocardiography for the morphology of the aorta. *Am J Card Imaging* 1995; 9:115-20.

32. Tunick PA, Kronzon I. Atheromas of the thoracic aorta: clinical and therapeutic update. *J Am Coll Cardiol* 2000; 35:545-54.

33. Erbel R. General cardiology. Diseases of the thoracic aorta. *Heart* 2001; 86:227-234.

34. Eggebrecht H, Baumgart D, Herold U, Jakob H, Erbel R. Multiple penetrating atherosclerotic ulcers of the abdominal aorta: treatment by endovascular stent-graft placement. *Heart* 2001; 85:526.

35. Pande A, Meier B, Fleisch M, Kammerlander R, Simonet F, Lerch R. Intravascular ultrasound for diagnosis of aortic dissection. *Am J Cardiol* 1991; 67:662-663.

36. Görge G, Erbel R, Gerber T, Ge J, Zamorano J, Mackowski T, Nixdorff U, Mohr-Kahaly S, Meyer J. Intravasaler Ultraschall bei Patienten mit Verdacht auf Aortendissektion: Vergleich zur transösophagealen Echokardiographie. *Z Kardiol* 1992; 81:37-43.

37. Weintraub AR, Erbel R, Görge G, et al. Intravascular ultrasound imaging in acute aortic dissection. *J Am Coll Cardiol* 1994; 24: 495-503.

38. Alfonso F, Goicolea J, Aragoncillo P, Hernández R, Macaya C. Diagnosis of aortic intramural hematoma by intravascular ultrasound imaging. *Am J Cardiol* 1995; 76: 735-8.

39. Yamada E, Matsumura M, Kyo S, Omoto R. Usefulness of a prototype intravascular ultrasound imaging in evaluation of aortic dissection and comparison with angiographic study, transesophageal echocardiography, computed tomography, and magnetic resonance imaging. *Am J Cardiol* 1995; 68: 642-51.

40. Görge G, Ge J, Baumgart D, von Birgelen C, Erbel R. In vivo tomographic assessment of the heart and blood vessels with intravascular ultrasound. *Basic Res Cardiol* 1998; 93: 219-240.

41. Cavaye DM, French WJ, White RA, Lerman RD, Mehringer CM, Tabbara MR, Kopchok GE. Intravascular ultrasound imaging of an acute dissecting aortic aneurysm-a case report. *J Vasc Surg* 1991; 13:510-512.

42. Walker PJ, Dake MD, Mitchell RS, Miller DC. The use of endovascular techniques for the treatment of complications of aortic dissection. *J Vasc Surg* 1993; 18:1042-1051.

43. Görge G, Erbel R. Intravasaler Ultraschall zur Steuerung der perkutanen Fenestration einer Aortendissektionsmembran. *Dtsch Med Wschr* 1996; 121:1598-1602.

44. Koschyk DH, Meinertz T, Nienaber CA. Intravascular ultrasound for stent implantation in aortic dissection: *Circulation* 2000; 102: 480-481.

45. Nesser J, Eggebrecht H, Baumgart D, Ebner C, Gschwendter M, Barkhausen J, Erbel R, Nienaber C. Emergency stent-graft placement for impending rupture of the descending thoracic aorta. *J Endovasc Ther* 2002 (in press).

46. Stock JH, Reller MD, Sharma S, Pavcnik D, Shiota T, Sahn DJ. Transballoon intravascular ultrasound imaging during balloon angioplasty in animal models with coarctation and branch pulmonary stenosis. *Circulation* 1997; 95:2354-57.

47. Nienaber CA, Fattori R, Kzbf G, et al. Nonsurgical reconstruction of thoracic aortic dissection by stent-graft placement. *N Engl J Med* 1999; 340:1539-45.

48. Dake MD, Miller DC, Mitchell RS, Semba CP, Moore KA, Sakai T. The «first generation» of endovascular stent-grafts for patients with aneurysms of the descending thoracic aorta. *J Thorac Cardiovasc Surg* 1998; 116:689-703.

49. Erbel R, Bednarczyk I, Pop T, Todt M, Henrichs KJ, Brunier A, Thelen M, Meyer J. Detection of dissection of the aortic intima and media after angioplasty of coarctation of the aorta. *Circulation* 1990; 81:805-814.

50. Buck T, Görge G, Hunold P, Erbel R. Three-dimensional imaging in aortic disease by lighthouse transesophageal echocardiography using intravascular ultrasound catheters. *J Am Soc Echocardiogr* 1998; 11:243-58.

51. Pandian NG, Weintraub A, Kreis A, Schwartz S, Konstam D, Salem N. Intracardiac, intravascular, two-dimensional high frequency ultrasound imaging of pulmonary artery and its branches in humans and animals. *Circulation* 1990; 81:2007-2012.

52. Pandian NG, Kreis A, Brockway B. Detection of intra-arterial thrombus by intravascular high frequency two-dimensional ultrasound imaging in vitro and in vivo studies. *Am J Cardiol* 1990; 65:1280-1283.

53. Kato C. Clinical evaluation of acute and chronic pulmonary thromboembolism using intravascular ultrasound and angioscopy. *J Cardiol (Japan)* 1999; 34:317-324.

54. Siegel RJ, Fishbein MC, Chae JS, Helfant RH, Hickey A, Forrester JS. Comparative

studies of angioscopy and ultrasound for the evaluation of arterial disease. *Echocardiography* 1990; 7:495-502.

55. Porter TR, Mohanty PK, Pandian NG. Intravascular ultrasound imaging of pulmonary arteries. Methodology, clinical applications, and future potential. *Chest* 1994; 106:1551-57.

56. Porter TR, Taylor DO, Cycan A, Fields J, Bagley CW, Pandian NG, Mohanty PK. Endothelium-dependent pulmonary artery responses in chronic heart failure: influence of pulmonary hypertension. *J Am Coll Cardiol* 1993; 22:1418-24.

57. Kravitz KD, Scharf GR, Chandrasekaran K. In vivo diagnosis of pulmonary atherosclerosis. Role of intravascular ultrasound. *Chest* 1994; 106:632-34.

58. Kawano T. Wall morphology of the pulmonary artery-intravascular ultrasound imaging and pathological evaluation. *Kurume Med* 1994; 41:221-32.

59. Erbel R, Schweizer P, Effert S. Direkter einund zweidimensionaler echokardiographischer Nachweis einer akuten Lungenarterienembolie. *Dtsch Med Wschr* 1981; 6:179-180.

60. Nixdorff U, Erbel R, Drexler M, Meyer J. Detection of thrombembolus of the right pulmonary artery by transesophageal two-dimensional echocardiography. *Am J Cardiol* 1988; 61:567-572.

61. Görge G, Erbel R, Schuster S, Ge J, Meyer J. Intravascular ultrasound in diagnosis of acute pulmonary embolism. *Lancet* 1991; 337:623-24.

62. Ricou F, Nicod PH, Moser KM, Peterson KL. Catheter-based intravascular ultrasound imaging of chronic thromboembolic pulmonary disease. *Am J Cardiol* 1991; 67: 749-52.

63. Tapson VF, Davidson CJ, Gurbel PA, Sheikh KH, Kisslo KB, Stack RS. Rapid and accurate diagnosis of pulmonary emboli in a canine model using intravascular ultrasound imaging. *Chest* 1991; 100: 1410-13.

64. Tapson VF, Davidson CJ, Kisslo KB, Stack RS. Rapid visualization of massive pulmonary emboli utilizing intravascular ultrasound. *Chest* 1994; 105:888-90.

65. Görge G, Schuster S, Ge J, Meyer J, Erbel R. Intravascular ultrasound in patients with acute pulmonary embolism after treatment with intravenous urokinase and high-dose heparin. *Heart* 1997; 77:73-77.

66. Bruch C, Othman T, Görge G, et al. Intensive medical monitoring with transesophageal echocardiography in fulminant pulmonary embolism. *Dtsch Med Wschr* 1996; 121:829-833.

SECTION IV

Coronary Angioscopy

19

Coronary Angioscopy: Technical Considerations. Image Interpretation. Diagnosis of Acute Coronary Syndromes

FERNANDO ALFONSO, MD

Technical Considerations. Imaging Protocol. Image Interpretation. Angioscopic Findings in Specific Angiographic Patterns. Coronary Angioscopy in Relation to Presenting Coronary Syndromes. Clinical Implications of Angioscopic Findings. References.

PERSPECTIVE

Percutaneous coronary angioscopy (CA) is a recently developed technique that provides unique insights about the luminal surface of the coronary arteries.[1-3] CA constitutes a very useful tool for readily visualizing in vivo the inner aspect of the vessel wall from within the coronary lumen. Real-time, full-motion, colored images of the coronary lumen and vessel wall can be easily obtained from patients undergoing percutaneous diagnostic or therapeutic procedures.[1-6] In contrast with other intracoronary techniques that may be more difficult to interpret, the direct visualization of the coronary vessel wall provided by CA generates in the observer a unique and amazing feeling of reality and dynamism. This feeling is not often obtained from the still pictures that are frequently required to illustrate major findings of this technique.

Clinical studies have demonstrated the usefulness of CA in readily visualizing the normal or abnormal coronary lumen, details of the vessel surface, intracoronary thrombi, the appearance (color, morphology, protrusion) of atherosclerotic plaques, and the presence of intimal flaps and coronary dissection.[1-6] Currently, CA is the technique of choice for the accurate diagnosis of intracoronary thrombus.[1-3] Therefore, it is important to emphasize that 1) most of this information is unique and cannot be obtained with any other available technique and 2) CA findings complement, with very comprehensive information «seeing is believing», data that can also be obtained with other techniques such as coronary angiography or intravascular ultrasound (IVUS). The complementary insights obtained from each imaging technique are most valuable for unraveling the pathologic substrate in especially challenging anatomic settings[1-6] (Fig. 19-1).

Although coronary angiography is widely available and still unsurpassed in providing a road map of the entire coronary tree and in identifying clinically relevant discrete luminal narrowing, some of its limitations soon became apparent and are now well established.[7-10] Currently, coronary angiography is no longer considered the gold standard for the precise and accurate diagnosis of coronary atherosclerosis. In this regard, while the extent and severity of coronary atherosclerosis (a disease of the vessel wall) is best

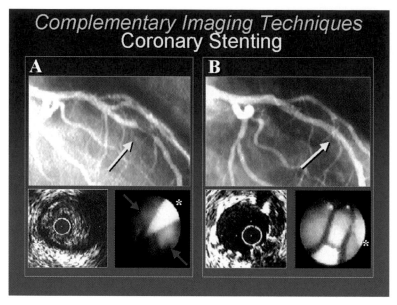

Figure 19-1. Importance of the complementary information provided by intracoronary diagnostic techniques. Patient with unstable angina and a severe lesion in the middle section of the left anterior descending coronary artery. A) Before intervention: Top, angiogram showing the severe narrowing. Bottom left, hypoechogenic plaque on intravascular ultrasound, with wedging of the imaging catheter. Bottom right, angioscopic examination of the «proximal aspect» of the lesion showing the lumen, red thrombus, and guidewire (asterisk). B) After coronary stenting: Top, final angiographic result. Bottom left, intravascular ultrasound image revealing a fully apposed and well expanded stent (the stent struts are readily recognized). Bottom right, angioscopic visualization of the implanted stent No residual thrombus is visualized at this spot (asterisk = guidewire).

depicted by IVUS,[11-15] the pathophysiology of acute coronary syndromes, where plaque fracture or erosion with superimposed thrombus formation play a major role, is best evaluated by CA.[1-6] In fact, angiographic characterization of complicated plaques is limited to a few indirect findings discernable in the lumen silhouette (Fig. 19-2). All these findings explain the considerable interest raised by the use of CA to fully elucidate the underlying pathologic substrate of patients with acute coronary syndromes for either clinical or research purposes.

In this chapter we will discuss the value of CA in the diagnosis of patients with coronary artery disease, with special emphasis on acute coronary syndromes, after briefly reviewing some technical aspects and the clues for CA image interpretation.

TECHNICAL CONSIDERATIONS. IMAGING PROTOCOL

Several commercially available, disposable, CA catheters have been widely used.[1-6] Herein, we will describe in detail one of these catheters, with which we have acquired clinical experience. The Baxter angioscope (Baxter Healthcare Corporation, Edwards LIS Division, Irvine, CA) has a polyethylene 4.5-French catheter with a length of 125 cm (Fig. 19-3). It can accommodate conventional 0.014-inch guidewires and can be advanced through 8-French guiding catheters. This angioscope has an integrated design of a flexible catheter jacket with 2 independent units that can move separately. The outer catheter contains the occlusion cuff, which is positioned proximally, adjacent to the flush

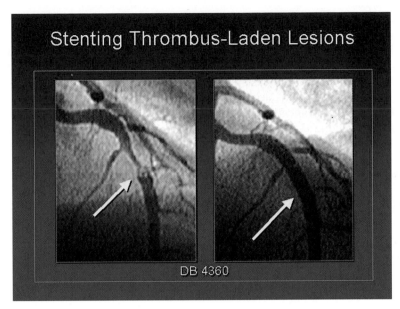

Figure 19-2. Angiographic image of a severe lesion on the proximal left anterior descending coronary artery immediately after the first septal perforator branch. An intraluminal filling defect (highly suggestive of intracoronary thrombus) is recognized distal to the lesion. After coronary stenting a «clean» angiographic result is obtained.

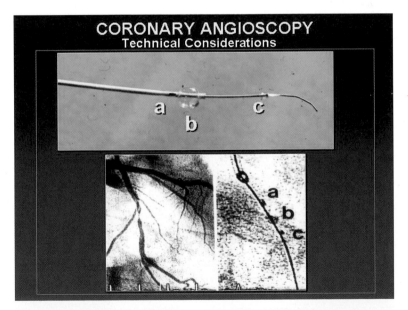

Figure 19-3. Top: Coronary angioscope. Fiber-optic bundle on the guidewire. The occlusion balloon is inflated, the inner catheter is advanced mid-way, and the xenon light is on. A) Proximal marker. B) Occlusion cuff, C) Distal tip radiopaque marker. Bottom: Angioscopic examination of a severe lesion on the left circumflex coronary artery. The radiopaque markers are easily identified on fluoroscopy.

port. The inner catheter has a 0.6-mm diameter shaft and contains the movable optic bundle, which telescopes independently of the cuff. The fiber-optic bundle consists of a 3000-pixel fused bundle surrounded by 10 light fibers with an objective lens at the tip.

The angioscope is advanced using a double monorail technique (inner and outer catheter respectively) over a radiopaque guidewire. Prior to use, angioscopes should be tested for balloon inflation, irrigation system, and flaws in the jacketing. Image sharpness should be optimized (dedicated focus knob), the intensity of light checked, and the white balance adjusted for color correction (automatically performed by imaging a reference white surface). Once within the coronary lumen, the region of interest is identified. Then, the cuff of the balloon (compliant, volumetric, rubber balloon) is gently inflated (up to 5 mm in diameter) with a mixed solution (50% saline and 50% contrast medium). Next, a power injector is used to infuse warm Ringer's lactate solution at rates of 30 to 48 ml per minute to clear blood from the area of interest. Subsequently, the fiber-optic bundle is advanced and tracked through up to 5 cm of the vessel length. Special care is required to document on fluoroscopy the positions of the radiopaque distal tip marker of the optic bundle with respect to angiographic landmarks.[1-6, 16-18]

Only patients with vessels ⩾2.5 mm by visual estimation and target lesions located in a relatively straight coronary segment should be considered for CA. Vessels with very proximal stenosis (location <20 mm from the ostium), heavy calcification, or excessive tortuosity are considered unsuitable for this technique. Imaging should be restricted to the proximal and mid-coronary segments.

Attempts should be made to obtain a circumferential (⩾3 quadrants) visualization of the target coronary segment. However, currently available angioscopes are relatively rigid and not steerable. Sometimes, circular visualization of the region of interest can be especially challenging. On rare occasions, the imaging catheter has to be completely retrieved from the vessel and rotated outside the guiding catheter. During the study, the intensity of illumination can be manually adjusted,

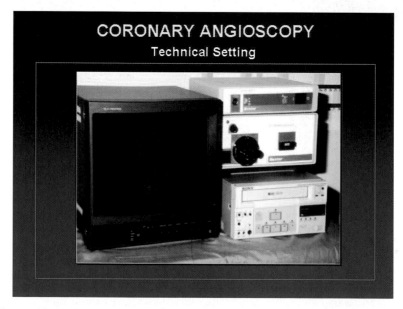

Figure 19-4. Image monitor, fiber-optic light source, video recording system.

according to the distance of the target lesion and the reflection of the vessel wall, to optimize color reproduction and to avoid halation. In general, we try to avoid crossing the lesion with the imaging catheter before intervention. Accordingly, only the proximal aspect of the culprit lesion is visualized so it is likely that certain lesion characteristics may be missed.

The angioscope is connected to a fiber-optic light source and to a miniature video camera. The image of the monitor is magnified and displayed online during the procedure and also recorded on a 0.5-inch super-VHS videotape for subsequent playback and analysis (Fig. 19-4). Online images are crisp and have excellent resolution and color quality. Super-VHS recordings suffer from image degradation but are still acceptable for diagnostic purposes. Still images are of poorer resolution and should never be interpreted without reviewing the motion picture.

Finally, it should be kept in mind that prolonged CA examination can cause transient angina, with concomitant electrocardio-graphic changes, that are quickly reversible after deflation of the occlusive cuff.[1-6, 16-18] CA-related ischemia may be more severe than that caused by IVUS interrogation or coronary angioplasty procedures. Experience and a meticulous technique are therefore mandatory. In rare cases, coronary spasm may be produced and complete withdrawal of the imaging catheter may be necessary. Transient episodes of complete A-V block may occur during studies of the right coronary artery. Manipulation of the relatively rigid imaging probe may also induce wall damage and angiographic changes have been documented after the insertion of the device.[19, 20]

IMAGE INTERPRETATION

Classification of Angioscopic Findings

Thrombi are visualized as red intraluminal structures that persist despite flushing, and

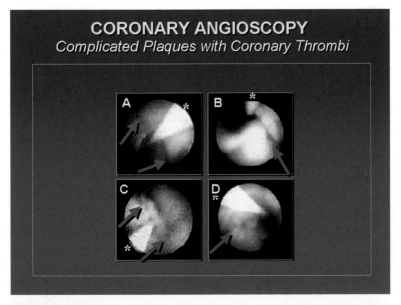

Figure 19-5. Angioscopic images of complicated lesions (A to D). The morphology of coronary lumen is smooth in A and irregular in B and D. C shows a total occlusion (no residual lumen) where the guidewire (asterisk) is wedged. Atherosclerotic yellow plaques can be appreciated (A-C). Red thrombi are also clearly visualized (red arrows).

are either mural (lining thrombus) or protrude into the coronary lumen (including occlusive thrombus)[1-6, 21-23] (Fig. 19-5). White thrombi usually show a cotton-like appearance, which may help in the differential diagnosis with coronary dissections or intimal flaps.[1-6, 21-23] Dissections consist of disrupted tissue that may be loose or immobile, but overhanging into the vessel's lumen. On CA dissection is visualized as large, sail-like, white protruding structure.[24-26] Intimal flaps are visualized as small, thin, faint, highly mobile fronds of white tissue (Fig. 19-6). Eventually, further clinical and anatomic information may be required to differentiate between white thrombus and coronary dissections. Atheromatous plaques may be categorized as flat (non-protruding) or protruding into the lumen. Plaque color should be evaluated according to its predominant chromatic characteristics.[21-23] Thus, plaques are classified as predominantly yellow, white, or mixed (patchy yellow and white plaques) (Fig. 19-7). Finally, after coronary intervention, the cuts caused by atherectomy[27] and stent struts after coronary stenting[28-29] may be also recognized.

Reproducibility of Angioscopic Findings

Since CA is a qualitative technique, there is concern about interpretation subjectivity and reproducibility. Classification systems that assess CA features exhaustively (i.e., multiple items subdivided into several categories) may be flawed by a low interobserver agreement.[21] However, good reproducibility has been observed when CA images are evaluated using relatively simple diagnostic criteria.[22, 30] To determine interobserver agreement in angioscopic findings, a random subset of 100 different coronary segments from our total patient population was selected and reviewed by two experienced observers.[22] Care was taken to include only short runs of angioscopic images for

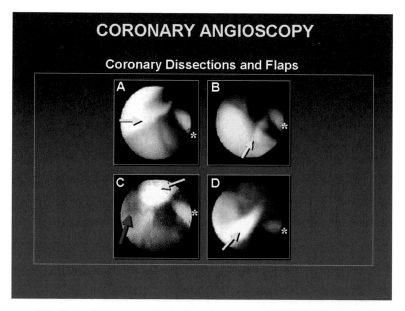

Figure 19-6.   A and B: Faint, highly mobile intimal flaps (yellow arrows) are visualized as white fronds of tissue on the coronary wall opposite to the location of the guidewire (asterisk). C and D: Non-mobile, relatively large dissections (yellow arrows) after coronary interventions. The disrupted atherosclerotic plaque can also be recognized with some residual thrombus (C, red arrow).

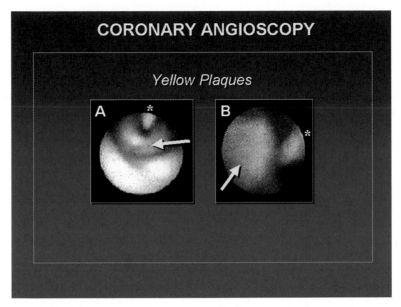

Figure 19-7.   A) Smooth, protruding yellow plaque (yellow arrow), almost completely occluding the coronary lumen. Proximal to the plaque a relatively normal whitish vessel wall is visualized. B) Eccentric yellow plaque. Asterisk denotes the guidewire.

analysis. Video recordings were interpreted blindly, without knowledge of the patient's clinical or procedural data. The items analyzed included the presence of a normal vessel wall, red thrombus, yellow plaque, intimal flaps, and side branches. Thrombi and yellow-plaques are both classified as either protruding or mural. Inter-rater agreement and kappa values (agreement in excess of what would be expected by chance) for these coronary segments are summarized in Table 19-1.[22,31] It should be emphasized that the use of

this relatively simple CA classification results in good interobserver reproducibility,[22] but is shadowed by the poor recognition of uncommon, yet potentially relevant, diagnoses.

Recently, quantitative colorimetric CA analysis has been developed to avoid hardware-induced chromatic distortion and the subjectivity of human color perception. Preliminary in vitro studies[32] suggest the potential value of this technique in assessing CA findings in a more objective and reproducible way. Further studies, however, are still

Table 19-1.   Agreement in Coronary Angioscopy Findings

	Normal Surface	Thrombus	Yellow plaque	Flap	Side-branches	Protruding*
Agreement	95%	95%	92%	94%	98%	77%
Kappa	0.88	0.89	0.81	0.82	0.92	0.66

* Protruding vs. parietal was considered only for thrombus and yellow plaques.

required to determine the value of this quantitative information during routine diagnostic imaging.

ANGIOSCOPIC FINDINGS IN SPECIFIC ANGIOGRAPHIC PATTERNS

Angiographically Normal Coronary Segments

It is well known that coronary angiography underestimates the extent and severity of atherosclerotic disease when compared with histopathological studies[7-10]. More recently, IVUS studies confirmed these observations, demonstrating that atherosclerotic plaque is generally visible on angiographically normal coronary segments of patients with coronary artery disease.[14, 15] However, the value of CA in this setting has been little evaluated. With CA, Annex et al.[33] were able to detect atheromatous changes in 10 of 12 angiographically normal vessels. They found either yellow atheromatous lesions or white lesions classified as «lipoid streaks.» To determine whether CA can detect the presence of atherosclerotic disease on proximal, angiographically normal coronary segments, we studied 52 patients before coronary angioplasty[31] (Fig. 19-8). Therefore, in contrast with the previous study,[33] the proximal coronary segments of vessels with severe distal lesions were studied. In 7 patients, angiography revealed luminal irregularities on the coronary segment proximal to the culprit lesion; all them also had proximal disease by CA. In the remaining 45 patients (87 %), angiography revealed a smooth vessel contour proximal to the target lesion. In 30 (67 %) of these patients, CA visualized proximal disease, including yellow plaque in 19 patients, mural thrombus in 5, mixed plaques in 4, and small flaps in 2 patients. Interestingly, all

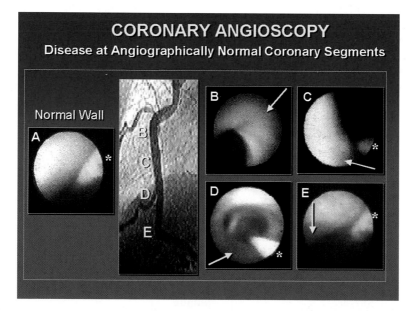

Figure 19-8. Coronary angioscopy findings on angiographically normal coronary segments. The right coronary artery is angiographically normal. At some locations (A), findings of coronary angioscopy are also normal. However, multiple sites (B to E) with non-protruding yellow plaques can be identified (yellow arrows) on angioscopy. A large smooth lumen is always present at these sites. Please notice the origin of a right ventricular branch on D. Asterisk denotes the guidewire location. Adapted from Alfonso et al.[31]

mural thrombi and the 2 flaps were seen in patients with unstable angina. In most patients, CA findings appeared to be discrete and well separated from the angiographic lesion site. All these plaques were relatively subtle and did not protrude into the coronary lumen.[31] Our findings suggest that CA is sensitive enough to visualize atherosclerotic disease at angiographically normal sites, confirming that atherosclerotic involvement of the arterial wall extends beyond the angiographic lesion site.[31, 33] In addition, it appears that the incidence and extent of atherosclerotic disease at angiographically silent sites detected with CA is slightly lower than that found with IVUS.[31] In this regard, CA appears to be better suited to depicting minor luminal surface irregularities, whereas near-field artifacts sometimes prevent accurate ultrasonic evaluation of such areas. These CA findings would represent the surface correlate (like an iceberg's peak) of underlying fully developed plaques. Therefore, it seems likely that the complementary information (tomographic study of the wall versus direct visualization of the luminal surface) that is obtained with each technique may provide further insights into the pathophysiology and clinical implications of atherosclerotic disease in angiographically normal coronary segments. In addition, the potential correlation of CA findings with information about endothelial dysfunction on angiographically normal coronary arteries[34] requires prospective evaluation.

CA also provides useful clinical insights in patients with cardiac allograft vasculopathy. In a preliminary study, Ventura et al.[35] suggested that in cardiac transplant recipients CA is more sensitive than angiography in detecting early allograft atherosclerosis. Subsequently, in an elegant study Mehra et al.[36] analyzed 107 consecutive heart transplant recipients using both IVUS and CA. Yellow (pigmented) intimal thickening was correlated with the presence of hyperlipidemia, prednisone dose, and time since transplantation. These patients also had increased intimal thickening and more frequent acute allograft rejection than the remaining patients.[36] They suggested that cardiac allograft vasculopathy is a heterogeneous disease with varied morphologic expression that has different clinical implications.

Angiographically Complex Lesions

Histopathological findings suggest that lipid-rich plaques with thin fibrous caps are vulnerable to rupture and thrombus formation.[37] Extensive clinical experience suggests that angiography may help to identify some markers of the disrupted plaque.[38-41] Patients with acute coronary syndromes frequently present with acutely occluded vessels, complex lesions, or lesions with intraluminal filling defects, all highly suggestive of a ruptured plaque with associated thrombus.[38-41] In addition, progression from stable to unstable angina has been reported to occur in some patients with eccentric lesions.[41] Lesions with these angiographic characteristics have been directly implicated in the genesis of acute coronary syndromes or, alternatively, are a harbinger of disease progression and clinical deterioration.[38-41] Nevertheless, the assessment of the underlying pathologic substrate in lesions with a complex angiographic appearance is currently a major limitation of angiography and further characterization of these lesions during coronary interventions appears to be especially warranted. With this aim, we used CA to study 47 patients with angiographically complex lesions before coronary intervention.[42] Complex angiographic lesions included coronary occlusions, lesions with intraluminal filling defects suggestive of thrombus or ulceration, and highly eccentric lesions (Ambrose Types I-II).[38-41] In all patients, CA visualized the protruding material causing the angiographic appearance. At this site, CA detected red thrombi in 34 patients (72 %) (14 protruding, 20 lining) and atherosclerotic plaque in 45 patients (96 %). Plaques were classified as predominantly yellow in 24 patients, mixed in

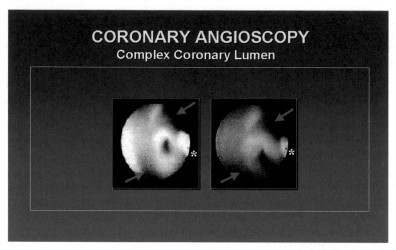

Figure 19-9.   Complex coronary lumen at sites with associated red thrombi (red arrows). The guidewire (asterisk) is not entering the true lumen.

12 and white in 9. The incidence of thrombi on CA was significantly higher for occluded vessels or lesions with intraluminal filling defects or ulceration than in eccentric lesions. However, plaque coloration was not significantly different in these angiographic subgroups. At these sites, most patients presented a raised plaque, yellow or mixed, associated with an intracoronary red thrombus (suggesting thrombi anchored on ruptured atherosclerotic plaques). In addition, in 2 of the 4 patients who presented ulcerated lesions, luminal narrowing was not very severe and the angioscope could gently cross the culprit lesion. As the optic fiber was withdrawn, a thin, white, sail-like structure protruded into the lumen. Just beneath it, a localized cavity with yellow plaque and associated red thrombus could be visualized. It is noteworthy that CA demonstrated that the underlying substrate may be different in lesions with a similar angiographic appearance (Fig. 19-9).

Total Occlusions

During coronary interventions, assessment of the underlying substrate in occluded vessels is a current limitation of angiography in which CA may prove useful. Percutaneous transluminal coronary angioplasty of occluded vessels is still a therapeutic challenge.[43, 44] The results of angioplasty in this setting are much worse than those obtained in other types of lesions and the restenosis rate is higher.[43, 44] The reason why the restenosis rate is higher is unknown, but a suboptimal initial result or the presence of angiographically unrecognized dissections or thrombi, may be involved.

Previous studies demonstrated the value of CA to define the nature of abrupt vessel closure complicating a previous coronary intervention.[45] In most cases, coronary dissection is considered the cause of vessel closure, but in 20% of patients intracoronary thrombosis appears to play a major role. Therefore, CA can be used to select appropriate therapy for these patients.[45] We also analyzed the value of CA in patients undergoing coronary interventions on occluded native coronary arteries.[46] In all patients, CA before dilation visualized protruding material that occluded the coronary lumen where the guidewire was wedged. The occlusion was a red thrombus in 90% of patients and a protruding yellow plaque in 10%. On angiography, however, only 33% of patients showed evidence of thrombus ($p < 0.01$ vs CA). After dilation,

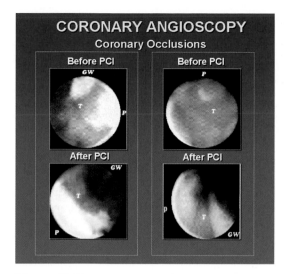

Figure 19-10. Angioscopic findings during coronary angioplasty of occluded vessels. Before coronary intervention (PCI), the vessel lumen is occluded by protruding red thrombi (T) and yellow plaques (P). After the procedure, residual thrombus (angiographically silent) is still visualized in most patients. GW denotes guidewire. Adapted from Alfonso et al.[46]

residual thrombus with plaque was seen in 89 % of patients and residual coronary dissections in 72 %. However, angiography only revealed dissection in 55 % and residual thrombus in 10 % of patients (both p < 0.001). Thus, an occlusive yellow plaque with red thrombus is the most common underlying substrate in occluded lesions (Fig. 19-10). After successful dilation, angiographically silent mural thrombi are still seen in most patients.[46] These findings make it tempting to speculate that patients with significant residual thrombus immediately after dilation may be at higher risk of thrombus progression. This could explain the higher risk for recurrent restenosis in these patients.

Saphenous Vein Grafts

Accelerated atherosclerosis may occur in saphenous vein grafts after coronary surgery.

Histopathological studies have suggested that lesions located on vein grafts may exhibit subtle morphologic differences compared with those of native arteries, and may be prone to disruption. Silva et al.[47] compared CA findings in the native coronary arteries of 42 patients with unstable angina to the corresponding findings in the saphenous vein grafts of 18 patients who also had unstable angina. There were no significant differences between the two groups in terms of plaque color, surface texture, or incidence of complex plaque morphology (ulceration or coronary thrombosis). However, loosely adherent, friable plaques were absent on the native coronary arteries but were detected with CA in 44 % of saphenous vein grafts. These findings may explain why many patients with diseased saphenous vein grafts present clinically with non-Q-wave myocardial infarction, as well as the increased risk of distal embolization during coronary interventions. In patients with old saphenous vein grafts and bulky lesions, CA has been used to guide therapy and visualize thrombus removal.[48] Some investigators have suggested the potential use of extractional atherectomy and intracoronary urokinase in selected patients with this adverse anatomy.[48]

CORONARY ANGIOSCOPY IN RELATION TO PRESENTING CORONARY SYNDROMES

Stable Angina and Unstable Angina

Pathological and experimental studies have demonstrated that plaque disruption with superimposed occlusive or non-occlusive thrombosis is the main cause of acute coronary syndromes.[37,49] Lipid-rich xanthomatous atherosclerotic plaques are rupture-prone and very thrombogenic after disruption.[37] The atheromatous core of the plaque is very rich in extracellular lipid, mainly cholesterol and its esters.[37] This atheromatous core has a distinct yellowish coloration and constitutes the most thrombogenic component of the plaque.[50]

In patients with unstable angina, CA is frequently able to visualize disrupted plaques and intracoronary thrombi that are frequently angiographically silent.[1-6] In most of these patients, a yellowish plaque is also visualized.[1-6, 51] Alternatively, most patients with stable angina have a smooth plaque surface without associated intracoronary thrombus. de Feyter et al.[30] evaluated ischemia-related lesion characteristics in patients with stable or unstable angina with IVUS and CA. They found a poor correlation between clinical status and angiographic features. In addition, probably due to the use of relatively low frequency transducers, the plaque composition determined by ultrasound was similar in patients with stable and unstable angina. However, CA was able to detect plaque rupture and thrombosis in 17 % of patients with stable angina versus 68 % of patients with unstable angina (p < 0.05). Thieme et al.[52] validated CA findings of patients with unstable angina performing histomorphological analyses of specimens removed by atherectomy. They found that 89 % of patients with unstable angina had yellow lesions. Alternatively, in patients with stable angina, gray-white and yellow plaques were similarly distributed. Histologically, gray-white lesions usually represented fibrous plaque without degeneration, whereas yellow lesions were more frequently associated with degenerated plaques or atheroma. In addition, some additional clinical factors also appear to play an important role in CA findings in patients with unstable angina. In this regard, Silva et al.[53] demonstrated that diabetic patients with unstable angina had a higher prevalence of plaque ulceration and intracoronary thrombus formation than non-diabetic patients with unstable angina. Finally, hyperlipidemia also appears to be a major determinant of plaque color.[23]

In an elegant study, Takano et al.[54] demonstrated that mechanical and structural characteristics of vulnerable plaques may also be related to CA findings. They used CA to visualize plaque characteristics and IVUS, with simultaneous intracoronary pressure recordings, to assess coronary distensibility. Yellow plaques, which are frequent in patients with acute coronary syndromes, had a pattern of positive remodeling and a relatively high distensibility index. Alternatively, lesions with white plaques more frequently had paradoxical vessel shrinkage and were relatively stiff. They suggested that yellow plaques, with a greater distensibility and degree of positive remodeling, may be mechanically and structurally weak. Mechanical fatigue caused by repetitive stretching may lead to rupture. Therefore they suggested that yellow plaques should be considered vulnerable. Likewise, Smits et al.[55] also studied coronary lesions before interventions with both CA and IVUS. They found that complex lesions on CA (irregular surface or thrombus) showed predominantly compensatory enlargement on ultrasound, whereas smooth lesions were found predominantly in shrunken arterial segments. These findings support and complement previous studies that suggest that positive remodeling is frequently detected by IVUS in patients with unstable angina, whereas negative remodeling occurs more often in patients with stable angina.[56]

Finally, the ability of CA to detect thrombi is of paramount importance in the study of patients with unstable angina.[1-6] Thrombi are frequently visualized in these patients whereas they are rare in patients with stable angina. The high sensitivity of CA for the precise diagnosis of intracoronary thrombus has been clearly demonstrated.[1-6] Several studies have suggested that in the early stages of coronary thrombosis a white, platelet-rich, thrombus may be the predominant pathologic substrate.[57] This would be the predominant pattern in patients with unstable angina studied «immediately» after the last episode of angina.[1, 3] Interestingly, thrombus color, as detected by CA, may predict its angiographic recognition. In this regard, Abela et al.[58] suggested that the sensitivity of angiography was lower for white than for red thrombi.

From a pragmatic point of view, thrombus recognition may also have clinical implications. De Zwaan et al.[59] demonstrated that, in unstable patients, thrombolysis was only of benefit in the presence of total or subtotal coronary occlusion. Theoretically speaking, CA findings may help to identify patients with acute coronary syndromes that could benefit from IIb/IIIa platelet inhibitors, coadjuvant antithrombotic, or even thrombolytic therapy. Bailey et al.[60] reported the value of CA to monitor the efficacy of local administration of glycoprotein IIb/IIIa receptor blockers. They were able to visualize a successful resolution of the thrombus in 11 out of 12 patients associated with a favorable clinical course. Alternatively, for patients with bulky red thrombi, other antithrombotic regimens would appear more appealing. However, the issue of thrombus color is still controversial and further complicated by recent histopathological studies in a porcine model,[61] suggesting that visual classification of thrombus color into white, mixed red and white, or red may not accurately reflect its histopathological morphology.

Myocardial Infarction

CA findings in the evolving phase of an acute myocardial infarction have also been established.[3] In this setting, a red thrombus, usually occlusive, is always present. These findings are in striking contrast to those found in patients with unstable angina when studied very few hours after the last episode of chest pain.[1-6] In the latter clinical scenario, a white thrombus, presumably platelet-rich, may be found at the site of the target lesion.[1-6] Such findings have been used to explain, at least in part, the effectiveness of thrombolytic therapy in acute myocardial infarction and the fact that this therapy does not benefit patients with unstable angina. However, the pathologic substrate of patients pre-

senting recurrent ischemia after an acute myocardial infarction is not as well established. In our own experience,[62] most of these patients still have a red, protruding or occlusive, thrombus in the infarct-related artery. Accordingly, our data suggest that residual red thrombus may be of paramount pathogenic importance in the appearance of recurrent ischemia after infarction[62, 63] (Fig. 19-11). These findings differ from those found in other patients with unstable angina where red thrombi are not so prevalent and occlusive thrombi are rare. A yellow or mixed (patchy yellow and white) plaque appears to be equally prevalent in patients with post-infarction angina and other types of unstable angina.[62] These results are in keeping with previous histopathological studies suggesting that two-thirds of patients with myocardial infarction present occlusive, fibrin-rich thrombi.[64] Other studies, however, have suggested a high prevalence of white thrombi even in patients studied some time after a myocardial infarction. Tabata et al.[65] used CA to evaluate 17 patients with postinfarction angina. Although intracoronary thrombus was visualized in every patient, only 5 had red thrombi whereas the remaining 12 patients presented a white or grayish-white thrombus at the lesion site. Differences in patient characteristics could help to explain such apparently conflicting results. In addition, as previously discussed in this chapter, the number of patients with occluded vessels and the time elapsed from the last episode of angina to CA examination may be relevant.[46, 62, 65]

After successful reperfusion of patients with myocardial infarction, Ueda el al.[66] demonstrated that thrombi were always recognized overlying yellow plaques. Thrombi and yellow plaques were visible up to one month after the episode of acute myocardial infarction. They suggested that in these patients red thrombi could form after blood flow was obstructed by a white thrombus. Van Belle et al.[67] also used CA to determine the natural history of infarct-related plaques

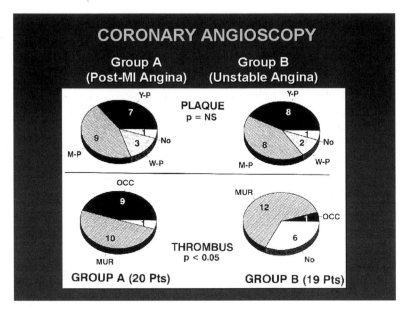

Figure 19-11. Coronary angioscopy findings in patients with post-infarction (post-MI) angina (Group A) versus those found in patients with unstable angina but without a previous myocardial infarction. Y-P = Yellow plaque. M-P = Mixed plaque. W-P = White plaque. OCC = Occlusive thrombus. MUR = Mural thrombus. Adapted from Alfonso et al.[62]

after myocardial infarction. They analyzed the morphological characteristics of the infarct-related lesion in 56 patients between 24 hours and 4 weeks after the infarction. Most lesions were complex, the predominant color was yellow (79%), and thrombi were found in 77% of patients. During the 1-month time window since the occurrence of myocardial infarction, they were unable to detect any significant difference except for a slight increase in the presence of uniformly white plaques. In addition, they also found that the initial use of a thrombolytic agent was associated with a reduction in thrombus size. It is clear that such findings suggest that the healing of a infarct-related lesion requires more than 1 month to be completed and that unstable yellow plaques with associated red thrombi are common during this period.[63, 67] Definitive evidence on this topic, however, comes from a subsequent report by Ueda et al.[68] in which 85 patients with acute myocardial infarction underwent serial (1, 6,

and 18 months) CA examinations to evaluate the healing process of infarct related plaques. As expected, the prevalence of thrombi and yellow plaques was high for a variable period following the infarction, but progressively decreased during follow-up. Interestingly, patients with diabetes and hyperlipidemia appear to have an impaired healing process.

More recently, Asakura et al.[69] studied the overall prevalence of yellow plaques in patients with recent myocardial infarction. They evaluated the culprit coronary lesion and non-infarct related coronary arteries in 20 patients. They found that in these patients with recent myocardial infarction, all three major coronary arteries were widely diseased and had multiple, yellow non-disrupted plaques. Accordingly, these investigators suggested that acute myocardial infarction may be a pan-coronary process of vulnerable plaque development eventually leading to coronary plaque rupture.

CLINICAL IMPLICATIONS
OF ANGIOSCOPIC FINDINGS

Several studies using CA have suggested the potential clinical implications of lesions containing yellow plaque. Recently, Uchida et al.[70] hypothesized that plaque characteristics could «predict» the occurrence of acute coronary syndromes during follow-up. In that study, acute coronary events occurred more frequently in patients with yellow plaques, and were especially prevalent among patients with «glistening» yellow plaques. However, care should be taken with attempts to subclassify yellow plaques since color brightness is strongly dependent on the degree of illumination and distance from the angioscope. On the other hand, the possible influence of yellow plaque on the restenosis risk after coronary interventions is controversial. While some investigators[71] have reported that the presence of a yellow plaque reduces the risk of restenosis, other groups[72] suggest that plaque color has no effect on the incidence of restenosis. As discussed previously, thrombus recognition by CA could potentially be used to select the best suited antiplatelet or antithrombotic therapy. Finally, the long-term clinical outcome after coronary interventions appears to be significantly worse in patients with thrombus-laden plaques. The risk of restenosis seems to be higher in these patients.[72] In the study by Feld et al.,[73] the presence of thrombi was an independent predictor of adverse outcome after interventions. In the study by White et al.[74] including 122 patients, patients with thrombi on CA had a 3-fold greater risk of an adverse clinical outcome. The use of CA during coronary interventions (Fig. 19-12) will be described in detail in the next chapter.

REFERENCES

1. Sherman TC, Litvack F, Grundfest W, Lee M, Hickey A, Chaux A, Kass R, Blanche C, Matloff J, Morgenstern L, Ganz W, Swan HJ, Forrester J. Coronary angioscopy in patients with unstable angina pectoris. *N Engl J Med* 1986; 315:913-919.
2. Uchida Y, Tomaru T, Nakamura F, Furuse A, Fujimori Y, Hasegawa K. Percutaneous coronary angioscopy in patients with coronary artery disease. *Am Heart J* 1987; 114:1216-1222.
3. Mizuno K, Satomura K, Miyamoto A, Ko A, Shibuya T, Tsunenori A, Kurita A, Nakamura H, Ambrose JA. Angioscopic evaluation of coronary-artery thrombi in

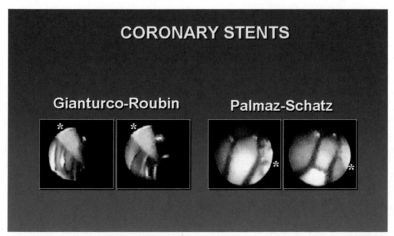

Figure 19-12.   Coronary angioscopy visualization of different stent designs. Left: coil-stent. Right: slotted-tube stent. Asterisk denotes the presence of the guidewire. The stents struts are clearly visualized, well apposed against the vessel wall, without residual dissections or thrombi.

acute coronary syndromes. *N Engl J Med* 1992; 326:287-291.

4. Lee G, Garcia JM, Corso PJ, Chan MC, Rink JL, Pichard A, Lee KK, Reis RL, Mason DT. Correlation of coronary angioscopic to angiographic findings in coronary artery disease. *Am J Cardiol* 1986; 58:238-241.

5. Siegel RJ, Ariani M, Fishbein MC, Chae JS, Park JC, Maurer G, Forrester JS. Histopathologic validation of angioscopy and intravascular ultrasound. *Circulation* 1991; 84;109-117.

6. Ramee SR, White CJ, Collins TJ, Mesa JE, Murgo JP. Percutaneous angioscopy during coronary angioplasty using a steerable microangioscope. *J Am Coll Cardiol* 1991; 17:100-105.

7. Marcus ML, Harrison DG, White CW, McPhearson DD, Wilson RF, Kerber RE. Assessing the physiological significance of coronary obstruction in patients: importance of diffuse undetected atherosclerosis. *Prog Cardiovasc Dis* 1988; 31:39-56.

8. Dietz WA, Tobis JM, Isner JM. Failure of angiography to accurately depict the extent of coronary artery narrowing in three fatal cases of percutaneous transluminal coronary angioplasty. *J Am Coll Cardiol* 1992; 19: 1261-1270.

9. Grondin CM, Dyrda I, Pasternac A, Campeau L, Bourassa MG, Lesperance J. Discrepancies between cineangiographic and postmortem findings in patients with coronary artery disease and recent coronary revascularization. *Circulation* 1974; 49: 703-708.

10. Arnett EN, Isner JN, Redwood DR, Kent KM, Baker WP, Ackerstein H, Roberts WC. Coronary artery narrowing in coronary heart disease: comparison of cineangiographic and necropsy findings. *Ann Intern Med* 1979; 91:350-356.

11. Nishimura RA, Edwards WD, Warnes CA, Reeder GS, Holmes DR, Tajik AJ, Yock PG. Intravascular ultrasound imaging: in vitro validation and pathologic correlation. *J Am Coll Cardiol* 1990; 16:145-154.

12. Hermiller JB, Tenaglia AN, Kisslo KB, Phillips HR, Bashore TM, Stack RS, Davidson CJ. In vivo validation of compensatory enlargement of atherosclerotic coronary arteries. *Am J Cardiol* 1993; 71:665-668.

13. Glagov S, Weisenberg E, Zarins CK, Stankunavicious R, Koletti GK. Compensatory enlargement of human atherosclerotic coronary arteries. *N Engl J Med* 1987; 316:1371-1375.

14. Nissen SE, Gurley JC, Grines CL, Booth DC, McClure R, Berk M, Fischer C, DeMaria AN. Intravascular ultrasound assessment of lumen size and wall morphology in normal subjects and patients with coronary artery disease. *Circulation* 1991; 84:1087-1099.

15. Alfonso F, Macaya C, Goicolea J, Iñiguez A, Hernández R, Zamorano J, Pérez-Vizcayno MJ, Zarco P. Intravascular ultrasound imaging of angiographically normal coronary segments in patients with coronary artery disease. *Am Heart J* 1994; 127:536-544.

16. Alfonso F, Goicolea J, Hernández R, Bañuelos C, Segovia J, Fernández-Ortiz A, Gonçalves M, Alonso L, Macaya C. Angioscopio Coronario: Experiencia inicial durante el intervencionismo coronario. *Rev Esp Cardiol* 1995; 48:798-806.

17. Uchida Y. Ed., Coronary Angioscopy. Futura Publishing Company. *Armonk*. New York 2001.

18. Spears JR, Spokojny AM, Marais HJ. Coronary angioscopy during cardiac catheterization *J Am Coll Cardiol* 1985; 6:93-97.

19. Alfonso F, Hernández R, Goicolea J, Silva JC, Segovia J, Bañuelos C, Zarco P, Macaya C. Angiographic deterioration of the previously dilated coronary segment induced by angioscopic examination. *Am J Cardiol* 1994; 74:604-606.

20. Lee G, Beerline D, Lee M, Wong W, Argenal AJ, Chan MC, Theis JH, Mason DT. Hazards of angioscopic examination: documentation of damage to the arterial intima. *Am Heart J* 1988; 116:1530-1536.

21. Den Heijer P, Foley DP, Hillege HL, Lablanche JM, Dijk RB, Franzen D, Morice MC, Serra A, Scheerder IK, Serruys PW, Lie KI. The «Ermenonville» classification of observations at coronary angioscopy-evaluation of intra- and inter-observer agreement. *Europ Heart J* 1994; 15;815-822.

22. Alfonso F, Silva JC, Goicolea J, Hernández R, Goncalves M, Segovia J, Fernández-Or-

tiz A, Bañuelos C, Macaya C. Reproducibility in the interpretation of coronary angioscopy findings. *Circulation* 1995; 92:I-600.

23. Kitamura K, Mizuno K, Miyamoto A, Nakamura H. Serum lipid profiles in the presence of yellow plaque in coronary lesions in vivo. *Am J Cardiol* 1997; 79:676-679.

24. Uchida Y, Hasegawa K, Kawamura K, Shibuya I. Angioscopic observations of the coronary luminal changes induced by percutaneous transluminal coronary angioplasty. *Am Heart J* 1989; 117;769-776.

25. Ramee SR, White CJ, Collins TJ, Mesa JE, Murgo JP. Percutaneous angioscopy during coronary angioplasty using a steerable microangioscope. *J Am Coll Cardiol* 1991; 17:100-105.

26. Larracet FS, Dupouy PJ, Rande JLD, Hirosaka A, Kvasnicka J, Geschwind HJ. Angioscopy after laser and balloon coronary angioplasty. *J Am Coll Cardiol* 1994; 23:1321-1326.

27. Umans VA, Baptista J, di Mario C, von Birgelen C, Quaedvlieg P, de Feyter P, Serruys PW. Angiographic, ultrasonic and angioscopic assessment of the coronary artery wall and lumen area configuration after directional atherectomy: the mechanism revisited. *Am Heart J* 1995; 130:217-227.

28. Ueda Y, Nanto S, Komamura K, Kodama K. Neointimal coverage of stents in human coronary arteries observed by angioscopy. *J Am Coll Cardiol* 1994; 23:341-346.

29. Teirstein PS, Schatz RA, Wong SC, Rocha-Singh J. Coronary stenting with angioscopic guidance. *Am J Cardiol* 1995;75:344-347.

30. de Feyter PJ, Ozaki Y, Baptista J, Escaned J, di Mario C, de Jaegere PPT, Serruys PW, Roelandt JR. Ischemia-related lesion characteristics in patients with stable or unstable angina. A study with intracoronary angioplasty and ultrasound. *Circulation* 1995; 92:1408-1413.

31. Alfonso F, Goicolea J, Hernández R, Segovia J, Silva JC, Pérez-Vizcayno MJ, Rollan MJ, Bañuelos P, Macaya C. Findings of coronary angioscopy in angiographically normal coronary segments of patients with coronary artery disease. *Am Heart J* 1995; 130:987-993.

32. Lehmann KG, van Suylen RJ, Stibbe J, Slager CJ, Oomen JA, Maas A, di Mario C,

de Feyter P, Serruys PW. Composition of human thrombus assessed by quantitative colorimetric angioscopic analysis. *Circulation* 1997; 96:3030-3041.

33. Annex BH, Larkin TJ, Hacala M, O'Neill W. Detection of atherosclerotic lesions in angiographically normal coronary arteries by percutaneous coronary angioscopy. *J Am Coll Cardiol* 1993; 88:I-589.

34. Werns SW, Walton JA, Hsia HH, Nabel EG, Sanz ML, Pitt B. Evidence of endothelial dysfunction in angiographically normal coronary arteries of patients with coronary artery disease. *Circulation* 1989; 79:287-291.

35. Ventura HO, Jain A, Mesa JE, White CJ, Ramee SR, Collins TJ, Murgo JP. Angioscopic and ultrasound in cardiac transplantation: assessment and comparison of intracoronary morphology. *J Am Coll Cardiol* 1992; 19:173A.

36. Mehra MR, Ventura HO, Jain SP, Ramireddy K, Ali A, Stapleton DD, Smart FW, Ramee SR, Collins TJ, White CJ. Heterogenicity of cardiac allograft vasculopathy: Clinical insights from coronary angioscopy. *J Am Coll Cardiol* 1997; 29:1339-1344.

37. Falk E, Shah PK, Fuster V. Coronary plaque disruption. *Circulation* 1995; 92:657-671.

38. Chen L, Chester MR, Redwood S, Huang J, Leatham E, Kaski JC. Angiographic stenosis progression and coronary events in patients with «stabilized» unstable angina. *Circulation* 1995; 91:2319-2324.

39. Capone G, Wolf NM, Meyer B, Meister SG. Frequency of intracoronary filling defects by angiography in angina pectoris at rest. *Am J Cardiol* 1985; 56:403-406.

40. Fuster V, Frye RL, Connolly DC, Danielson MA, Elveback LR, Kurland LT. Arteriographic patterns early in the onset of the coronary syndromes. *Br Heart J* 1975; 37:1250-1255.

41. Ambrose JA, Winters SL, Arora RR, Eng A, Riccio A, Gorlin R, Fuster V. Angiographic evolution of coronary artery morphology in unstable angina. *J Am Coll Cardiol* 1986; 7:472-478.

42. Alfonso F, Fernández-Ortiz A, Goicolea J, Hernández R, Segovia J, Phillips P, Bañuelos C, Macaya C. Angioscopic evaluation of angiographically complex lesions. *Am Heart J* 1997; 134:703-711.

43. Ivanhoe RJ, Weintraub WS, Douglas JS, Lembo NJ, Furman M, Gershony G, Cohen CL, King III SB. Percutaneous transluminal coronary angioplasty of chronic total occlusions. Primary success, restenosis and long term clinical follow-up. *Circulation* 1992; 85:106-115.

44. Bell MR, Berger PB, Bresnahan JF, Reeder GS, Bailey KR, Holmes DR. Initial and long-term outcome of 354 patients after coronary balloon angioplasty of total coronary occlusions. *Circulation* 1992; 85:1003-1011.

45. White CM, Ramee SR, Collins TJ, Jain SP, Escobar A. Coronary angioscopy study of abrupt occlusion after angioplasty. *J Am Coll Cardiol* 1995; 25:1681-1684.

46. Alfonso F, Goicolea J, Hernández R, Gonçalves M, Segovia J, Bañuelos C, Zarco P, Macaya C. Angioscopic findings of coronary angioplasty of coronary occlusions. *J Am Coll Cardiol* 1995; 26;135-141.

47. Silva JA, White CJ, Collins TJ, Ramee SR. Morphologic comparison of atherosclerotic lesions in native coronary arteries and saphenous vein graphs with coronary angioscopy in patients with unstable angina. *Am Heart J* 1998; 136:156-163.

48. Kaplan BM, Safian RD, Goldstein JA, Grines CL, O'Neill WW. Efficacy of angioscopy in determining the effectiveness of intracoronary urokinase and TEC atherectomy thrombus removal from occluded saphenous vein graft prior to stent implantation. *Cathet Cardiovasc Diagn* 1995; 36:335-337.

49. Davies MJ, Thomas A. Thrombosis and acute coronary lesions in sudden cardiac ischemic death. *N Engl J Med* 1984; 310:1137-1140.

50. Fernández-Ortiz A, Badimon JJ, Falk E, Fuster V, Meyer B, Mailhac A, Weng D, Shah PK, Badimon L. Characterization of the relative thrombogenicity of atherosclerotic plaque components. Implications and consequences of plaque rupture. *J Am Coll Cardiol* 1994; 23:1562-1569.

51. Alfonso F. Aportaciones de las nuevas técnicas invasivas de imagen al conocimiento de la biopatología de la angina inestable. *Rev Esp Cardiol* 1999; 52:Sup1:23-38.

52. Thieme T, Wernecke KD, Meyer R, Brandenstein E, Habedank D, Hinz A, Felix SB, Baumann G, Kleber FX. Angioscopic evaluation of atherosclerotic plaques: validation by histomorphologic analysis and association with stable and unstable coronary syndromes. *J Am Coll Cardiol* 1996; 28:1-6.

53. Silva JA, Escobar A, Collins TJ, Ramee SR, White CJ. Unstable angina. A comparison of angioscopic findings between diabetic and nondiabetic patients. *Circulation* 1995; 92:1731-1736.

54. Takamo M, Mizuno K, Okamatsu K, Yokoyama S, Ohba T, Sakai S. Mechanical and structural characteristics of vulnerable plaques: analysis by coronary angioscopy and intravascular ultrasound. *J Am Coll Cardiol* 2001; 38:99-104.

55. Smits PC, Pasterkamp G, de Jaegere PP, de Feyter PJ, Borst C. Angioscopic complex lesions are predominantly compensatory enlarged: an angioscopy and intracoronary ultrasound study. *Cardiovasc Res* 1999; 41:458-464.

56. Nakamura M, Nishikawa H, Mukai S, Setsuda M, Nakajima K, Tanade H, Suzuki H, Ohnishi T, Kakatua Y, Yeung AC. Impact of coronary artery remodelling on clinical presentation of patients with coronary artery disease. *J Am Coll Cardiol* 2001; 37: 63-69.

57. Chesebro JH, Webster MW, Zoldhelyi P, Roche PC, Badimon L, Badimon JJ. Antithrombotic therapy and progression of coronary artery disease. Antiplatelet versus antithrombins. *Circulation* 1992; 86; 1992; 86; III:100-110.

58. Abela GS, Eisenberg JD, Mittleman MA, Nesto RW, Leeman D, Zarich S, Waxman S, Prieto AR, Manzo KS. Detecting and differentiating white from red thrombus by angiography in angina pectoris and in acute myocardial infarction. *Am J Cardiol* 1999; 83:94-97.

59. De Zwaan C, Bar FW, Janssen JA, de Swart HB, Vermeer F, Wellens HJ. Effects of thrombolytic therapy in unstable angina: Clinical and angiographic results. *J Am Coll Cardiol* 1988; 12:301-309.

60. Bailey SR, O'Leary E, Chilton R. Angioscopic evaluation of site-specific administration of ReoPro. *Cathet Cardiovasc Diagn* 1997; 42:181-184.

61. Maegn M, den Heijer P, Olesen PG, Emmertsen NC, Nielsen TT, Falk E, Andersen HR. Histopathologic validation of in-vivo angioscopic observation of coronary thrombus after angioplasty in a porcine model. *Coron Artery Dis* 2001; 12:53-59.

62. Alfonso F, Segovia J, Goicolea J, Hernández R, Fernández-Ortiz A, Bañuelos C, Macaya C. Angioscopic characteristics of coronary narrowing in patients with recurrent myocardial ischemia after myocardial infarction. *Am J Cardiol* 1997; 79:1394-1396.

63. Alfonso F. Natural history of infarct-related lesions. *Circulation* 1998; 98:1825-1826.

64. Kragel AH, Gertz SD, Roberts WC. Morphologic comparison of frequency and types of acute lesions in the major epicardial coronary arteries in unstable angina pectoris, sudden coronary death and acute myocardial infarction. *J Am Coll Cardiol* 1991; 18:801-808.

65. Tabata H, Mizuno K, Arakawa K, Satomura K, Shibuya T, Kurita A, Nakamura H. Angioscopic identification of thrombus in patients with postinfarction angina. *J Am Coll Cardiol* 1995; 25:1282-1285.

66. Ueda Y, Asakura M, Hirayama A, Komamura K, Hori M, Komada K. Intracoronary morphology of culprit lesions after reperfusion in acute myocardial infarction: serial angioscopic observations. *J Am Coll Cardiol* 1996; 27:606-610.

67. Van Belle E, Lablanche JM, Bauters C, Renaud N, McFadden EP, Bertrand ME. Coronary angioscopic findings in the infarct related vessel within 1 month of acute myocardial infarction. Natural history and effect of thrombolysis. *Circulation* 1998; 97:26-33.

68. Ueda Y, Asakura M, Yamaguchi O, Hirayama A, Hori M, Kodama K. The healing process of infarct-related plaques. Insights from 18 months serial angioscopic follow-up. *J Am Coll Cardiol* 2001; 38:1916-1922.

69. Asakura M, Ueda Y, Yamaguchi O, Adachi T, Hirayama A, Hori M, Kodama K. Extensive development of vulnerable plaques as a pan-coronary process in patients with myocardial infarction: an angioscopic study. *J Am Coll Cardiol* 2001; 37:1284-1288.

70. Uchida Y, Nakamura F, Tomaru T, Morita T, Oshima T, Sasaki T, Morizuki S, Hirose J. Prediction of acute coronary syndromes by percutaneous coronary angioscopy in patients with stable angina. *Am Heart J* 1995; 130:195-203.

71. Itoh A, Miyazaki S, Nonogi H, Daikoku S, Haze K. Angioscopic prediction of successful dilation and of restenosis in percutaneous transluminal coronary angioplasty. Significance of yellow plaque. *Circulation* 1995; 91:1389-1396.

72. Bauters Ch, Lablanche JM, McFadden EP, Hamon M, Bertrand ME. Relation of coronary angioscopic findings at coronary angioplasty to angiographic restenosis. *Circulation* 1995; 92:2473-2479.

73. Feld S, Ganim M, Carell ES, Kjellgren O, Kirkeeide RL, Vaughn WK, Kelly R, McGhie AI, Kramer N, Loyd D, Anderson HV, Schoroth G, Smalling RW. Comparison of angioscopy, intravascular ultrasound imaging and quantitative coronary angiography in predicting clinical outcome after coronary interventions in high risk patients. *J Am Coll Cardiol* 1996; 28:97-105.

74. White CJ, Ramee SR, Collins TJ, Escobar AE, Karsan A, Shaw D, Jain SP, Bass TA, Heuser RR, Teirstein PS, Bonan R, Walter PD, Smalling RW. Coronary thrombus increases PTCA risk. Angioscopy as a clinical tool. *Circulation* 1996; 93:253-258.

20

Coronary Angioscopy: Therapeutic Implications. Value During Coronary Interventions

PIM J. DE FEYTER, MD
JURGEN LIGTHART, MD
KENGO TANABE, MD

Introduction. Angioscopic Observations after Coronary Intervention. Angioscopy to Predict In-Hospital Major Complications or Late Restenosis after Balloon Angioplasty. Angioscopy of Proximal Coronary Segment. Angioscopy to Assess Abrupt Periprocedural Occlusion after Balloon Angioplasty. Angioscopy to Select Device for Treatment of Saphenous Vein Bypass Graft Lesions. Coronary Angioscopy and Thrombolysis. Angioscopy and Pharmacological Stabilization of the Vulnerable Coronary Plaque. Conclusion. Recommended Reading. References.

INTRODUCTION

Coronary angiography is, and in the near foreseeable future will continue to be, the gold standard for coronary imaging as a guide for percutaneous coronary interventions.

Yet, the interpretation of coronary angiographic images is not always straightforward. It can sometimes be misleading or certain features may not be detectable, such as the color of intracoronary thrombi. Two other catheter-based coronary imaging modalities, intracoronary ultrasound and coronary angioscopy, may offer additional valuable diagnostic information. In this chapter we will focus on the diagnostic and prognostic value of coronary angioscopy during percutaneous coronary interventions. Pioneering studies have shown that coronary angioscopy is safe and feasible *in vivo* in both animals and humans.[1-15]

The greatest strength of angioscopy is its ability to provide a full-color, three-dimensional perspective of the coronary surface morphology and intracoronary structures. Consequently, angioscopy is suitable for distinguishing between a smooth or disrupted plaque surface, yellow or white plaques, red or white thrombi, and presence of intimal flaps or dissections. Therefore, angioscopy may be helpful in selecting treatment, such as antiplatelet or thrombolytic therapy, or in monitoring coronary interventions, such as balloon angioplasty, stent implantation, atherectomy, or laser treatment.

ANGIOSCOPIC OBSERVATIONS AFTER CORONARY INTERVENTION

Angiography severely underestimates the presence of flaps, dissections, or thrombi during balloon angioplasty in patients with either stable or unstable angina[16-19] (Table 20-1) (Figs. 20-1, 20-2).

Angioscopy revealed additional information, often undetected by angiography, in patients with acute coronary syndromes who underwent balloon angioplasty. Uchida et

Table 20-1. Angiographic and Angioscopic
Findings in Acute Coronary Syndromes after
Balloon Angioplasty in 21 Patients

	Angiography	Angioscopy
Flap	5	15
Dissection	0	2
Thrombus	3	11

From Uchida, Coronary Angioscopy, pp. 131-164.

al.[19] studied 36 patients with acute coronary syndrome. All the patients had an occlusive thrombus before angioplasty. After angioplasty, occlusive thrombi were no longer present, but 33 patients had a mural thrombus and, most interestingly, there was evidence of distal thrombotic embolization in 7 patients, underscoring the fact that these patients require intense anti-platelet treatment with GP IIb/IIIa inhibitors.

Serial angioscopy in patients with stable angina who underwent balloon angioplasty

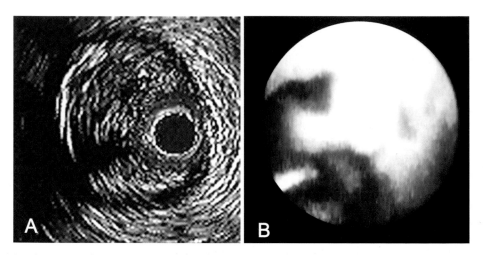

Figure 20-1. IVUS post balloon angioplasty revealing a large dissecting flap within the lumen extending from 01 o'clock to 09 o'clock. The flap is clearly visible with angioscopy. Angiographic findings were inconclusive.

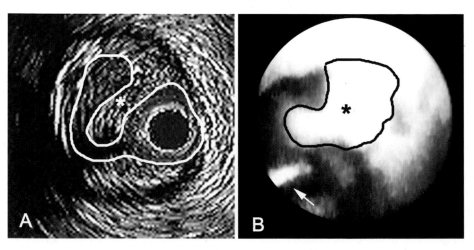

Figure 20-2. Schematics of Figure 20-1A, B. * = flap, arrow = guidewire.

Table 20-2. Serial Angioscopic Findings after Angioplasty of Stable Plaques

	Before angioplasty	Immediately after angioplasty	1 month	6 months	12 monts
N of plaques	30	30	26	20	20
Flap	0	21	2	0	0
White	18	7	12	16	15
Yellow	12	23	14	4	5

From Uchida, Coronary Angioscopy, pp. 131-164.

demonstrated the high incidence of flaps immediately after the procedure, which all were virtually healed 1 month following angioplasty[19] (Table 20-2). Angioscopy clearly demonstrated that, following angioplasty, the color of the plaques changed from yellow to white, due to the formation of neointimal hyperplasia, suggesting that plaque sealing and stabilization may have occurred.[19] Angioscopic evaluation of prolonged versus standard balloon inflation during coronary angioplasty in a randomized study revealed that prolonged balloon inflation results in a larger lumen and lower incidence of intimal flaps in comparison with standard inflation.[20]

Angioscopic evaluation after directional atherectomy revealed the presence of a thrombus in 61 % of the patients, the majority of which were newly formed thrombi at the atherectomy site undisclosed by angiography.[21] Flaps and dissections occurring in 83 % of the patients were detected almost exclusively by angioscopy (Figs. 20-3, 20-4).

Angioscopy after laser angioplasty revealed that laser treatment does not result in thermal injury and that irregular channels with significant tissue remnants were created, which explained the suboptimal angiographic result often observed after laser treatment.[22, 23]

Angioscopy after laser and balloon coronary angioplasty showed that balloon angioplasty was associated with a higher incidence of dissections (43 % vs. 17 %) and subintimal hemorrhage (53 % vs. 17 %) than laser angioplasty.[24]

Angioscopic evaluation after stent implantation demonstrated that balloon-induced dissection was successfully tackled by stent implantation and that plaque protrusion through the stent struts was often observed immediately after stent implantation[25] (Figs. 20-5, 20-6). It appears that the coronary stent acts as an anchor for thrombus formation, which may be caused by flow disturbances. The stent struts become covered by layers of fibrin, which then catch red blood cells that become incorporated, thus forming a mural or globular red thrombus. We have observed a few cases where incomplete stent expansion was associated with a total red clot occlusion.

Stent coverage by neointimal hyperplasia can be observed by serial angioscopy.[19, 26] It was shown that stent coverage is achieved in many cases in stable plaques after 1 month, but it is often still incomplete (Table 20-3). After 3 months, the stents were almost completely covered with neointimal hyperplasia. Almost similar findings were observed after stenting of unstable plaques (Table 20-4). These findings may affect the duration of post-stent implantation treatment with thienopyridines.

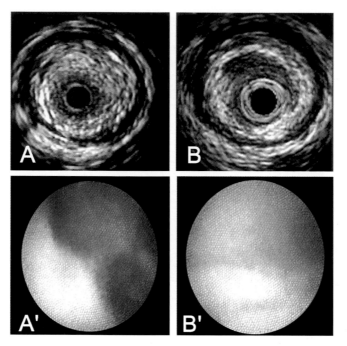

Figure 20-3. IVUS before (A) and after (B) directional coronary atherectomy. Angioscopy before (A′) showing a significant red thrombus on a yellow plaque, and after removal of plaque and thrombus, (B′) after atherectomy, showing a white flap unnoticed by angiography.

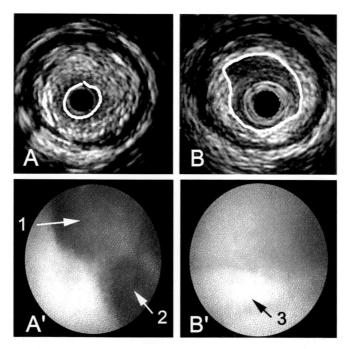

Figure 20-4. Schematics of Figure 20-3. Red thrombus: arrow 1, lumen: arrow 2, white flap: arrow 3.

Table 20-3. Angioscopic Observations of Neo-Intimal Coverage of Stents in Stable Patients

Serial angioscopy	Uchida		Ueda	
	1 month	**6 months**	**8-45 days**	**65-142 days**
N. of stents	20	15	11	13
Complete coverage	15	14	2	11
Incomplete coverage	5	1	9	0

From Uchida, Coronary Angioscopy, pp. 131-164 and Ueda, JACC 1994; 23:341.

Table 20-4. Serial Angioscopic Findings after Stenting of Unstable Plaques

	1 month	6 months
N. of stents	21	21
Complete coverage	13 (61%)	18 (86%)
Incomplete coverage	8 (39%)	3 (14%)

From Uchida, Coronary Angioscopy pp. 131-164.

ANGIOSCOPY TO PREDICT IN-HOSPITAL MAJOR COMPLICATIONS OR LATE RESTENOSIS AFTER BALLOON ANGIOPLASTY

Several studies have indicated that various angioscopic variables were associated with an increase in major in-hospital complications (death, non-fatal myocardial infarction, or emergent revascularization).[27-30] It appeared that the presence of a thrombus, a yellow plaque, or a disrupted surface were pre-

Table 20-5. Angioscopy to Predict Major in-hospital Complications*

Authors	N. of patients	Angioscopy	Occurrence of complication
Itoh[27]	47	No thrombus/thrombus White/yellow	2% vs. 14% 0% vs. 7%
White[28]	74	No thrombus/thrombus	2% vs. 14%
Waxman**[29]	32	No thrombus/thrombus White/yellow No disruption/disruption No complex/complex lesion	4% vs. 36% 4% vs. 33% 4.5% vs. 30% 0% vs. 33%
Feld**[30]	33	No thrombus/thrombus White/yellow No disruption/disruption	10% vs. 62% 0% vs. 41% 17% vs. 70%

* Major in-hospital complication: death, non-fatal myocardial infarction, emergent revascularization.
** High risk patients.

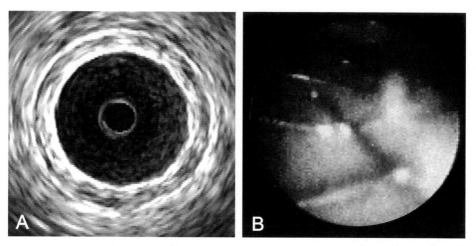

Figure 20-5.   Post stent implantation. IVUS (A) demonstrates complete apposition of stent. Angioscopy (B) shows nice apposition of the stent and a white flap protruding through the stent struts.

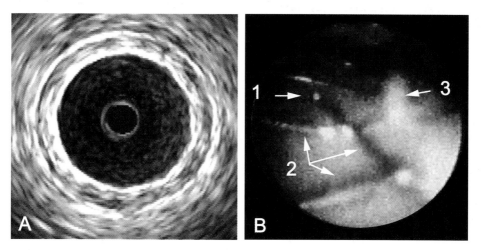

Figure 20-6.   Air bubble: arrow 1, stent struts: arrow 2, protruding flap: arrow 3.

dictive of a higher likelihood of in-hospital cardiac adverse events (Table 20-5).

Although angioscopy after balloon angioplasty revealed intimal flaps in more than 60 % of cases, these findings were not predictive for an adverse event.[30] It is worth mentioning that 1) angiography significantly under-diagnosed the presence of coronary thrombi (20 % versus 60 % for angioscopy) and 2) that angiographic variables were much less powerful predictors of major in-hospital complications.

The findings in relation to the predictive value of angioscopic variables to predict late restenosis are somewhat conflicting. Itoh et al.[27] demonstrated that yellow plaques were associated with a restenosis rate of 17 % versus 58 % in the case of white plaques. Bauters et al.[31] found the opposite results; yellow plaques had a restenosis rate of 49 % versus a restenosis rate of 37 % in white plaques. However, Bauters et al.[31] showed that absence of any thrombus or the presence of a lining thrombus or a protruding thrombus was associated with restenosis rates of 38 %, 47 %, and 65 %, respectively, whereas the late loss was 0.47 ± 0.54 mm, 0.59 ± 0.67 mm, and 1.07 ± 0.77 mm, respectively.

These results indicate that coronary angioscopy may be helpful in predicting the risk of major in-hospital complication or late restenosis after balloon angioplasty. Unfortunately, no data are available on predictive angioscopic findings after coronary stent implantation.

ANGIOSCOPY OF PROXIMAL CORONARY SEGMENT

Angioscopy can detect damage of the coronary segments proximal to the treated lesion caused by passage of the balloon. The damage may consist of endothelial exfoliation, intimal flaps and mural bleeding. Mechanical damage was observed in 63 % of the patients.[16]

ANGIOSCOPY TO ASSESS ABRUPT PERIPROCEDURAL OCCLUSION AFTER BALLOON ANGIOPLASTY

Abrupt periprocedural coronary occlusion after balloon angioplasty is caused by thrombi, dissection, or plaque disruption with extrusion of the plaque components.

Coronary angiography cannot reliably identify the exact underlying cause of abrupt occlusion in individual cases. However, coronary angioscopy was successful in distinguishing between these different causes.[32, 33] White et al.[34] performed coronary angioscopy in 17 patients with angiographic confirmation of post-angioplasty vessel occlusion. Angioscopy demonstrated that the primary cause was dissection in 82 % of patients and intracoronary thrombi in 18 % of patients. Angiography was much less accurate and only correctly identified the exact cause of abrupt occlusion in 29 % of cases.

The importance of the use of angioscopy in this particular setting is now much less relevant because stent implantation, irrespective of the underlying cause, will almost always remedy the problem.

ANGIOSCOPY TO SELECT DEVICE FOR TREATMENT OF SAPHENOUS VEIN BYPASS GRAFT LESIONS

Angiographically, it is often difficult to comprehensively assess complex intra-graft lesions with regard to friability, the presence of thrombi, or ulcerations.

Angioscopy may be helpful to identify features that may be useful in selecting the appropriate treatment modality.[35] White et al.,[36] in a study of 21 patients, showed that angioscopy identified thrombi in 71 %, dissection in 66 %, and friability in 52 % of cases vs. angiography in 19 %, 9.5 %, and 19 % of cases, respectively.

Thus, similar to the situation in native coronary arteries, angioscopy is superior to angiography in assessing complex intragraft lesion morphology. Accurate assessment of underlying graft disease with angioscopy may assist in the selection of the appropriate percutaneous treatment approach. The presence of red thrombi may lead to pre-treatment with a thrombolytic agent which, in the case of a totally occluded graft, may be infused in the graft over a period of 24 to 48 hours. In the presence of soft, friable material, one may preferentially select a covered stent or use a distal embolic protection device to prevent the deleterious effects of embolization.

CORONARY ANGIOSCOPY AND THROMBOLYSIS

Coronary angioscopy showed that intracoronary thrombi in patients with unstable angina were white, whereas red thrombi were predominantly observed in patients

SECTION V

Intracoronary Doppler

21

Technical Considerations. Diagnostic Patterns. Clinical Applications

JAVIER SORIANO, MD
JAVIER BOTAS, MD
JAIME ELIZAGA, MD

Introduction. Coronary Physiology and Doppler Patterns in coronary blood flow velocity. Clinical applications of the Doppler Guidewire. Safety and complications of the technique. Conclusions. References.

INTRODUCTION

In the last few years, angiographic and intravascular ultrasound techniques have seen considerable development, which has lead to tremendous progress in our knowledge of coronary anatomy. Even so, these techniques are still limited. The eccentric nature of the lesions (75 % are eccentric), as well as the presence of diffuse disease and sequential lesions, complicate treatment decisions that are based solely on morphological assessment of the lesions. Doppler velocimetry studies of myocardial blood flow contribute significant functional information about coronary disease that cannot be obtained with morphological techniques. Given the current technical simplicity of Doppler imaging studies, the technique can be easily applied in diagnostic and therapeutic procedures in daily practice.

The physiological bases and technical aspects of intracoronary Doppler, and its clinical applications in intravascular diagnostics are reviewed in this chapter.

TECHNICAL CONSIDERATIONS

Principles of Doppler Velocimetry

Basic Principles

Flow evaluation using Doppler velocimetry is based on a relatively simple physical principle. When a receiver and source of sonic energy move, it originates a change in frequency between them. Movement that reduces the distance between the source and receiver increases the frequency, and movement that increases this distance decreases the frequency. This phenomenon is known as the Doppler effect and was described by the Austrian physicist Christian Johann Doppler (1803-53). The relative movement between energy source and the receptor is called the Doppler shift and is proportional to the speed and direction of movement. Electronic processing of signals can measure this effect and precisely determine the velocity at which two objects move relative to each other.

Application to Blood Flow

In practice, the Doppler principle is applied to blood flow using a piezoelectric crystal mounted on the tip of an intravascular catheter to transmit and receive high-frequency sounds in order to measure the speed at which the red blood cells move through an artery. The transducer transmits and receives ultrasound at a known frequency, and the instrument measures the Doppler shift produced by the movement of the red blood cells (Fig. 21-1). The operator manipulates the transducer and positions it exactly using fluoroscopy while electronic circuits analyze the signal that allows continuous determinations to be made of the changes in Doppler frequency and blood flow velocity, thereby identifying different flow patterns.

Blood flow velocity is obtained by calculating the difference between the frequency of transmission and reception (Doppler frequency shift), using the following equation:

$$V = \frac{(F_1 - F_0) \times (C)}{2F_0 \times (\cos\Phi)}$$

V = blood flow velocity
F_0 = transmission frequency (transducer)
F_1 = return frequency
C = constant of the speed of sound in blood
Φ = angle of incidence

This formula has several ratios that must be taken into account if the Doppler technique is to be applied optimally to coronary circulation. The measurement of velocity (V) depends on the angle of incidence (Φ), so it is essential that the transducer be lined up parallel to the direction of the bloodstream to obtain an angle of incidence of 0° and a cosine of 1. Under these conditions, the changes in the Doppler frequency of the blood flow are faithfully reflected.[1]

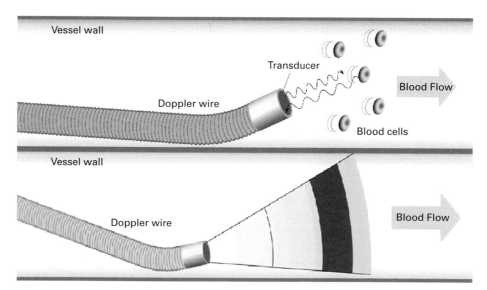

Figure 21-1. *Top*: Diagram of the Doppler concept. An intravascular piezoelectric transducer emits high-frequency ultrasonic waves that bounce off the moving red blood cells. The difference between the transmission frequency and reception frequency is the Doppler shift, a value directly related to the velocity and direction of the moving red blood cells. *Bottom*: Diagram of the ultrasonic beam transmitted by the Doppler guidewire transducer. The volume of the blood stream under examination is relatively large, as it produces a wide ultrasound beam that diverges 45° forwards, thus obtaining a wide sample of the flow velocities at a preset distance from the transducer. (Courtesy of Jomed.)

Doppler systems can measure velocity with continued or pulsed ultrasound waves. In continuous-wave Doppler systems, the transducer detects the maximum velocity at any point along the ultrasound beam. In intracoronary use, the maximum velocity is of less interest than knowing the flow velocity at a predetermined distance from the transducer. This can be done using pulsed-wave Doppler systems, which also measure the magnitude and direction of flow changes. This is why pulsed-wave technology is used on all intracoronary Doppler devices.

The narrow space between the position of the transducer and the sample volume are both an advantage and disadvantage with pulsed-wave Doppler. Only a small sample of blood is examined and it may not precisely reflect the velocity of the whole bloodstream in the area studied. This problem is particularly relevant in areas of turbulent flow (such as areas distal to severe stenoses) or in geometrically complicated coronary segments, where different strata of the bloodstream can move at different velocities.

Blood flow velocity measured in the coronary arteries is a function of instantaneous volumetric flow. These two parameters are related by the following formula

$Q = k \times A \times V$
Q = flow volume in ml/s
V = velocity in cm/s
A = cross-section of the vessel in cm^2
k = constant applied to the mean velocity

Therefore, volumetric blood flow can be calculated as the product of the vessel cross-section, measured angiographically, multiplied by the flow velocity and a correction factor for the parabolic profile of flow through the vessel. When the cross-section of the vessel remains constant, changes in Doppler flow velocity can be used to represent the changes in absolute coronary flow. Conservation of the flow velocity along the entire length of the epicardial artery is the result of a gradual decrease in vascular section as volumetric flow is distributed towards the lateral branches.[2] The severity of resting coronary stenosis can be assessed by applying these principles, as well as the relative increase in flow in response to vasodilators.

Doppler Signal. Techniques of analysis

The flow signal obtained with intracoronary Doppler is analyzed using two different methods. The zero-crossing method calculates the Doppler frequency shift from the interval between each pair of adjacent zero crossing signals of the same polarity. Although this technique is simple and precise in laminar flow areas, it is imprecise in areas of turbulent flow and for the determination of peak velocities. This method obtains a Doppler shift value that represents only an approximation to the many flow components.

The second Doppler signal processing method is more sophisticated and uses spectral analysis of the signal with fast Fourier transform (FFT). This method analyzes the frequency components to distinguish turbulent flow from laminar flow and correctly weigh the contribution of each flow pattern to the integrated value. Animal and human values have shown that the zero-crossing method underestimates the mean velocity in comparison with FFT. Large differences have been observed between the measurements of flow velocity obtained with each of these methods.[2] For this reason, FFT is the method of choice in the latest models of intracoronary Doppler devices, for the reliability and precision of its measurements in the assessment of coronary flow physiology.

Doppler equipment

Initial Prototypes

The first model designed to measure intracoronary flow velocity consisted in a transducer mounted on a Sones[3] or Judkins[4] angiographic catheter. With these systems it was not possible to make selective measurements in the vessel of interest and there was contamination in the flow due to aortic components. Smaller devices were subsequently developed for sub-selective intracoronary placement.[5] The initial devices were relatively large (diameter 3F, 1 mm) and could measure the velocities only in the proximal segments of the coronary arteries. All of these Doppler catheters used the zero-crossing method for signal processing, which limited their ability to differentiate laminar flow from turbulent flow. In addition, the early transducer models used a pulse frequency of 20 MHz with a pulse repetition frequency of 62.5 kHz, thus limiting the detection to peak velocities of 110 cm/s, which are lower than those that occur in severely stenotic arteries.

Current equipment.
Doppler guidewire

Technical advances finally led to the development of a guidewire equipped with a miniaturized Doppler transducer (Flowire, Cardiometrics Inc., California). This device consists of a flexible, steerable guidewire measuring 175- 300 cm, with a tip-mounted piezoelectric 12-MHz to 15-MHz ultrasonic transducer. The profile (0.014 inches) is small and its handling is similar to that of regular angioplasty guidewires. With a cross-section of 0.164 mm², the guide has an almost negligible effect on coronary flow and can advance to the segments distal to the coronary stenosis to record post-stenotic velocity, as it is not obstructive even in the most severe lesions nor does it produce any alteration in the flow distal to the tip even in small-caliber arteries. The guidewire adapts to monorail or coaxial angioplasty systems, allowing diagnostic and therapeutic procedures to be carried out without changing the wire (Fig. 21-2).

The Doppler flowire uses a pulsed-wave transducer which places the sample volume 4.2 mm distal to the tip of the guidewire. The volume of blood examined is relatively large using a wide ultrasound beam that diverges,

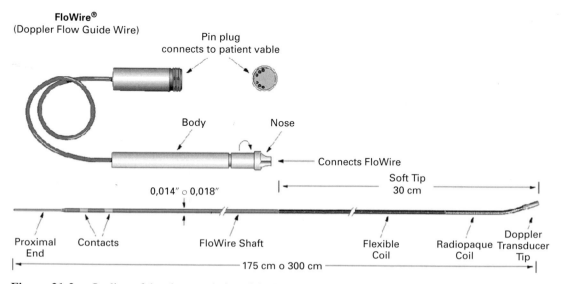

Figure 21-2. Outline of the characteristics of the Doppler FloWire guidewire, which has a miniaturized 12-MHz transducer in the tip. The guide is connected to the console by means of two cables, the first of which is a rotating connector fitted directly to the distal end of the guidewire that can be used as a rotor. The second connects the guidewire body cable to the console. (Courtesy of Jomed.)

in the latest model, at an angle of 45° forward to allow a large part of the flow velocity profile to be sampled (Figure 21-1, bottom). The signal transmitted by the transducer is processed using the square of the Doppler audio signal obtained by a real-time spectral analyzer using FFT. An adjustable pulse-repetition frequency of 12 to 94 kHz, a pulse duration of 0.83 μs and a sampling delay of 0.5 μs are satisfactory technical aspects for the spectral analysis of the signal. The frequency response of this system calculates approximately 90 spectra per second. The flowire is connected to a console with a monitor to display the patient's demographic and hemodynamic parameters (heart rate and arterial blood pressure), an ECG signal, and the spectrum flow signal as processed by the

FFT, generating a phased-spectrum tracing on the monitor using a grayscale that allows assessment of the relative contribution of the systole and diastole to the coronary flow.

In some cases, the movement of the vessel wall and signals from vein structures produce artifacts that can be eliminated by repositioning the guide in a more central area or by adjusting the J shape of the wire tip. It can occasionally be difficult to obtain an appropriate distal signal and it may be deduced that this reduction is due to stenosis. For this reason, the signal must be sought using different guide-tip alignments until the spectrum with the greatest velocity and intensity is obtained (Fig. 21-3). In tortuous segments or in complex lesions, additional manipulation may be required.

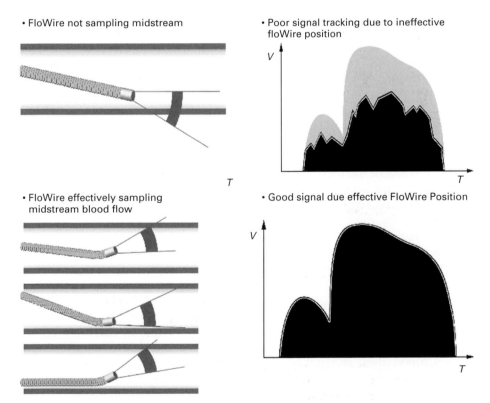

Figure 21-3. Diagram of the capture of a good Doppler signal, ensuring the clinical effectiveness of the measurement of coronary flow. *Top*: When sampling of the central area of the blood flow is not achieved, then a low-quality spectrum signal is obtained. *Bottom*: By repositioning the guide or shaping the tip in the form of a J, a good, dense, regular and reproducible signal is obtained. (Courtesy of Jomed.)

The Doppler flowire has been validated experimentally in dogs by measuring the coronary velocity in the proximal segment of the coronary arteries. An excellent correlation ($r^2 = 0.936$) has been found between the Doppler flow velocity spectrum and electromagnetic flow probes.[6]

CORONARY PHYSIOLOGY AND DOPPLER PATTERNS IN CORONARY BLOOD FLOW VELOCITY

Characteristics of Coronary Blood Flow

Coronary blood flow has a distinctive phase characteristic, which is higher during diastole. In addition, there are differences between the right (RC) and left (LC) coronary arteries. The LC is subject to the pressure transmitted by the left ventricle during systole, whereas the RC receives a much lower level of pressure. For this reason, the blood flow in the LC and its branches occurs primarily during diastole, whereas the RC has a much more continuous flow throughout the cardiac cycle.[7] Saphenous vein grafts have a predominantly diastolic pattern, similar to that of the native arteries, although there may be acuminate systolic waves in the proximal segment reflecting the great capacity for distension of these grafts. In the proximal segment of grafts of internal mammary artery, the flow velocity is similar to that of the subclavian, with systolic dominance. The pattern changes distally, close to the anastomosis, and shows the dominance of the diastolic component and velocities similar to those of the native coronary artery.[8]

Myocardial blood flow is regulated by changes in vascular resistance at the level of the coronary arterioles, with a self-regulation mechanism determined by oxygen consumption, sympathetic stimulation, and endothelial production of nitric oxide.[9] Coronary vascular resistance may be con-

sidered to be the sum of three different components. The first of these components lies in the large epicardial arteries, whose main function is as capacitance vessels with a minimal contribution to total coronary resistance in the absence of fixed or dynamic stenosis. The second, and most important, component lies in the precapillary arterioles. The last component is located in the intramural coronary capillaries, where resistance rises considerably during systole, due to the mechanical compression produced by ventricular contraction.[7]

Gould et al,[10] originally described the principle of coronary flow reserve (CFR) in the 1970s. During exercise, and in the absence of stenosis, coronary flow may increase by 4 to 6-fold to satisfy the oxygen demands of the myocardium. This effect is mediated by the vasodilation of the arterioles, or resistance vessels, which are tonically constrained at rest. The term CFR refers to the maximum capacity of the coronary vessel bed to increase the blood flow in response to an increase in demand or to a stimulus producing a maximal hyperemia response. This capacity is generally expressed as the ratio between the maximum flow in hyperemia with respect to the baseline flow, that is to say the coronary reserve flow ratio (range of 4 to 7 in laboratory animals and 2 to 5 in humans).[9] Although the physiological stimulus for an increase in coronary flow is a greater oxygen demand, this stimulus is difficult to reproduce in the catheterization laboratory so hyperemia is usually induced pharmacologically. To improve the reliability of CFR measurements, intracoronary nitroglycerin (NTG i.c., 100-200 μg) should be administered before the determination to set the epicardial tone and minimize differences in the vessel size under baseline conditions and with hyperemia.[11] This prevents the vasodilator effect of the drugs used to induce hyperemia, thus permitting the isolation of the changes in velocity due to microvascular vasodilation.

Determination of the Doppler coronary flow patterns

The assessment of coronary flow physiology with a Doppler guidewire is performed after administering sodium heparin (5000-10,000 IU i.v.), as for any interventional procedure. The technique for the assessment of coronary lesions and microvascular function requires several steps to obtain the Doppler parameters included in Table 21-1. The Doppler flowire is advanced until it is 1 cm proximal to the lesion to be assessed. Once a good, stabilized signal is obtained, the average peak velocity (APV) is measured, together with the diastolic-systolic velocity ratio (DSVR), which gives information on the flow pulsatility characteristics. Afterwards, the wire is advanced distally to the lesion and the same measurements (APV and DSRV) are repeated. With both APV values, the proximal-distal (P/D) APV ratio[12] is calculated. The distal determinations must be made far enough from the lesion, at a distance equivalent to 4 to 6 times the vessel diameter (1-2 cm),[12] to avoid recording the increase in velocity associated with the turbulent flow produced by stenosis. The evaluation of the coronary flow reserve (CFR) with Doppler flowire requires the determination of the ratio between the baseline and hyperemic flow after pharmacological stimulation of the maximum coronary flow. With the transducer placed distally to the lesion, 12 to 18 μg of adenosine is injected into the coronary ostium. APV is recorded before and after injection. Adenosine is an endothelium-independent arteriolar vasodilator that, if preceded by the administration of i.c. NTG (100-200 kg), has a negligible effect on the cross-sectional area of the conductance vessels.[11] An appropriate increase in the flow velocity during hyperemia (>2:1) defines CFR as normal.

APV has been measured in normal human coronary arteries to define its normal limits, which are similar in all three vessels.[13] The intra —and interobserver variability was less than 5 % and the results were highly variable, with APV values of 23 ± 11 cm/s (mean ± SD of all arterial segments) with very wide limits (9 to 61 cm/s). The maximum velocity of the blood flow was 42 ± 17 cm/s (limits of 14 to 82 cm/s).[13] In another study of angiographically normal coronary arteries, hyperemia was produced with i.c. adenosine. The APV in the LC (LAD and Cx) was 25 to 30 cm/s, with a diastolic peak of 40-50 cm/s and a systolic peak of 10-20 cm/sec. In the RC and in certain distal locations of the LC, these APVs were 15-20 % lower. There were no differences between the proximal and distal velocities during hyperemia, and there was a dominant diastolic flow pattern in all of the arterial segments (DSVR >1.5), although this pattern

Table 21-1. Doppler guidewire-defined coronary flow parameters

APV (Average Peak Velocity). This represents an average of the instantaneous peak velocities in cm/s.

DSVR (Diastolic Systolic Velocity Ratio). An ECG signal is necessary to assess this ratio, the quotient of the diastolic and systolic mean velocities. It is an indicator of the pulsatility of flow.

CFR (Coronary Flow Reserve) is the quotient of the hyperemic and baseline APV values, calculated after i.c. or i.v. administration of adenosine. It gives an approximation of vascular reactivity, assessing the flow reserve capacity of the coronary bed. This capacity may be compromised by functionally significant lesions or by microvascular disease.

P/D (acronym of the ratio between the Proximal APV and Distal APV). It requires the presence of arterial branches between the proximal assessment site and the stenosis. It evalues the degree of flow impairment produced by a coronary stenosis.

was less notable in the RC. The CFR was similar in all 3 arteries.[14] Figure 4 shows two examples of a normal pattern for coronary flow velocity as assessed with a Doppler guidewire.

Diastolic-Systolic Velocity Ratio (DSVR)

The DSVR is the quotient of the mean diastolic and systolic velocities and is an indicator of flow pulsatility. In the LC, its value is >1.5 with predominantly diastolic flow (Figs. 21-4 and 21-5), whereas it is ~1.0 in the RC with an almost equal contribution to the flow.

The reduction in the normal diastolic pattern and DSVR has been demonstrated after experimental induction of stenosis,[15] and these results have been confirmed by intraoperative studies during graft occlusion.[16] Coronary arteries with lesions show a reduced DSVR, with a dominant systolic pattern in over 50% of cases.[14,17] Figure 21-6 illustrates two examples of abnormal coronary flow velocity patterns.

Proximal and Distal Velocity Ratio (P/D)

The translesional flow velocity can be used to assess the hemodynamic significance of coronary lesions by assuming two facts: 1) That changes in flow velocity reflect changes in the blood volume flow and require that the vessel section remains constant. 2) That the epicardial artery area diminishes in proportion to the volumetric flow as the main vessels branch out, so that the flow velocity remains constant throughout the artery. In the branches, there is a gradual reduction in vessel section, in such a way that the proportion of the flow channeled to a particular branch will have a velocity similar to that of the flow in the main branch.[18] The continuity equation requires that be flow present in the proximal vessels to reach the distal segment.

The P/D velocity ratio determined using Doppler is 1 in normal coronary arteries.[14] Significant epicardial lesions increase resistance and redirect the flow to branches proximal to the lesion, with the volume and flow velocity diminishing in the post-stenotic region. This is reflected by an abnormally high P/D ratio.[17,19] Based on clinical trials assessing the pressure gradient and the results of myocardial scintigraphy, a cut-off point of 1.7 for the P/D ratio has been proposed to identify hemodynamically significant lesions (Fig. 21-7). A reduction in post-stenotic velocity leading to a P/D ratio >1.7 is related to a translesional gradient >30 mm Hg in branched arterial systems.[14,19]

The greatest limitations to the clinical use of this index are that the flow velocity proximal to the stenosis can only be measured in two out of three patients, and that the absence of important collateral branches in the RC and in the vein grafts means that there is no significant flow redistribution.[2] Furthermore, in cases of diffuse distal disease or serial lesions, the distal velocity may increase, thus giving a falsely normalized value for the P/D ratio, so this quotient should not be used in these cases.

Coronary Flow Reserve (CFR)

This is the most useful Doppler parameter, and the one mainly used to assess the physiological significance of epicardial coronary stenoses and the functional status of the distal microcirculation. In laboratory animals, as epicardial stenosis increases there is a predictable drop in the CFR which begins at about 60% of stenosis in the vessel diameter. With stenosis in excess of 80-90%, all of the coronary reserve is exhausted and the flow at rest begins to decline.[10,20] Animal models have described how the reserve flow diminishes with severity of the stenosis, reaching ratios of 1:1 for the most severe lesions.[21] it

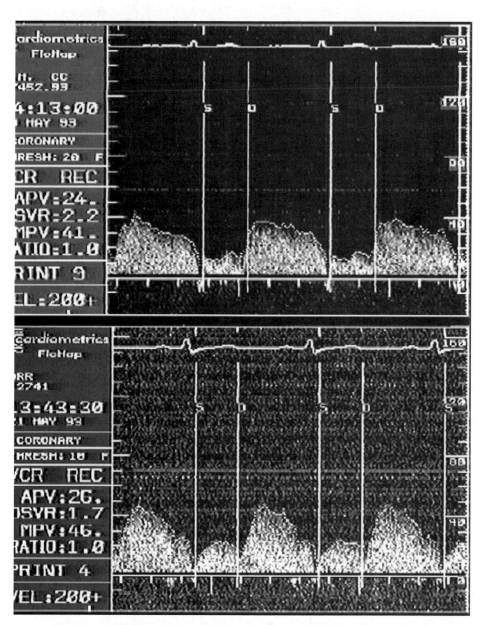

Figure 21-4. Doppler spectrum signal of the coronary flow velocity obtained with a Doppler flowire in two patients whose coronary arteries have no significant lesions. Close to the upper part of each record, there is a simultaneous display of the electrocardiogram and heartbeat. S and D indicate the systolic and diastolic periods. In both, the velocity scale is shown on the right in cm/s. On the left is the average peak velocity (APV) and the diastolic to systolic velocity ratio (DSVR). In both cases, the flow has diastolic dominance with normal APV and DSVR values.

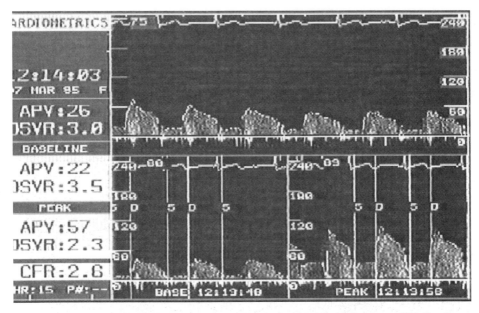

Figure 21-5. Record of the flow velocity spectrum, obtained with a Doppler guidewire in a coronary artery without angiographic lesions, captured under baseline conditions (*lower left box*) and at maximum hyperemia induced with intracoronary adenosine (*lower right box*). The *upper box* shows the spectrum of the flow velocity moving onscreen in real time. Close to the upper part of each box, there is a simultaneous display of the electrocardiogram and heartbeat. To the left or right of each box is the velocity scale in cm/s. The left edge shows the average peak velocity (APV), the diastolic-to-systolic velocity ratio (DSVR), and coronary flow reserve (CFR), or the ratio of average peak velocity of the baseline (Base) divided by the average peak velocity during hyperemia (Peak). S and D indicate the systolic and diastolic periods. Note the phasic normal flow velocity pattern, which predominates during diastole (DSVR 3.0). The coronary flow reserve is calculated from the hyperemic APV of 57 cm/s and the baseline APV of 22 cm/s to give a normal CFR of 2.6.

is therefore assumed that a reduction in the hyperemic flow through the lesion would be indicative of the stenosis severity, and is linearly related to the pressure gradient.[21] CFR would be the functional equivalent of the morphological description of epicardial coronary lesions.

When there is a coronary lesion in a human being, CFR must be measured post-stenotically as it is lower than the proximal value in arteries with lesions where the gradient is greater than 20 mm Hg. In addition, the measurement of proximal CFR is influenced by branching and the pre-stenotic deviation of the blood to regions with lower resistance.[19] In that study, Donohue et al.[19]

compared the angiographic findings with those of a Doppler flowire and translesional gradients, with a statistically significant abnormality being detected in the distal APV, DSVR and CFR in patients with a lesion-related gradient in excess of 20 mm Hg.

Pharmacological induction of hyperemia

Iodine contrast media were used in the past but they are not very effective because they do not produce maximal vasodilation.[22] NTG is a vasodilator that predominantly acts on the epicardial coronary vessels, so the in-

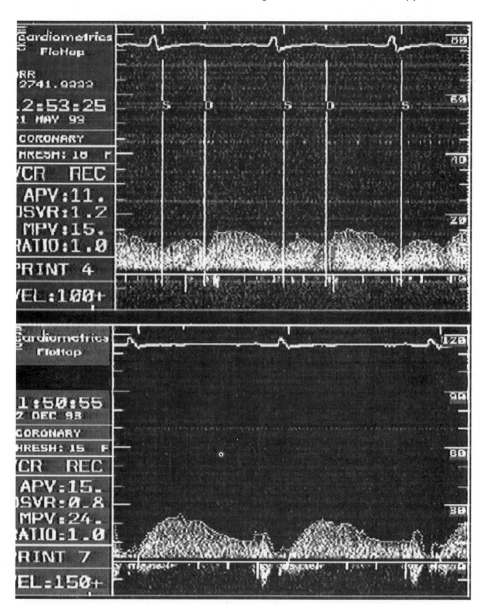

Figure 21-6. Doppler spectrum signal of the coronary flow velocity obtained with a Doppler guidewire in two patients whose coronary arteries have significant lesions. The abbreviations are the same as in Figure 21-4. In both cases there is a reduction in the baseline flow velocity with a low APV and an abnormal phasic pattern without a clear diastolic predominance (abnormal DSVR of 1.2 and 0.8.)

crease in flow velocity is lower as it is counteracted by the large simultaneous increase in the section of the proximal arterial segments.[9]

The coronary vasodilators most common-ly used to produce hyperemia are dipyridamole, papaverine and adenosine. All of these substances have very little effect on the largest-caliber epicardial arteries after treatment with i.c. NTG.

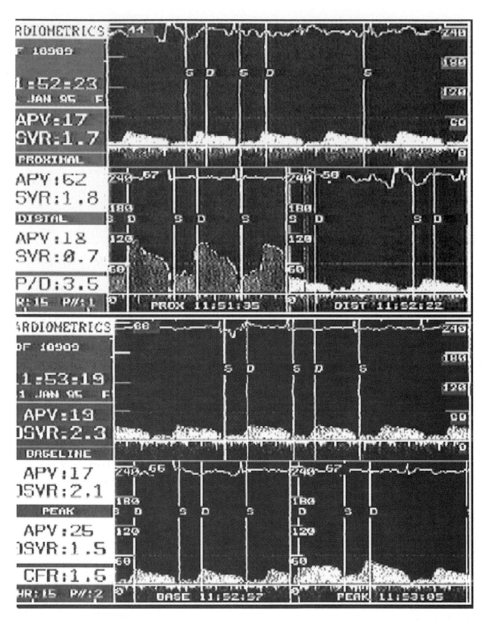

Figure 21-7. Composition of records obtained with the Doppler flowire showing the blood flow velocities in a coronary artery with a hemodynamically significant lesion. The abbreviations are the same as in Figure 21-5. *Figure on the top:* The upper part records the velocity distal to the stenosis. The lower boxes illustrate the coronary flow velocity proximal (left) and distal (right) to the lesion. The ratio of the proximal to distal (P/D) value is calculated from the proximal APV of 62 cm/s and the distal APV of 18 cm/s to give an abnormal P/D of 3.5. *Figure below:* the lower boxes show the baseline post-stenotic (17 cm/s) and hyperemic (25 cm/s) velocities to calculate the coronary flow reserve, which is also abnormal at 1.5. The flow distal to a significant lesion shows a reduction in the baseline velocity, an abnormal phasic pattern, and a lack of hyperemic response.

An intravenous (i.v.) infusion of dipyridamole (0.56-0.84 mg/kg/min) produces maximal coronary vasodilation, but it is relatively long lasting, making it impossible to assess CFR repeatedly during the same procedure.[23]

The intracoronary injection of a bolus of adenosine at a dose of 8-18 μg (usually 12) into the RC and 12-18 μg (usually 18 μg) in the LC or papaverine (8-12 μg)[24] produces maximal hyperemia, leading to an increase in the distal coronary flow similar to that following the occlusion of a coronary artery in dogs for 15 seconds.[22] Papaverine and dipyridamole have similar effects on the occasional production of ventricular arrhythmias.[23]

Adenosine has effects that are similar in magnitude to those of papaverine and it can be administered as an i.c. bolus or as an i.v. infusion (dose of 140 μg/kg/min).[25] The time interval between the bolus and the peak effect and duration of hyperemia are lower (up to 4 times lower) with adenosine than with papaverine.[26] In addition, i.c. adenosine does not induce changes in heartbeat or , blood pressure, nor does it prolong the QT interval, as has been seen with papaverine.[27] It may rarely produce mild hypotension, bradycardia or first and second-degree AV blocking, or symptoms such as flushing, chest discomfort, dyspnea, and headache. In view of its greater safety, ease of use, and scant side effects, adenosine administered as an i.c. bolus or as an i.v. perfusion is the agent of choice for the induction of hyperemia.

Normal CFR Values

Intracoronary papaverine increases coronary flow velocity by 4 to 6 times in individuals with normal coronary arteries.[24] In unselected patients subjected to coronary interventions, the CFR in arteries without significant lesions was 2.9 ± 0.95, with relatively large individual variations (range 2.1 to 4.2).[2] Similar results have been obtained with i.c. adenosine (12-18 μg in a bolus, CFR between 2.5 and 3.5) in a serie of 490 patients that included patients with normal coronary arteries, vessels without significant stenoses, and heart transplant recipients.[28, 29] Values > 2 are normal (Fig. 21-5) and values < 2 suggest the presence of a significant functional or organic coronary obstruction (Fig. 21-7).

Limitations on CFR

Any interpretation of CFR must take into account the variable hemodynamic conditions under which it is obtained. As CFR is a quotient, changes in the resting flow without changes in the hyperemic flow, or vice versa, will considerably affect the result.[21] Increases in resting or baseline flow will reduce the CFR in the absence of other disturbances, such as those caused by factors that drive up myocardial oxygen consumption (thyrotoxicosis, for instance), or by factors such as anemia, increases in heartbeat, ventricular pre-load, or contractility.[9] On the other hand, variations in blood pressure do not change CFR as both resting and hyperemic flow increase similarly.[30] Furthermore, other factors, such as myocardial hypertrophy or microvascular disease (hypertension, diabetes, heart transplant, etc.), will lower the CFR and modify the assessment of the severity of lesions regardless of their specific factors.[31] CFR is less useful in assessing the functional significance of a residual stenosis after myocardial infarction in patients treated with primary angioplasty, since CFR is lower in this context due to abnormalities in microcirculation.[32, 33] Scarred myocardium has a tendency to give an abnormal vasodilation response because of structural damage to the vessel bed.[21] Despite these limitations, CFR provides valuable information and may be the only reliable Doppler parameter for RC and other unbranched segments.

Relative Coronary Flow Reserve (rCFR)

Absolute CFR is the sum of the conduit and microcirculation responses. To improve the diagnostic precision and identify false-positive results in the determination of CFR, it has been proposed that CFR be determined in a second artery, without significant lesions, to obtain a relative coronary flow reserve (rCFR) equal to the ratio of CFR in the problem vessel to CFR in the reference vessel. CFR is similar in the three vascular territories and, providing no regional differences exist, rCFR is 1.0 ± 0.2.[28, 29]

Relative CFR improves specificity for the study of the lesion and gives more reliable information about the status of the microvascular function.[34, 35] Due to unpredictable anomalies in microcirculation, rCFR has a better correlation with myocardial reserve flow fraction (RFFmyo) than the absolute CFR when coronary stenoses are 50-95 %.[36]

The presence of diffuse epicardial disease may invalidate rCFR as a way to assess stenosis since it will be diminished, so there is a risk of underestimating the severity of the problem lesion.[35] It should also be remembered that the determination of this parameter prolongs the examination procedure and is not possible in many patients because they do not present any normal coronary artery for comparison.

CLINICAL APPLICATIONS OF THE DOPPLER GUIDEWIRE

Assessment of Intermediate Lesions

The functional assessment of intermediate coronary lesions (diameter reduced by 30 % to 70 %) is an important clinical problem. The characterization of hemodynamically significant lesions is associated with three major alterations in the post-stenotic coronary flow determined using Doppler:

1. Reduction in velocity (APV generally less than 20 cm/s) (Fig. 21-6) and P/D ratio > 1.7 (Fig. 21-7) for lesions in branched systems are associated with a translesional gradient of more than 30 mm Hg.[19] In some studies, Doppler has been used to calculate, through the continuity equation, the percentage section of the stenosis. However, the application of this equation has considerable theoretical and practical limitations, the most important being the scant likelihood of obtaining appropriate records for quantification purposes (only in 16 % of the population under study).[37]

2. Reduction in the phased flow pattern DSVR < 1.5.[16, 17] This abnormality in the pulsed flow pattern has been used to assess coronary stenoses (Fig. 21-6). The «systolization» of coronary flow (lowering of diastolic velocity with relative conservation of systolic velocity) occurs in arteries with significant lesions and is reversible after a successful angioplasty procedure.[2, 14, 17, 38, 39] The DSVR is not as reliable as CFR for the functional diagnosis of lesions, but it is useful for checking their return to normal after angioplasty.

   The use of DSVR to assess the significance of lesions is limited by the large degree of variability in this index, which is influenced by changes in myocardial contractility and the measurement site. The predictive value of DSVR in determining the significance of the lesion is 80 %, versus 95 % for CFR. Consequently, CFR is used for making therapeutic decisions.[2, 9]

3. Reduction in CFR < 2.0 (Fig. 21-7). CFR is a reliable method for assessing the physiological significance of intermediate coronary lesions.[19, 20, 25, 40, 41] Various groups have demonstrated a close correlation between CFR measured by Doppler and CFR found with thallium[201] radionuclide scanning, or

sestamibi SPECT-Tc[99] in patients with intermediate coronary lesions. A cutoff point between 1.7 and 2.0 for CFR identifies over 90% of patients with abnormal radionuclide scans.[40-42] The sensitivity, specificity, and predictive value of CFR were 94%, 95%, and 94%, respectively, in the study made by Joey et al.[41] CFR can often identify the culprit lesion in patients with multivessel disease presenting unstable angina without ECG alterations. It can also identify moderate lesions requiring intervention. In a comparative study using angiography, Doppler, and stress test in 225 patients with a single vessel disease, prior to and 6 months after angioplasty, distal CFR showed the best correlation with the percentage stenosis and minimal lumen diameter with respect to other Doppler parameters such as DSVR and the P/D ratio. Logistic regression showed that only CFR and the percentage of stenosis or the minimal lumen diameter were independent predictors of the outcome of the stress test.[43]

In short, DSVR < 1.5 for the LC, P/D ratio > 1.7, and CFR < 2.0 are considered indicators of hemodynamically significant coronary lesions in clinical practice.

Importantly, intracoronary Doppler measurements have also been able to identify patients who do not require revascularization. A normal translesional velocity gradient and/or normal CFR suggest the presence of non-flow-limiting lesions, so intervention can be deferred without risk.[44,45]

Assessment of Endothelial Function

The interaction between vasoconstriction and vasodilation produced by the endothelium helps to determine vascular tone and the response to changes in metabolic requirements.[46,47] Healthy endothelium releases nitric oxide that, in addition to being a powerful vasodilator, has an anti-aggregant effect on platelets and inhibits the proliferation of smooth muscle cells. An endothelial lesion leads to a drop in the production and release of nitric oxide (from its precursor, L-arginine), and a minimal penetration of this substance due to subendothelial thickening. These are possible explanations for the endothelium-mediated vasodilation disorder observed in patients with hypertension,[46] diabetes mellitus,[48] hyperlipidemia, and atherosclerosis.[47]

Acetylcholine (ACh) is the drug most commonly used to study endothelial function. Vasoconstriction or vasodilation after the administration of ACh are the net effect of the opposing actions of this substance on endothelial cells (vasodilation due to stimulation of nitric oxide release) and on smooth muscle cells (vasoconstriction caused by the direct effect on cholinergic receptors). At doses between 10^{-8} and 10^{-6}M, ACh produces vasodilation by stimulating normally reactive endothelium, whereas it produces paradoxical vasoconstriction of the epicardial vessels in patients with significant endothelial dysfunction.[49]

Adenosine is an endothelium-independent vasodilator, i.e., it does not require a healthy endothelium or the production of nitric oxide to induce arteriolar dilation.[50] The serial administration of ACh and adenosine may differentiate between a reduction in CFR due to anatomical defects (lack of response to either agent) from a reduction in CFR due to endothelial dysfunction (normal response to adenosine and abnormal response to acetylcholine). Endothelial dysfunction is seen in diffuse atherosclerotic vasculopathy in transplants[51] and in metabolic diseases such as diabetes mellitus[48] or hyperlipidemia,[47] in which there is endothelial dysfunction in the resistance vessels.

Assessment of Microcirculation

Microvascular Angina. Syndrome X

In syndrome X (myocardial ischemia due to a dysfunction in coronary microcirculation), the gold standard for diagnosis if the demonstration of a low CFR in the presence of angiographically normal epicardial arteries.[52] Before establishing this diagnosis, other causes of angina with normal coronary results, and low CFR must be excluded, such as those causing left ventricular hypertrophy (aortic stenosis,[53] hypertension,[54] etc.).

Microvascular disease with reduction of CFR has been shown in some patients with syndrome X, although the findings are discrepant because the studies differed in their inclusion criteria and methodology.[55, 56, 57] In this population, the flow velocity response is heterogeneous and may reflect both the intrinsic response mediated by the endothelium and diminishment of the response to an endothelium-independent vasodilator such as adenosine.[57]

Microvascular Disease in Cardiac Transplant

Autopsy studies have defined cardiac transplant vasculopathy as a diffuse disease affecting vessels of less than 400 μ in diameter.[2] CFR may be useful in identifying graft rejection and diffuse vascular disease, thus providing guidance for treatment in transplanted patients.[58] More recent studies have shown a decline in CFR without disease of the epicardial vessels and a dissociation between the degree of flow reduction and the severity of the intimal thickening of the coronary arteries as assessed by intravascular ultrasound.[59, 60] In accordance with these studies, more and more patients with heart transplants are being assessed with Doppler as a means to detect small vessel disease at an early stage.

Doppler Coronary flow in acute and chronic myocardial infarction

It is known that in patients with myocardial infarction, the semi-quantitative flow degree TIMI ≤ 2 has prognostic implications. In patients treated with primary angioplasty, it has been shown that a TIMI degree ≤ 2 correlates with low coronary flow velocities.[9, 33, 61, 62] Although the Doppler velocity cannot differentiate between TIMI degrees 1 and 2,[33, 61, 62] and there is an overlap between degree 2 and the lowest values of TIMI 3, the measurement of this velocity in the artery responsible for infarction might identify the patients who could benefit from additional mechanical or pharmacological measures aimed at improving coronary flow.

After infarction, CFR is altered by disturbances in microcirculation and it is not easy to discern whether this alteration is linked with residual stenosis or with potential myocardial viability. It is less useful for the functional assessment of residual stenosis.[32] In the absence of residual stenosis, the maintenance of CFR might indicate myocardial viability.[2] If there is a residual lesion at a similar angiographic stenosis, CFR is much lower in patients with prior infarction when compared with control subjects,[63] and after angioplasty it remains abnormal in 80 % of patients with infarction and only in 44 % of patients without it.[63] Furthermore, the CFR assessed after primary angioplasty has not predictive value for the prognosis of subsequent cardiac events.[64]

Other clinical applications of the Doppler guidewire are related to coronary interventions and are discussed in the following chapter.

SAFETY AND COMPLICATIONS OF THE TECHNIQUE

The risks and complications of using the Doppler guidewire are similar to those of other forms of coronary instrumentation.

Transient atrioventricular block has been reported in 2 % of the assessments of the RC (normally asymptomatic and more frequent in transplant recipients), as well as angina due to coronary steal in less than 1 %, and coronary vasospasm and dissection in connection with the guidewire.[65] In a recent study of 906 unselected patients in which i.c. adenosine or papaverine were used, a total of 2.9 % adverse cardiac events were reported, distributed as follows: 15 (1.6 %) cases of severe transient bradycardia (asystole or 2nd-3rd degree block) following administration of adenosine, 9 cases (0.99 %) of vasospasm as the guidewire was advanced, 2 (0.22 %) ventricular fibrillation, and 1 (0.11 %) hypotension with bradycardia and extrasystole. The incidence of complications was significantly greater in transplanted patients with respect to those subjected to coronary arteriography or angioplasty. Doppler assessment in the RC is associated with a greater incidence of complications, particularly bradycardia, when compared with the LC. All complications resolved with medical treatment.[66]

CONCLUSIONS

The study of coronary flow velocity with a Doppler guidewire has become a routine process over the last few years and is accessible to all hemodynamics laboratories. Its technical development has led to the functional assessment of moderate coronary lesions and the results of interventional procedures, and to the study of coronary circulation at the microvascular and endothelial levels. Because of the high correlation between post-stenotic CFR and radionuclide stress imaging, this assessment in the catheterization laboratory might be useful before intervention. These and other advances in our knowledge of coronary physiology have been useful in expanding the evidence available for therapeutic decision-making.

Acknowledgements: Our gratitude to Ms. Belen Moya, shelf manager at Jomed for Spain and Portugal, for her valuable assistance in the preparation of this chapter.

REFERENCES

1. Hatle L, Angelsen B. Physics of blood flow. In Hatle L, Angelsen B, eds. Doppler Ultrasound in Cardiology: Philadelphia, Lea & Febiger,1982:8-31.
2. Carlier SG, Di Mario C, Kern MJ, Serruys PW. Intracoronary Doppler and pressure monitoring. In Topol EJ, ed. Textbook of Interventional Cardiology, 3rd ed. WB Saunders Co. 1999:748-81.
3. Hartley CJ, Cole JS. An ultrasonic Doppler system for measuring blood flow in small vessels. J Appl Physiol 1974; 37:626-9.
4. Kern MJ, Courtois M, Ludbrook PA. A simplified method to measure coronary blood flow velocity in patients: Validation and application of a new Judkins-style Doppler-tipped angiographic catheter. Am Heart J 1990; 120:1202-12.
5. Sibley DH, Millar HD, Hartley CJ, Whitlow PL. Subselective measurement of coronary blood flow velocity using a steerable Doppler catheter. J Am Coll Cardiol 1986; 8:1332.
6. Doucette JW, Corl PD, Payne HM, et al. Validation of a Doppler guide wire for intravascular measurement of coronary artery flow velocity. Circulation 1992; 85:1899-911.
7. Sabiston DC Jr, Gregg DE. Effect of cardiac contraction on coronary blood flow. Circulation 1957; 15:14-23.
8. Bach RG, Kern MJ, Donohue TJ, et al. Comparison of arterial and venous coronary bypass conduits. Analysis of intravessel blood flow velocity characteristics. Circulation 1992; 86:I-181.
9. Chou TM, Zellner C, Kern MJ. Evaluation of myocardial blood flow and metabolism. In Baim D &Grossman W eds. Grossman's Cardiac Catheterization, Angiography and Intervention. 6th ed. Lippincott, Williams &Wilkins de Philadelphia. 2000:393-421.
10. Gould KL, Lipscomb K, Hamilton GW. Physiologic basis for assessing critical coronary stenosis. Instantaneous flow response and regional distribution during coronary

hyperemia as measures of coronary flow reserve. Am J Cardiol 1974; 33:87-94.

11. Shammas NW, Thondapu V, Gerasimou EM, et al. Effect of pretreatment with nitroglycerine on coronary flow reserve measured using bolus of intracoronary adenosine. Circulation 1995; 92:I-264.

12. Kern MJ, Donohue TJ, Aguirre FV, et al. Assessment of angiographically intermediate coronary artery stenosis using the Doppler flowire. Am J Cardiol 1993; 71:26D-33D.

13. Ofili EO, Labovitz AJ, Kern MJ. Coronary flow dynamics in normal and diseased artery. Am J Cardiol 1993; 71:3D-9D.

14. Ofili EO, Kern MJ, Labovitz AJ, et al. Analysis of coronary blood flow velocity dynamics in angiographically normal and stenosed arteries before and after endolumen enlargement by angioplasty. J Am Coll Cardiol 1993; 21:308-16.

15. Wiesner TF, Levesque MJ, Rooz E, Nerem RM, Epicardial coronary flow including the presence of stenosis and aorto-coronary bypasses. II: Experimental comparison and parametric investigations. J Biomech Eng 1988; 110:144.

16. Kajiya F, Tsujioka K, Ogasawara Y, et al. Analysis of flow characteristics in poststenotic regions of the human coronary artery during bypass graft surgery. Circulation 1987; 76:1092-1100.

17. Segal J, Kern MJ, Scott NA. Alteration of phasic coronary artery flow velocity in human during percutaneous coronary angioplasty. J Am Coll Cardiol 1992; 20:276-86.

18. Seiler C, Kirkeeide RL, Gould KL. Basic structure-function relations of the epicardial coronary vascular tree. Basis of quantitative coronary arteriography for diffuse coronary artery disease. Circulation 1992; 85:1987-2003.

19. Donohue TJ, Kern MJ, Aguirre FV, et al. Assessing the hemodynamic significance of coronary artery stenoses: analysis of translesional pressure-flow velocity relations in patients. J Am Coll Cardiol 1993; 22:449-58.

20. Gould KL, Kirkeeide R, Buchi M. Coronary flow reserve as a physiologic measure of stenosis severity. Part I: Relative and absolute coronary flow reserve during changing aortic pressure. Part II: Determination of ar-teriographic stenosis dimensions under standardized conditions. J Am Coll Cardiol 1990; 15:459-74.

21. Klocke FJ. Measurements of coronary flow reserve: defining pathophysiology versus making decisions about patient care. Circulation 1987; 76:1183-9.

22. Bookstein JJ, Higgins CB. Comparative efficacy of coronary vasodilatory methods. Invest Radiol 1977; 12:121-7.

23. Rossen JD, Simonetti I, Marcus ML, Winniford MD. Coronary dilation with standard dose dipyridamole and dipyridamole combined with handgrip. Circulation 1989; 79:566-72.

24. Wilson RF, White CW. Intracoronary papaverine: an ideal coronary vasodilator for studies of the coronary circulation in conscious humans. Circulation 1986; 73:444-51.

25. Kern MJ, Dilegonul U, Aguirre FV, Hilton TCl. Intravenous adenosine: continuous infusion and low dose bolus administration for determination of coronary vascular reserve in patients with and without coronary artery disease. J Am Coll Cardiol 1991; 18:718-29.

26. Wilson RF, Wyche K, Christensen BV, Zimmer S, Laxson DD. Effects of adenosine on human coronary arterial circulation. Circulation 1990; 82:1598-606.

27. Wilson RF, White CW. Serious ventricular dysrhythmias after intracoronary papaverine. Am J Cardiol 1988; 62:1301-2.

28. Kern MJ, Donohue TJ. Doppler assessment of coronary blood flow. Am J Cardiol 1996; 77:520-5.

29. Kern MJ, Bach RG, Mechem CJ, et al. Variations in normal coronary vasodilatory reserve stratified by artery, gender, heart transplantation and coronary artery disease. J Am Coll Cardiol 1996; 28:1154-60.

30. McGinn AL, White CW, Wilson RF. Interstudy variability of coronary flow reserve. Circulation 1990; 81:1319-30.

31. Strauer BE. The significance of coronary reserve in clinical heart disease. J Am Coll Cardiol 1990; 15:775-83.

32. Caleys MJ, Vrints CJ, Bosmans JM, et al. Coronary flow reserve measurement during coronary angioplasty in the infarct-related vessel. Circulation 1995; 92:I-326.

33. Moore JA, Kern MJ, Donohue TJ, et al. Disparity of TIMI grade flow and directly

measured flow velocity during direct angioplasty for acute myocardial infarction. Cathet Cardiovasc Diagn 1994; 32:86.

34. Kern MJ, Donohue TJ, Bach RG, Aguirre FV, Caracciolo ES, Wolford TL. Assessment of intermediate coronary stenosis by relative coronary flow velocity reserve. J Am Coll Cardiol 1997; 29(suppl A):21A.

35. Baumgart D, Haude M, George G, et al. Improved assessment of coronary stenosis reserve using the relative flow velocity reserve. Circulation 1998; 98:40-6.

36. Baumgart D, Haude M, Liu F, et al. Fractional velocity reserve a new index for stenosis severity assessment with good correlation to fractional flow reserve. J Am Coll Cardiol 1997; 29(suppl A):126A.

37. Di Mario C, Meneveau N, Gil R, et al. Maximal blood flow velocity in severe coronary stenosis measured with a Doppler guidewire. Am J Cardiol 1993; 71:54D-61D.

38. Heller LI, Silver KH, Villegas BJ, Balcom SJ, Weiner BH. Blood flow velocity in the right coronary artery: assessment before and after angioplasty. J Am Coll Cardiol 1994; 24:1012-7.

39. Serruys PW, Di Mario C, Meneveau N, et al. Intracoronary pressure and flow velocity with sensor-tip guidewires: a new methodologic approach for assessment of coronary hemodynamics before and after coronary interventions. Am J Cardiol 1993; 71:41D-53D.

40. Miller DD, Donohue TJ, Younis IT, Bach RG, et al. Correlation of pharmacologic Tc99-Sestamibi myocardial perfusion imaging with post-stenotic coronary flow reserve in patients with angiographically intermediate coronary stenoses. Circulation 1994; 89:2150-60.

41. Joey JD, Schulman DS, Lasorda D, Farah T, Donohue BC, Reichek N. Intracoronary Doppler guide wire versus stress single-photon emission computed tomographic thallium-201 imaging in assessment of intermediate coronary stenoses. J Am Coll Cardiol 1994; 24:940-7.

42. Donohue TJ, Miller DD, Bach RG, et al. Correlation of poststenotic hyperemic coronary flow velocity and pressure with abnormal stress myocardial perfusion imaging in coronary artery disease. Am J Cardiol 1996; 77:948-54.

43. Piek JJ, Boersma E, Di Mario C, et al. Angiographical and Doppler flow-derived parameters for assessment of coronary lesion severity and its relation to the result of exercise electrocardiography. DEBATE study group. Eur Heart J 2000; 21:466-74.

44. Kern MJ, Donohue TJ, Aguirre FV, et al. Clinical outcome of deferring angioplasty in patients with normal translesional pressure flow velocity measurements. J Am Coll Cardiol 1995; 25:178-87.

45. Moses J, Shaknovich A, Kreps E, et al. Clinical follow-up of intermediate lesions not hemodynamically significant by Doppler flow wire criteria. Circulation 1994; 90:I-227.

46. Panza JA, Quyyumi AA, Brush JE, Epstein SE. Abnormal endothelium-dependent vascular relaxation in patients with essential hypertension. N Engl J Med 1990; 323:22-7.

47. Forstermann U, Mugge A, Alheid U, Averich A, Frolich JC. Selective attenuation of endothelium-mediated vasodilation in atherosclerotic human coronary arteries. Circ Res 1988; 62:185-90.

48. Johnstone MT, Gallagher SJ, Scales KM, et al. Endothelium-dependent vasodilation is impaired in patients with insulin-dependent diabetes mellitus. Circulation 1992; 68:I-168.

49. Hodgson JM, Marshall JJ. Direct vasoconstriction and endothelium-dependent vasodilation. Mechanisms of acetylcholine effects on coronary flow and arterial diameter in patients with nonstenotic coronary arteries. Circulation 1989; 79:1043-51.

50. Zijlstra F, Juilliere Y, Serruys PW, et al. Value and limitations of intracoronary adenosine for the assessment of coronary flow reserve. Cathet Cardiovasc Diag 1988; 15:76-80.

51. Gagliardi G, Crea F, Polleta B. et al. Coronary microvascular endothelial dysfunction in transplanted children. Eur Heart J 2001; 22:254-60.

52. Cannon ROIII, Camici PG, Epstein SE. Pathophysiological dilemma of Syndrome X. Circulation 1992; 85:883-92.

53. Marcus ML, Doty DB, Hirratzka LF, Wright CB, Enpthan CD. Decreased coronary reserve as mechanism of angina pectoris in patients with aortic stenosis and normal coron-

ary arteries. N Engl J Med 1982; 37:1362-6.

54. Houghton JL, Prisant LM, Carr AA, van Dohlen W, Frank MJ. Relationship of left ventricular mass to impairment of coronary vasodilator reserve in hypertensive heart disease. Am Heart J 1991; 21:1107-12.

55. Chauhan A, Mullins PA, Petch MC, Schofield PM. Is coronary flow reserve in response to papaverine really normal in syndrome X? Circulation 1994; 89:1998-2004.

56. Rosen SD, Uren NG, Kaski JC, Tousoulis D, Davies GJ, Camici PG. Coronary vasodilator reserve, pain perception and sex in patients with syndrome X. Circulation 1994; 90:50-60.

57. Quyyumi AA, Cannon RO, Panza JA, Diodati JG, Epstein SE. Endothelial dysfunction in patients with chest pain and normal coronary arteries. Circulation 1992; 86:1864-71.

58. McGinn AL, Wilson RF, Olivari MT, Homans DC, White CW. Coronary vasodilator reserve after human orthotopic cardiac transplantation. Circulation 1988; 78:1200-9.

59. Wolford T, Kern MJ. Assessment of transplant arteriopathy by intracoronary two-dimensional ultrasound imaging and coronary flow velocity. Cathet Cardiovasc Diag 1995; 35:335-42.

60. Caracciolo EA, Wolford TL, Underwood RD, et al. Influence of intimal thickening on coronary blood flow responses in orthotopic heart transplant recipients. Circulation 1995; 92:II-182-II-190.

61. Kern MJ, Moore JA, Aguirre FV, et al. Determination of angiographic (TIMI grade) blood flow by intracoronary Doppler flow velocity during acute myocardial infarction. Circulation 1996; 94:1545-52.

62. Aguirre FV, Donohue TJ, Bach RG, et al. Coronary flow velocity of infarct-related arteries. Physiologic differences between complete (TIMI III) and incomplete (TIMI 0, I, II) angiographic coronary perfusion. J Am Coll Cardiol 1995; 25:401A.

63. Claeys MJ, Vrintz CJ, Bosmans J, et al. Coronary flow reserve during coronary angioplasty in patients with a recent myocardial infarction. Relation to stenosis and myocardial viability. J Am Coll Cardiol 1996; 28:1712-9.

64. Miller DD, Nallamothu RB, Shaw LJ, et al. Does intracoronary Doppler assessment of post-stenotic reperfusion flow enhance cardiac event prediction as compared to other post-myocardial infarction risk markers? J Am Coll Cardiol 1997; 29(suppl A):71A.

65. Mechem C, Kern MJ, Aguirre FV, et al. Safety and outcome of angioplasty guidewire Doppler instrumentation in patients with normal or mildly diseased coronary arteries. Circulation 1992; 85:I-323.

66. Qian J, Baumgart D, Oldenburg O, Haude M, Sacj S, Erbel R. Safety of intracoronary Doppler flow measurement. Am Heart J 2000; 140:502-10.

22

Value of Doppler During Coronary Interventions. Predictors of Restenosis

Carlo Di Mario, MD
Kostantinos Toutouzas, MD
Flavio Airoldi, MD

Introduction. Coronary Flow Reserve. Flow Alterations Following Balloon Angioplasty. Guidance to Provisional Stenting. Flow Velocity Changes after Stent Implantation. Alternative Indices of Functional Stenosis Severity During Coronary Interventions. Conclusions. References.

INTRODUCTION

The miniaturization of intracoronary devices fitted with a Doppler flow transducer has made physiological assessment of coronary blood flow *in vivo* during diagnostic and therapeutic catheterization feasible. Doppler flow probes are commonly used to evaluate ambiguous lesions and to determine the success of coronary interventions at restoring normal flow reserve. The Doppler guidewire (Jomed Endosonics, Rancho Cordova, CA) is a 0.014-inch steerable, 175-cm long, flexible guidewire with handling characteristics similar to commonly used angioplasty wires and a 12-MHz piezoelectric transducer integrated into the tip. The small profile allows the operator to advance the device into distal coronary segments and beyond stenoses. In addition, the guidewire device accommodates over-the-wire or monorail balloon angioplasty systems, thus enabling diagnostic and therapeutic procedures without having to change the wire. The Flowire™ transducer uses a pulsed-waveform Doppler that samples

5.2 mm beyond the guidewire tip. It samples a relatively large blood volume by using an ultrasound beam that diverges at an angle of 14° to either side of the centerline of flow. The Doppler guidewire is attached via a sterile cable to a console that displays the flow signal pattern and generates a superimposed envelope tracing that depicts the relative contributions of systolic and diastolic flow and continuously updates the measurements of peak velocity, averaged over 2 consecutive beats (APV). This system has been validated by *in vitro* and *in vivo* models, by comparison with electromagnetic quantitative volumetric analysis[1] and its safety has been tested in 906 patients. Most of the complications (bradycardia, atrioventricular block) were rapidly reversible and due to the concomitant use of adenosine.[2]

CORONARY FLOW RESERVE

The principle of flow reserve was established by the original work of Gould, Lipscomb, and Hamilton.[3] In the absence of a significant coronary lesion, the distal arteriolar bed actively dilates in response to increased metabolic demands (such as exertion), producing a two-fold to six-fold increase in coronary blood flow. In the presence of a hemodynamically significant stenosis, distal vasodilation occurs in a progressive fashion at rest, thus maintaining a stable level of coronary blood flow. However, in the presence of a significant stenosis, continuous tonic vasodilation impairs the ability to further dilate in response to increased demands, thus leading to inducible myocardial ischemia. The term coronary flow reserve refers to the maximum capacity of the coronary vascular bed to increase blood flow in response to demand. This capacity is expressed as the ratio of maximum hyperemic to basal flow. If all measurements are obtained during maximal vasodilatation (i.e., after nitrates), the cross-sectional area does not change so the ratio of velocities is equal to the ratio of coronary flows and the terms coronary flow reserve (CFR) or coronary velocity reserve (CFVR) can be used interchangeably.

An increase in coronary blood flow, reactive hyperemia, can be induced by transient coronary occlusion or using pharmacological agents, such as papaverine or adenosine and adenosine triphosphate (ATP). Intracoronary adenosine or ATP do not induce significant changes in heart rate or blood pressure and do not prolong the QT interval, avoiding the potentially dangerous ventricular arrhythmias that are occasionally observed after papaverine.[4] However, the time from intracoronary injection of adenosine to peak effect and the total duration of the hyperemic response is much shorter.[5] A continuous intravenous infusion of 140 μg/kg/min of adenosine also induces maximal coronary vasodilatation, but may produce mild hypotension, bradycardia, flushing, chest discomfort, headache, dyspnea or atrioventricular block.[6] In view of the high safety profile, absence of side effects and ease of use, low-dose intracoronary adenosine is the most frequently used method (24-60 μg for the LCA, 12 μg for the right coronary artery as starting bolus to reduce the risk of sinus node or AV-node depression). If a guiding catheter with side-holes must be used, practical advice is to triple the dose of adenosine injected.[7]

Using intracoronary adenosine in a large control group of 490 subjects, including patients with chest pain and angiographically normal arteries, non-stenotic vessels in patients with known coronary artery disease, and cardiac transplantation recipients, CFR was similar in men and women and in the left anterior descending, left circumflex, and right coronary arteries. The lowest values were observed in the group with significant atherosclerotic involvement of other arteries (2.5 ± 0.95).[8] After coronary interventions, even with complete elimination of the epicardial stenosis by successful stent implantation, similar CFR values are observed (final CFR of 2.59 ± 0.87 in 132 patients).[9] The large individual variability and low average values measured in arteries without significant epicardial stenoses, but in patients with coronary artery disease, is due to the presence of many other variables that affect CFR in this patient population. For example, left ventricular hypertrophy is associated with abnormal CFR due to the increased resting demands of greater muscle mass.[10] Corrective factors for basal flow velocity and age have been proposed and calculated from measurements made in 141 patients with angina-like symptoms and angiographically unobstructed coronary arteries (corrected CFR for LAD = 2.85 × CFR × 10 × (0.48 × log bAPV) + (0.025 × Age in years) − 1.16).[11] Since flow reserve is a ratio, changes in resting flow without changes in hyperemic flow will considerably influence the result. Furthermore, factors such as heart rate, preload, myocardial hypertrophy, or disease of the microvasculature will alter the hyperemic pressure flow relationship and modify the flow reserve.[12] The experience gained with i.c. Doppler is important because these last limitations also apply to new techniques able to measure coronary velocity and CFR non-invasively.[13-16]

FLOW ALTERATIONS FOLLOWING BALLOON ANGIOPLASTY

Doppler can replace other non-invasive functional methods for the assessment of lesion severity in the evaluation of angiographically intermediate lesions. It is a valuable alternative to gain time and reduce cost and patient discomfort, allowing the performance of PTCA immediately after angiography. During interventions, however, no other non-invasive methods of functional assessment are applicable and Doppler has the potential to become an indispensable functional tool for judging the results of percutaneous coronary interventions (PCI). Unfortunately the use of i.c. Doppler is challenged by the development of major hemodynamic changes and the presence of microvascular dysfunction and distal embolism, especially during coronary interventions, which may interfere with the ability of Doppler to detect the effect of PCI on epicardial stenoses. Angiographically successful coronary revascularization is usually associated with the restoration of normal Doppler flow characteristics,[17-19] but the persistence of impaired CFR after PTCA cannot be due only to the limitations of angiography in detecting true luminal gain after treatment.[20] Hemodynamic changes during the procedure, microembolization, or transient or persistent changes in the distal microvascular response may explain part of this discrepancy, as indicated by the later normalization of CFR in some lesions.[21]

Large studies have demonstrated that a post-intervention impairment in flow reserve is more frequently associated with persistent or recurrent angina and that the patients are also more likely to have a positive exercise test at 1 month and/or to require target lesion revascularization (TLR) by 6 months.[22,23] In

the DEBATE (Doppler Endpoints Balloon Angioplasty Trial Europe) trial, the combination of an optimal angiographic result (<35 % residual diameter stenosis) and CFR > 2.5 was associated with a favorable clinical outcome at 6 months (16 % incidence of major adverse cardiac events).[22] which had independent predictive value of the results of stress testing before and 6 months after treatment with PTCA.[24] Piek et al.[25] also showed in a subgroup of these patients undergoing 6 months measurement of CFVR that patients with recurrence of angina and target lesion revascularization maintained a low coronary flow reserve at follow-up due to restenosis and/or persistent elevated baseline blood flow velocity. Patients without restenosis showed a decrease or increase of coronary flow reserve during follow-up, determined by changes in hyperemic blood flow velocity. In a subanalysis of 183 patients, suboptimal coronary flow reserve was associated with a chronically elevated baseline average peak velocity, a transient deficit in the hyperemic average peak velocity, old age, and female gender.[26]

In the DEBATE trial the patients were also monitored for 15 min after the last balloon inflation: if CFR remained stable and no cyclical flow velocity variations were observed (a rare but ominous phenomenon related to recurrent platelet emboli[27,28]), no abrupt closure was observed in the 24 hours after PTCA.[29]

GUIDANCE TO PROVISIONAL STENTING

Based on these results, three randomized trials were developed to test the hypothesis that angiographic and Doppler parameters can detect lesions after PTCA at low risk of events, similar to the risk observed after stent implantation.[30-32] In DEBATE II, only short lesions in >2.75-mm vessels were included and patients underwent an unbalanced randomization with 97 patients treated with elective stenting and 523 divided according to whether they met a predetermined residual DS of <35% and CFR >2.5. These patients underwent a second randomization to stenting or PTCA. The study confirmed the high risk of MACE in PTCA patients who did not meet the angiographic and Doppler criteria and were not treated with a stent and observed a similar overall event-free survival in the groups of elective and provisional stenting (86.6 and 85.6%, respectively). Separate analysis of the subgroup that achieved the optimal endpoints after PTCA, however, showed that stenting could further decrease the number of events at follow-up (1-year event-free survival, 93.5% versus 84.1%; P = 0.066). This difference was not statistically significant but casts doubts on the provisional stenting strategy, especially when the higher cost of this strategy after one year of follow-up is considered (EUR 6573 versus EUR 5885; P = 0.014). The other two trials (FROST, French Randomized Optimal Stenting Trial, and DESTINI, Doppler Endpoints Stent International Investigation) enrolled 251 and 723 patients, respectively, and differed from DEBATE II because they had a simple 1:1 randomization protocol, lower threshold of CFR (2.0 DESTINI and 2.2 FROST), and broader inclusion criteria. DESTINI also enrolled patients with multivessel disease provided that all lesions were suitable for stent implantation. Both studies showed a similar clinical outcome at 1 year (in DESTINI the incidence of MACE was 17.8% in the elective stenting group and 18.9% in the guided PTCA group, and the incidence of repeat TLR at 1 year was 14.9% in the elective stent group and 15.6% in the guided PTCA group). In FROST a follow-up angiogram was also performed, showing similar MLD (1.90 ± 0.79 mm vs. 1.99 ± 0.70 mm, p = 0.39) and binary restenosis (27.1% vs. 21.4%, p = 0.37) in the groups with provisional and elective stenting, respectively. In the DESTINI trial, possibly because of the greater complexity of the lesions treated, a higher cost and procedure

duration was observed in the elective stenting arm and a significant difference persisted at 1 year in the US study patients.[33] In a subanalysis of DEBATE II, 45 patients with dissection after PTCA showed a CFVR similar to that of the patients without dissection: in this subgroup randomization to stenting did not improve immediate CFVR or long-term outcome.[34]

Two recent reviews on provisional stenting[35, 36] have stressed the fact that in these trials only a minority of the patients in a provisional stenting strategy guided by Doppler and QCA were treated with balloon angioplasty alone and that 50 to 60% of these patients received a stent anyway. Under these circumstances, it is unlikely that this strategy could be less expensive and time-consuming than elective stenting which, with modern stents, can be performed in 30 to 60% of cases without predilation.[37]

FLOW VELOCITY CHANGES AFTER STENT IMPLANTATION

Conceptually, there is limited value in the use of CFR when the presence of a stent has reduced the residual narrowing to <30% and created a regular circular lumen, sealing wall dissections. In reality, angiographically unapparent dissections, severe stent underexpansion, inappropriate comparison of the stent expansion with a diffusely diseased reference segment and residual untreated lesions may justify the use of a functional method of assessment of stenosis severity after stent implantation. In a comparative study of 33 patients treated with implantation of coil or tubular stents, Vrints et al.[38] reported that CFVR was higher in the group treated with tubular stents (2.46 ± 0.13 vs 1.96 ± 0.14, p < 0.05) despite similar angiographic final diameter stenosis (11 ± 2% vs 13 ± 2%, ns). To confirm that severe residual underexpansion was the main cause of this difference, a major increase in flow velocity was measured during pullback of the Doppler wire in coil stents (83 ± 24 % velocity increase) but not in tubular stents (5 ± 5 % velocity increase, p < 0.05) (Fig. 22-1).

When the analysis is limited to patients who underwent successful single tubular stent implantation (417 patients in the DES-TINI trial), a CFVR ≤2.0 (109 patients, 26 %) had a risk of new revascularization that was twice as high (22 % vs 11 %, p = 0.01) as that of patients with a normal (>2.0) CFVR. This difference remained significant after adjustment for all other clinical and angiographic variables correlated with the incidence of target lesion revascularization.[39]

ALTERNATIVE INDICES OF FUNCTIONAL STENOSIS SEVERITY DURING CORONARY INTERVENTIONS

Fractional flow reserve (FFR) is a measure of the maximum flow capacity for a stenotic vessel in comparison to the same vessel without stenosis. Unlike Doppler methods, FFR is unaffected by any increase in basal flow because all measurements are performed in a pharmacologically induced state of maximum vasodilation. It is also unaffected by changes in hemodynamic conditions at the

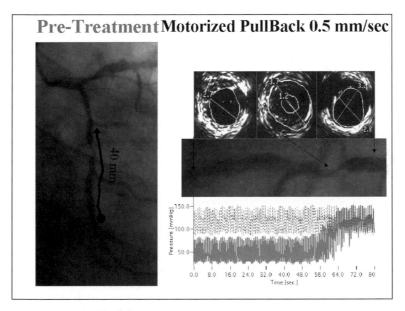

Figure 22-1.   *Left panel*: Angiographic frame in the right inferior oblique view of a severe lesion of the middle segment of the left circumflex artery. The black line indicates the length of the segment examined with motorized pullback of the Endosonics 0.014-inch WaveWire and the arrow shows the direction of recording (during pullback). *Right panel:* Three ultrasound cross-sections of the distal reference (right), mid-lesion (middle) and proximal reference (left) of the diseased segment. Arrows indicate the position of each cross-section in the corresponding angiographic image, rotated to facilitate comparison. Please note that plaque accumulation is also present at both reference sites, apparently disease-free on angiography. Both plaques are eccentric, more fibrous at the distal end, with a layer of subendothelial calcification with shadowing at the proximal site. A large, subocclusive, soft concentric plaque with moderate positive remodeling is observed at the site of the lesion. In the lower tracing, the top line follows the phasic changes of aortic pressure measured through the guiding catheter while the lower line measures the distal intracoronary pressure measured at the level of the microsensor of the WaveWire. Note that only the only sharp decrease in pressure is present at the level of the most severe lesion, indicating that pressure measurements can only detect functionally significant lesions.

time of assessment (arterial pressure, inotropic state, heart rate).[12] Uniquely, FFR allows calculation of both the antegrade and collateral components of flow.[40]

The value of FFR for the guidance of coronary interventions has been assessed in a large observational trial in patients with single-vessel disease treated with PTCA.[41] A cut-off value of 0.90 in combination with a residual diameter stenosis <35 % showed a significant difference in outcome, with 88 % of patients without major adverse cardiac events at 24 months in the group meeting these criteria and 59 % of patients event-free in the group with lower FFR and/or higher residual diameter stenosis.

FFR has also been proposed as an alternative to IVUS for assessing stent expansion, with FFR >0.94 recommended as an endpoint. Despite the good correlation, the pressures and type of stent used do not reflect current practice and suggest that the method can be applicable only for rather severe residual stenoses.[42] In a recent *in vitro* experiment using FFR, QCA, and IVUS a clear superiority of the imaging techniques over FFR was observed in the detection of moderate stent underexpansion.[43]

COMBINED PRESSURE-FLOW PARAMETERS

Simultaneous assessment of pressure and flow may overcome the limitations of both indices, but the use of two sensor-tipped wires makes this assessment very difficult in clinical practice.[44] Still, new indices based on the instantaneous relationship between pressure and flow in diastole, which have been shown to be highly correlated with stenosis severity in animal models,[45] have been applied in man.[46] Simplified indices based on the ratio between pressure gradient and flow velocity in basal and hyperemic conditions have been proposed. The combination of a wire-based pressure sensor and thermodilution system is another possible alternative to

overcoming the limitations of CFR.[47] A simple method for deriving CFR from the square root of the ratio between pressure measurements in hyperemic and basal conditions is under clinical evaluation.[48]

CONCLUSIONS

The usefulness of physiologic parameters to assess the functional severity of lesions of intermediate severity is confirmed by the guidelines of the ACC/AHA on cardiac catheterization. The application of these indices to guide coronary interventions is more questionable. Aside from the specific limitations of some indices proposed, the problem is the practical value of this assessment if a standard method of treatment (stent implantation) is applicable in most conditions and is able to achieve a good predictable immediate result. Another convincing element in favor of stent implantation is the potential use of this mechanical scaffold as a vehicle for powerful and effective antiproliferative substances.[49, 50]

REFERENCES

1. Doucette JW, Corl PD, Payne HM, Flynn AE, Goto M, Nassi M, Segal J. Validation of a Doppler guide wire for intravascular measurement of coronary artery flow velocity. *Circulation* 1992; 85:1899-911.
2. Qian J, Ge J, Baumgart D, Oldenburg O, Haude M, Sack S, Erbel R. Safety of intracoronary Doppler flow measurement. *Am Heart J* 2000; 140:502-10.
3. Gould KL, Lipscomb K, Hamilton GW. Physiologic basis for assessing critical coronary stenosis. Instantaneous flow response and regional distribution during coronary hyperemia as measures of coronary flow reserve. *Am J Cardiol* 1974; 33:87-94.
4. Wilson RF, White CW. Serious ventricular dysrhythmias after intracoronary papaverine. *Am J Cardiol* 1988; 62:1301-2.
5. Wilson RF, Wyche K, Christensen BV, Zimmer S, Laxson DD. Effects of adenosine

on human coronary arterial circulation. *Circulation* 1990; 82:1595-606.

6. Kern MJ, Deligonul U, Tatineni S, Serota H, Aguirre F, Hilton TC. Intravenous adenosine: continuous infusion and low dose bolus administration for determination of coronary vasodilator reserve in patients with and without coronary artery disease. *J Am Coll Cardiol* 1991; 18:718-29.

7. Abizaid A, Kornowski R, Mintz GS, Hong MK, Picahrd AD, Kent KM, Satler LF, Popma JJ, Bramwell O, Leon MB. Influence of guiding catheter selection on the measurement of coronary flow reserve. *Am J Cardiol* 1997; 79:703-4.

8. Kern MJ, Bach RG, Mechem CJ, Caracciolo EA, Aguirre FV, Miller LW, Donohue TJ. Variations in normal coronary vasodilatory reserve stratified by artery, gender, heart transplantation and coronary artery disease. *J Am Coll Cardiol* 1996; 28:1154-60.

9. Qian J, Ge J, Baumgart D, Sack S, Haude M, Erbel R. Prevalence of microvascular disease in patients with significant coronary artery disease. *Herz* 1999; 24:548-57.

10. Hamasaki S, Al Suwaidi J, Higano ST, Miyauchi K, Holmes DR, Jr., Lerman A. Attenuated coronary flow reserve and vascular remodeling in patients with hypertension and left ventricular hypertrophy. *J Am Coll Cardiol* 2000; 35:1654-60.

11. Wieneke H, Haude M, Ge J, Altmann C, Kaiser S, Baumgart D, von Birgelen C, Welge D, Erbel R. Corrected coronary flow velocity reserve: a new concept for assessing coronary perfusion. *J Am Coll Cardiol* 2000; 35:1713-20.

12. de Bruyne B, Bartunek J, Sys SU, Pijls NH, Heyndrickx GR, Wijns W. Simultaneous coronary pressure and flow velocity measurements in humans. Feasibility, reproducibility, and hemodynamic dependence of coronary flow velocity reserve, hyperemic flow versus pressure slope index, and fractional flow reserve. *Circulation* 1996; 94:1842-9.

13. Caiati C, Montaldo C, Zedda N, Bina A, Iliceto S. New noninvasive method for coronary flow reserve assessment: contrast-enhanced transthoracic second harmonic echo Doppler. *Circulation* 1999; 99:771-8.

14. Lepper W, Hoffmann R, Kamp O, Franke A, de Cock CC, Kuhl HP, Sieswerda GT, Dahl

J, Janssens U, Voci P, Visser CA, Hanrath P. Assessment of myocardial reperfusion by intravenous myocardial contrast echocardiography and coronary flow reserve after primary percutaneous transluminal coronary angioplasty [correction of angiography] in patients with acute myocardial infarction. *Circulation* 2000; 101:2368-74.

15. Caiati C, Zedda N, Montaldo C, Montisci R, Iliceto S. Contrast-enhanced transthoracic second harmonic echo Doppler with adenosine: a noninvasive, rapid and effective method for coronary flow reserve assessment. *J Am Coll Cardiol* 1999; 34:122-30.

16. Sakuma H, Koskenvuo JW, Niemi P, Kawada N, Toikka JO, Knuuti J, Laine H, Saraste M, Kormano M, Hartiala JJ. Assessment of coronary flow reserve using fast velocity-encoded cine MR imaging: validation study using positron emission tomography. *AJR Am J Roentgenol* 2000; 175:1029-33.

17. Segal J, Kern MJ, Scott NA, King SBd, Doucette JW, Heuser RR, Ofili E, Siegel R. Alterations of phasic coronary artery flow velocity in humans during percutaneous coronary angioplasty. *J Am Coll Cardiol* 1992; 20:276-86.

18. Ofili EO, Kern MJ, Labovitz AJ, St. Vrain JA, Segal J, Aguirre FV, Castello R. Analysis of coronary blood flow velocity dynamics in angiographically normal and stenosed arteries before and after endolumen enlargement by angioplasty. *J Am Coll Cardiol* 1993; 21:308-16.

19. Serruys PW, Di Mario C, Meneveau N, de Jaegere P, Strikwerda S, de Feyter PJ, Emanuelsson H. Intracoronary pressure and flow velocity with sensor-tip guidewires: a new methodologic approach for assessment of coronary hemodynamics before and after coronary interventions. *Am J Cardiol* 1993; 71:41D-53D.

20. Kern MJ, Dupouy P, Drury JH, Aguirre FV, Aptecar E, Bach RG, Caracciolo EA, Donohue TJ, Rande JL, Geschwind HJ, Mechem CJ, Kane G, Teiger E, Wolford TL. Role of coronary artery lumen enlargement in improving coronary blood flow after balloon angioplasty and stenting: a combined intravascular ultrasound Doppler flow and imaging study. *J Am Coll Cardiol* 1997; 29:1520-7.

21. Wilson RF, Johnson MR, Marcus ML, Aylward PE, Skorton DJ, Collins S, White CW. The effect of coronary angioplasty on coronary flow reserve. *Circulation* 1988; 77:873-85.

22. Serruys PW, di Mario C, Piek J, Schroeder E, Vrints C, Probst P, de Bruyne B, Hanet C, Fleck E, Haude M, Verna E, Voudris V, Geschwind H, Emanuelsson H, Muhlberger V, Danzi G, Peels HO, Ford AJ, Jr., Boersma E. Prognostic value of intracoronary flow velocity and diameter stenosis in assessing the short- and long-term outcomes of coronary balloon angioplasty: the DEBATE Study (Doppler Endpoints Balloon Angioplasty Trial Europe). *Circulation* 1997; 96:3369-77.

23. Dupouy P, Pelle G, Garot P, Kern MJ, Kane G, Woscoboinick J, Aptecar E, Belarbi A, Pernes JM, Dubois Rande JL, Teiger E. Physiologically guided angioplasty in support to a provisional stenting strategy: immediate and six-month outcome. *Catheter Cardiovasc Interv* 2000; 49:369-75.

24. Piek JJ, Boersma E, di Mario C, Schroeder E, Vrints C, Probst P, de Bruyne B, Hanet C, Fleck E, Haude M, Verna E, Voudris V, Geschwind H, Emanuelsson H, Muhlberger V, Peels HO, Serruys PW. Angiographical and Doppler flow-derived parameters for assessment of coronary lesion severity and its relation to the result of exercise electrocardiography. DEBATE study group. Doppler Endpoints Balloon Angioplasty Trial Europe [see comments]. *Eur Heart J* 2000; 21:466-74.

25. Piek JJ, Boersma E, Voskuil M, di Mario C, Schroeder E, Vrints C, Probst P, de Bruyne B, Hanet C, Fleck E, Haude M, Verna E, Voudris V, Geschwind H, Emanuelsson H, Muhlberger V, Peels HO, Serruys PW. The immediate and long-term effect of optimal balloon angioplasty on the absolute coronary blood flow velocity reserve. A subanalysis of the DEBATE study. Doppler Endpoints Balloon Angioplasty Trial Europe. *Eur Heart J* 2001; 22:1725-32.

26. Albertal M, Regar E, Van Langenhove G, Carlier SG, Serrano P, Boersma E, Bruyne B, di Mario C, Piek J, Serruys PW. Flow velocity and predictors of a suboptimal coronary flow velocity reserve after coronary balloon angioplasty. *Eur Heart J* 2002; 23:133-8.

27. Anderson HV, Kirkeeide RL, Stuart Y, Smalling RW, Heibig J, Willerson JT. Coronary artery flow monitoring following coronary interventions. *Am J Cardiol* 1993; 71:62D-69D.

28. Kern MJ, Donohue T, Bach R, Aguirre F, Bell C. Monitoring cyclical coronary blood flow alterations after coronary angioplasty for stent restenosis with a Doppler guide wire. *Am Heart J* 1993; 125:1159-61.

29. Sunamura M, di Mario C, Piek JJ, Schroeder E, Vrints C, Probst P, Heyndrickx GR, Fleck E, Serruys PW. Cyclic flow variations after angioplasty: a rare phenomenon predictive of immediate complications. DEBATE Investigator's Group. *Am Heart J* 1996; 131:843-8.

30. Serruys PW, de Bruyne B, Carlier S, Sousa JE, Piek J, Muramatsu T, Vrints C, Probst P, Seabra-Gomes R, Simpson I, Voudris V, Gurne O, Pijls N, Belardi J, van Es GA, Boersma E, Morel MA, van Hout B. Randomized comparison of primary stenting and provisional balloon angioplasty guided by flow velocity measurement [In Process Citation]. *Circulation* 2000; 102:2930-7.

31. di Mario C, Moses JW, Anderson TJ, Bonan R, Muramatsu T, Jain AC, Suarez de Lezo J, Cho SY, Kern M, Meredith IT, Cohen D, Moussa I, Colombo A. Randomized comparison of elective stent implantation and coronary balloon angioplasty guided by online quantitative angiography and intracoronary Doppler. *Circulation* 2000; 102:2938-44.

32. Lafont A, Dubois-Rande JL, Steg PG, Dupouy P, Carrie D, Coste P, Furber A, Beygui F, Feldman LJ, Rahal S, Tron C, Hamon M, Grollier G, Commeau P, Richard P, Colin P, Bauters C, Karrillon G, Ledru F, Citron B, Marie FN, Kern M. The French Randomized Optimal Stenting Trial: a prospective evaluation of provisional stenting guided by coronary velocity reserve and quantitative coronary angiography. F.R.O.S.T. Study Group. *J Am Coll Cardiol* 2000; 36:404-9.

33. Cohen D, Taira D, di Mario C, Moses J, Colombo A. In-hospital and 6 month follow-up costs of universal vs provisional stenting: results from the DESTINI trial. *Circulation* 1998; 98:I-499.

34. Albertal M, Van Langenhove G, Regar E, Kay IP, Foley D, Sianos G, Kozuma K, Beijsterveldt T, Carlier SG, Belardi JA, Boersma E, Sousa JE, de Bruyne B, Serruys PW. Uncomplicated moderate coronary artery dissections after balloon angioplasty: good outcome without stenting. *Heart* 2001; 86:193-8.

35. Cantor WJ, Peterson ED, Popma JJ, Zidar JP, Sketch MH, Jr., Tcheng JE, Ohman EM. Provisional stenting strategies: systematic overview and implications for clinical decision-making [In Process Citation]. *J Am Coll Cardiol* 2000; 36:1142-51.

36. Anderson HV, Carabello BA. Provisional versus routine stenting: routine stenting is here to stay. *Circulation* 2000; 102:2910-4.

37. Briguori C, Sheiban I, de Gregorio J, Anzuini A, Montorfano M, Pagnotta P, Marsico F, Leonardo F, di Mario C, Colombo A. Direct coronary stenting without predilation. *J Am Coll Cardiol* 1999; 34:1910-5.

38. Vrints CJ, Claeys MJ, Bosmans J, Conraads V, Snoeck JP. Effect of stenting on coronary flow velocity reserve: comparison of coil and tubular stents. *Heart* 1999; 82:465-70.

39. Nishida T, di Mario C, Kern M, Anderson T, Moussa I, Bonan R, Muramatsu T, Jain A, Suarez de Lezo J, Cho S, Meredith I, Moses J, Colombo A. Impact of final coronary flow velocity reserve on late outcome following stent implantation. *Eur Heart J* 2002; In press.

40. Pijls NH, van Son JA, Kirkeeide RL, de Bruyne B, Gould KL. Experimental basis of determining maximum coronary, myocardial, and collateral blood flow by pressure measurements for assessing functional stenosis severity before and after percutaneous transluminal coronary angioplasty. *Circulation* 1993; 87:1354-67.

41. Bech GJ, Pijls NH, De Bruyne B, Peels KH, Michels HR, Bonnier HJ, Koolen JJ. Usefulness of fractional flow reserve to predict clinical outcome after balloon angioplasty. *Circulation* 1999; 23; 99(7): 883-888.

42. Hanekamp CE, Koolen JJ, Pijls NH, Michels HR, Bonnier HJ. Comparison of quantitative coronary angiography, intravascular ultrasound, and coronary pressure measurement to assess optimum stent deployment. *Circulation* 1999; 99:1015-21.

43. Matthys K, Carlier S, Segers P, Ligthart J, Sianos G, Serrano P, Verdonck PR, Serruys PW. In vitro study of FFR, QCA, and IVUS for the assessment of optimal stent deployment. *Catheter Cardiovasc Interv* 2001; 54:363-75.

44. di Mario C, Gil R, de Feyter PJ, Schuurbiers JC, Serruys PW. Utilization of translesional hemodynamics: comparison of pressure and flow methods in stenosis assessment in patients with coronary artery disease. *Cathet Cardiovasc Diagn* 1996; 38:189-201.

45. Mancini GB, Cleary RM, DeBoe SF, Moore NB, Gallagher KP. Instantaneous hyperemic flow-versus-pressure slope index. Microsphere validation of an alternative to measures of coronary reserve. *Circulation* 1991; 84:862-70.

46. di Mario C, Krams R, Gil R, Serruys PW. Slope of the instantaneous hyperemic diastolic coronary flow velocity-pressure relation. A new index for assessment of the physiological significance of coronary stenosis in humans. *Circulation* 1994; 90:1215-24.

47. Pijls N, de Bruyne B, Smith L, Aarnoudse W, Barbato E, Bartunek J, Bech G, van de Vosse F. Coronary thermodilution to assess flow reserve: validation in humans. *Circulation* 2002; In press.

48. di Mario C, Liistro F, Colombo A. A new method for calculation of CFR from pressure measurements: initial clinical applications (abstract). *J Am Coll Cardiol* 2001; in press (March).

49. Sousa JE, Costa MA, Abizaid AC, Rensing BJ, Abizaid AS, Tanajura LF, Kozuma K, van Langenhove G, Sousa AG, Falotico R, Jaeger J, Popma JJ, Serruys PW. Sustained suppression of neointimal proliferation by sirolimus-eluting stents: one-year angiographic and intravascular ultrasound follow-up. *Circulation* 2001; 104:2007-11.

50. Sousa JE, Costa MA, Abizaid A, Abizaid AS, Feres F, Pinto IM, Seixas AC, Staico R, Mattos LA, Sousa AG, Falotico R, Jaeger J, Popma JJ, Serruys PW. Lack of Neointimal Proliferation After Implantation of Sirolimus-Coated Stents in Human Coronary Arteries : A Quantitative Coronary Angiography and Three-Dimensional Intravascular Ultrasound Study. *Circulation* 2001; 103:192-195.

SECTION VI

Pressure Wire

23

Technical Considerations. Basic Principles of Fractional Flow Reserve

JAVIER ESCANED, MD

Introduction. Some Relevant Physiological Aspects of Coronary Circulation. Physiological Information Obtained from Intracoronary Pressure Measurements. Practical Aspects of Fractional Flow Reserve. Potential Pitfalls during FFR. References.

INTRODUCTION

It has been stated several times in the preceding chapters that soon after its introduction as a diagnostic technique, the limitations of coronary angiography in assessing the underlying atherosclerotic involvement of the vessel studied became evident. We have also seen how these limitations led to the development during the late 1980s and through the 1990s of intracoronary ultrasound as a complement to coronary angiography, both as a diagnostic tool and as an aid in coronary interventions. During the same period, and in an attempt to overcome the poor relationship between angiographic and functional measurements of stenosis severity, intracoronary guidewires fitted with Doppler and pressure sensors were developed.[1-4] Eventually, they came to be used routinely in the catheterization laboratory for diagnostic and interventional purposes.[5]

The most common question, by far, raised during the review of a coronary angiogram is whether a given stenosis is hemodynamically significant and, therefore, is a cause of myocardial ischemia. An ideal physiological test to answer this question should 1) provide information which incorporates different aspects of coronary physiology and 2) be accurate, 3) independent of changing hemodynamic conditions, 4) easy to perform, 5) safe, and 6) easy to interpret. These ideal characteristics have been virtually fulfilled by a pressure-derived index of coronary flow reserve, namely fractional flow reserve (FFR).[6] To its credit, FFR has created unprecedented expectations among interventional cardiologists[7, 8] and has boosted interest in intracoronary physiology among interventional and non-interventional cardiologists alike.

In this chapter, we will focus on the theoretical background of FFR and on practical aspects of its use in the catheterization laboratory. We will also review, in the first place, the basic concepts of coronary physiology that are required for an adequate understanding of intracoronary physiology techniques.

SOME RELEVANT PHYSIOLOGICAL ASPECTS OF CORONARY CIRCULATION

An understanding of the physiological principles underlying intracoronary physiology techniques is essential for the adequate use of these techniques and correct interpretation of the results obtained with them. It is customary to describe coronary circulation in terms of analogies with simple electrical or hydraulic circuits. However, these analogies are far from capable of integrating the complexity of the phenomena that occur during the cardiac cycle. For this reason,we will combine this approach with specific comments about aspects which require an alternative description to the ones provided by that model.

Heart function is highly dependent on the maintenance and modulation of coronary blood flow. The myocardium, particularly the subendocardium, is the tissue with the highest baseline aerobic demands in the body (8-10 ml O^2/min/100 g vs 0.15 ml O^2/min/100 g in the skeletal muscle). The three main determinants of this demand are wall stress, inotropic state, and heart rate.[9, 10]

Coronary blood flow is influenced by extravascular compression. Throughout the cardiac cycle, variations in intramyocardial and intracavitary pressure modify coronary vascular resistance drastically.[11] Coronary blood flow is modulated by variations in the resistance of the vascular bed. Whereas blood flow is predominantly diastolic in the left coronary artery, in the right coronary artery there is also systolic blood flow due to the low extravascular compression exerted by the right ventricle and atria.[11, 12] As a result of this, the phasic characteristics of the trans-stenotic gradient are also different, paralleling the blood flow pattern through the stenosis.

In baseline circumstances, the relation between blood pressure and flow in the coronary arteries is not linear. If the only situation considered from now on is analogous to the mid end-diastole, that is to say, a situation in which extravascular compression is minimal and constant and there are no variations in coronary conductance, coronary blood flow remains stable over a broad range of pressures. This phenomenon receives the name of coronary self-regulation and is the result of

intrinsic myogenic tone, a response by the smooth muscle cells of the coronary arterioles to pressure variations.[13-15] Coronary self-regulation is only effective within the range of pressures indicated: when the perfusion pressure falls below this pressure, coronary blood flow decreases.

During maximum coronary hyperemia, the relation between coronary blood pressure and flow is linear. In contrast to the situation just described, complete vasodilation of resistance vessels induced by a maximum physiological or pharmacological hyperemic stimulus (increased myocardial metabolism) establishes a fixed relation between coronary perfusion pressure and blood flow. The slope of this relation is influenced by the resistance of the system: the lower this slope (conductance) is, the greater the resistance of the system will be.[16, 17] The pressure-flow relation during maximum hyperemia constitutes a ceiling of expected coronary flow values for different perfusion pressures.[18]

The increase in blood flow from the self-regulation to the maximum hyperemia situation constitutes an indicator of the functional state of the coronary system. This concept constitutes the coronary flow reserve, a

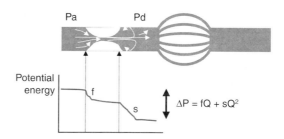

Figure 23-1. The development of an intracoronary gradient results from the loss of coronary flow energy as a result of friction (f) across the stenosis and the development of turbulence (s) during the separation of flow lines at the distal aspect of the stenosis. Since coronary flow is also modulated by the status of microcirculation, it can be inferred from the formula that the trans-stenotic gradient is also influenced by microcirculatory status.

functional indicator of the state of coronary circulation that is widely used in diagnostic techniques.[3, 18, 19] In Figures 23-1 through 23-3, this principle is illustrated schematically. It is important to remember that in normal conditions the coronary reserve is transmurally heterogeneous: in the subendocardium, the coronary reserve is smaller because there is a greater baseline degree of arteriolar vasodilation as a result of greater subendocardial metabolic requirements.

The presence of epicardial stenosis causes a loss of energy associated with blood flow that is expressed as a fall in effective perfusion pressure. Stenoses cause two types of resistance, one related with friction (f) and the other related with turbulence and the dispersion of blood flow after passing the stenosis (s) (Fig. 23-1). The trans-stenotic pressure gradient, ΔP, has a nonlinear relation with the f and s components and flow, Q, in accordance with the expression $\Delta P = fQ + sQ^2$. The resistive components of friction and turbulence are influenced by characteristics of the blood (viscosity and density) and the geometry of the stenosis (reduction of luminal area, length, and the inflow and outflow angles).[14, 18, 19] The complex interrelation between these factors contrasts with the simplicity of the indices of angiographic severity commonly used in clinical practice (e.g., the percentage of luminal diameter), and illustrates the limitations of angiography for evaluating the functional repercussions of stenosis.[1-3]

Coronary self-regulation compensates for the fall in blood pressure caused by stenosis in order to maintain constant coronary blood flow. The mechanism of self-regulation, which in physiological conditions adjusts microcirculatory resistance to myocardial energy requirements, has a chronic compensatory function in response to the fall in intracoronary pressure secondary to stenosis. As the stenosis increases in severity, sustained arteriolar vasodilation increasingly compromises the self-regulatory function to maintain an adequate myocardial blood flow. In other words, the compensatory function of

coronary self-regulation in a stenotic vessel is at the expense of reducing coronary reserve. The compromised coronary reserve is first evident in the subendocardium, where baseline arteriolar vasodilation is greater due to higher energy demands.

The hemodynamic effect of a stenosis is manifested in the smaller slope of the pressure-flow relation. The diagnostic utility of the coronary reserve concept derives from this finding. The potential increase in coronary blood flow from a given pressure at baseline to maximum hyperemia (that is, the coronary reserve) decreases in the presence of stenosis. This effect is quantifiable in absolute terms if measurements obtained at baseline and in hyperemia are available. In addition, because adjacent vascular beds have a conserved coronary reserve, the induction of maximum hyperemia tends to increase the heterogeneity of myocardial perfusion, a phenomenon that constitutes the basis for different diagnostic techniques. In this sense, pure arterial vasodilators (adenosine, papaverine, dipyridamole), administered systemically, enhance the heterogeneity of regional and transmural myocardial perfusion (inducing the theft phenomenon when the vessels of the epicardial layers dilate). Dobutamine exhausts coronary reserve in the stenotic vessel as a result of metabolically increasing myocardial demand (it increases contractility and myocardial oxygen consumption more than physical exercise) and specifically inducing vasodilation of the microcirculation (doses of 30-40 μg/kg/min produce an overall coronary vasodilation similar to that of adenosine administered systemically).[20] Finally, physical exercise is the most physiological stimulus, since it combines metabolic stimuli with neural modulation of the coronary circulation.

Microcirculatory dysfunction is also manifested as a smaller slope of the pressure-flow relation. This is important for the correct interpretation of diagnostic techniques based on coronary reserve, and explains the development of techniques for the specific assessment of epicardial and micro-circulatory resistance.[4-6, 21] Many clinical entities that cause remodeling of the coronary microcirculation also participate in the development of epicardial stenoses, such as diabetes mellitus, arterial hypertension, smoking, and hypercholesterolemia, as well as heart transplantation vasculopathy.[21] Likewise, microcirculatory resistance can increase in relation to alpha-adrenergic stimulation (e.g., in relation to physical exercise or mental stress),[22] during acute myocardial ischemia,[23] or as a result of microembolization (platelet or thrombotic aggregates, particles resulting from rotational atherectomy).[24] Another important observation for diagnostic techniques, particularly fractional flow reserve, is that microcirculatory dysfunction reduces the gradient of trans-stenotic pressure in an epicardial stenosis that, as discussed above, is dependent on coronary blood flow. This phenomenon can lead to an incorrect interpretation of diagnostic tests that are based on the Bernouilli formula or measurement of the translesional gradient.[5, 25] This again explains the importance of tests that allow independent assessment of the severity of an epicardial stenosis and the state of microcirculation.

PHYSIOLOGICAL INFORMATION OBTAINED FROM INTRACORONARY PRESSURE MEASUREMENTS

Use of Absolute Intracoronary Pressure Gradients

From a historical point of view, coronary pressure measurements were used to assess the severity of coronary stenoses or the result of percutaneous interventions,[26, 27] and even to predict the development of cardiac events.[28, 29] However, this approach was unsuccessful for several reason. In the first place, the relatively large diameter of the intracoronary or balloon catheters used in those studies interfered with the measurements made, to the point that significant gradients could be documented in coronary arteries without stenoses.[30] In the second place, the theoretical framework in which translesional pressure gradients were used to estimate stenosis severity was incorrect. The trans-stenotic pressure gradient is influenced by translesional blood flow, which is modulated by the degree of distal microvascular resistance and is highly variable.[25] Even when complete hyperemia is achieved, or when the vasodilatory reserve of the distal microvascular bed is exhausted by a severe stenosis, the absolute value of the transstenotic pressure gradient varies with head pressure. For these reasons, the reliability of intracoronary pressure measurements for the assessment of coronary stenoses was poor, and never reached widespread use in clinical practice. A major breakthrough in the use of intracoronary pressure gradients for functional assessment of coronary stenoses came from the introduction of a different theoretical framework, which was named fractional flow reserve (FFR).[6, 31-33] The principles and characteristics of this index will be discussed separately.

Myocardial Fractional Flow Reserve

Fractional flow reserve constitutes a link between intracoronary pressure measurements and the assessment of stenosis severity in terms of flow impairment. The cornerstone principle underlying this technique is that the pressure-flow relation in the coronary tree becomes linear during hyperemia. When such linearity is achieved, it becomes true that the proportion between two intracoronary pressures is identical to the proportion between the coronary flows corresponding to these pressures (Fig. 23-2). If this concept is applied to the pressures proximal (Pa) and distal (Pd) to a stenosis, we will be able to calculate the percentage fall in coronary flow caused by the stenosis: for

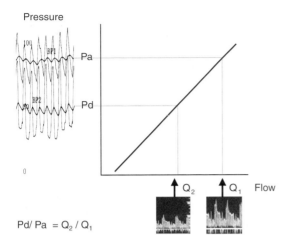

Pressure

Pd/ Pa $= Q_2 / Q_1$

Figure 23-2. Physiological principles of FFR. During maximal hyperemia, there is a linear relationship between pressure and flow. Let us consider two pressure measurements (Pa and Pd) with their corresponding coronary flows Q1 and Q2. Since Pd results from the effect of a coronary stenosis, it is possible to infer that the relative loss of intracoronary pressure is proportional to the loss in coronary flow induced by the same stenosis. See text for details.

example, Pd/Pa ratio = 0.5 will be interpreted as a 50% reduction in blood flow in the dependent myocardial territory caused by the stenosis in relation to a non-stenotic situation (in which case there would be no difference between Pa and Pd, and Pd/Pa = 1). This Pd/Pa ratio obtained during maximum hyperemia constitutes the myocardial fractional flow reserve. The term myocardial FFR, (FFRmyo) refers to the fact that the reduction in blood flow is estimated as that occurring in the myocardial territory vascularized by that vessel, and that therefore takes into consideration other sources of blood flow, such as collateral support. In recent years, the terms FFR and FFRmyo have become synonyms, although in the original work by Pijls et al a distinction between myocardial (FFRmyo) and coronary (FFRcor) fractional flow reserve was made, the latter calculated by subtracting the collateral contribution to myocardial blood flow from FFRmyo.

Two aspects that are critical in the success of fractional flow reserve are its ease of performance and interpretation. For the former, only two mean pressures (obtained from the guiding catheter and the pressure guidewire) recorded during maximal hyperemia induced pharmacologically are required. The latter is facilitated by a clear cut-off value for the identification of significant coronary stenoses (that is, those which are associated with inducible myocardial ischemia in noninvasive tests). The identification of this cut-off point, which equals 0.75, and its application under different clinical situations will be discussed in detail in the following chapters of this book.

The interpretation of FFR relies critically, however, on a number of specific features of this technique that stem from the previously described physiological characteristics of coronary circulation (Fig. 23-3). First, FFR is a specific technique for the hemodynamic assessment of stenoses. Unlike intracoronary Doppler, its use in coronary arteries without epicardial stenosis will not provide information on coronary microcirculation, and will only show that coronary conductance is maximal (an FFR = 1 would be documented). Second, FFR performs an assessment of the stenosis which is relative to a theoretical hemodynamic situation in which that stenosis would be absent. This characteristic makes FFR an especially useful index for assessing the need for percutaneous revascularization. It is also in marked contrast with coronary flow velocity reserve, in which the reference element is flow velocity before induction of hyperemia. Third, as anticipated above, the information provided by FFR refers to blood flow in the myocardial area of distribution of the studied vessel, and incorporates not only anterograde flow through the stenosis, but also collateral circulation from other vessels. In vessels with important collateral support, the relative effect of stenosis on the perfusion of the territory is smaller and, consequently, higher FFR values would be expected. Fourth, the status

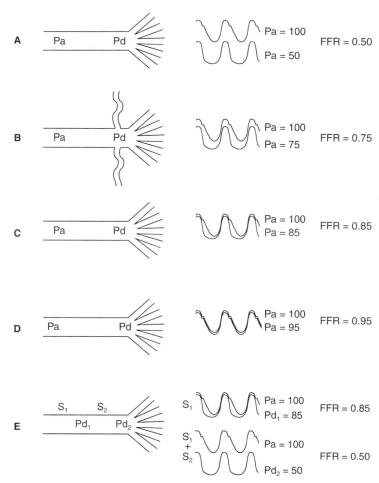

Figure 23-3. Fractional flow reserve is an index of stenosis that incorporates different variables with a net effect on coronary circulation. This figure illustrates some of these factors. Panel A shows the effect of coronary stenosis on the hyperemic pressure gradient in the presence of normal microcirculation. In panel B the same stenosis is depicted under circumstances of good collateral support. As a consequence of the collateral supply, Pd and, consequently, FFR are higher than in situation A. In panel C, the effect of microcirculatory dysfunction on FFR is shown. Since the increase in microvascular resistance decreases coronary blood flow, and since the hyperemic gradient is a function of trans-stenotic blood flow, Pa and FFR are higher. This does not constitute in itself a problem for clinical applications of FFR since, from a pragmatic point of view, it produces valid information for judging whether revascularization is needed in that vessel. Figure D shows what one should expect if coronary stenting is performed in that situation. From a hemodynamic point of view, a small increase in FFR would be noticed but, more importantly, no significant net benefit would be obtained since treatment would be limited to the epicardial vessel, but would not improve the underlying problem in the microcirculation. Figure E shows the effect of serial stenoses on FFR measurements. Even when the severity of the stenosis located upstream, S1, is similar to that shown in panel A, FFR measurements obtained when the pressure transducer is left between both stenoses (Pd1) would show a lower value, since the stenosis located downstream is limiting trans-stenotic flow. If FFR is performed across the 2 serial stenoses (Pd2), their combined effect would be assessed, but the severity of S1 might be underestimated. The issue of serial stenoses will be treated in detail in following chapters.

of coronary microcirculation is also incorporated in the assessment of a stenosis with FFR. Since the trans-stenotic pressure gradient is a function of coronary flow, attenuation of the hyperemic response by microcirculatory impairment will be associated with higher FFR values than those obtained in cases of normal microcirculation. From a practical viewpoint, this may not constitute a limitation of the technique: the finding of a normal FFR value in a stenosis with important underlying microcirculatory involvement would make it possible to anticipate a small percentage increment in myocardial blood flow if this vessel is revascularized. And fifth, an important aspect of FFR is its applicability under variable hemodynamic conditions, since it is relatively unaffected by them.[34] The superiority of FFR over 2 different indices of stenosis severity, coronary flow velocity reserve and hyperemic pressure-flow slope index, becomes evident.

tion between the radiopaque guidewire tip and the non-radiopaque stem, thus allowing accurate positioning of the pressure transducer under fluoroscopy (Figure 23-4). The interface consoles for the two guidewires are different. The WaveWire console (WaveMap) displays the aortic, intracoronary pressures, and FFR in a digital format, the latter being calculated automatically following intracoronary administration of adenosine or during continuous intravenous adenosine administration. It requires an external polygraph for the visualization and recording of pressure tracings. The RadiAnalyzer is a self-contained unit that allows visualization of aortic and intracoronary pressure, as well as instantaneous FFR, on a screen. The complete pressure tracing obtained during the induction of hyperemia is digitally recorded and can be post-processed to overcome artifacts which might have led to an erroneous estimation of FFR in the automatic mode.

PRACTICAL ASPECTS OF FRACTIONAL FLOW RESERVE

In the following paragraphs, the basic aspects of the performance of fractional flow reserve will be covered.

Hardware and Software for Intracoronary Pressure Measurement

Two solid-state pressure guidewires fitted with microtransducers are currently available: the PressureWire (Radi Medical Systems, Uppsala, Sweden) and the WaveWire (Endosonics, Rancho Cordoba, California). The torqueability and steerability of these wires and the stability of the pressure signal of these guidewires has improved considerably since the first versions, and virtually equals that of a conventional floppy guidewire for PTCA. In both guidewires, the pressure transducer is located at the transi-

Performance of the Procedure

It is advisable to use pressure guidewires in conjunction with coronary guiding catheters. This recommendation stems mainly from the potential need for performing an in-

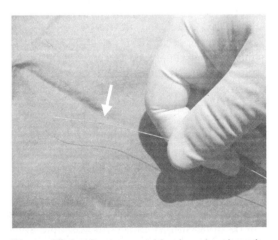

Figure 23-4. Pressure guidewire showing the location of the pressure microsensor.

terventional procedure should a complication derived from guidewire manipulation occur. Diagnostic coronary catheters have a smaller lumen and its inner coating is less smooth, which may interfere with guidewire manipulation. The available 0.014" pressure guidewires are compatible with regular interventional devices, such as balloon catheters, IVUS catheters, etc. As with other guidewires with floppy tips, pressure guidewires should be used with caution in single operator exchange (SOE) devices with a short monorail segment, like some IVUS catheters, since kinking and entanglement of the wire by the device may occur.[35] Guidewire manipulation in the coronary vessels is only performed following heparin administration, either after administration of a minimum of 5,000 units or adjusting the heparin dose to achieve an ACT of more than 250 seconds.

Pressure Calibration

As a pressure-derived index, one of the critical aspects of FFR measurement is an adequate handling of pressures through the procedure. Thorough flushing of the fluid line used for Pa is performed to eliminate air bubbles that might dampen the pressure signal. The pressure transducer and guidewire should be zeroed before introducing the guidewire in the guiding catheter.

Verification or Equalization of Pressures

To perform adequate equalization of pressures, the guidewire should be advanced until the pressure sensor is located exactly at the tip of the guiding catheter. Since the pressure sensor is located at the transition point between the opaque and non-radiopaque segments of the guidewire, this can be done simply under fluoroscopic control. In modern interfaces (RadiAnalyzer and WaveMap), an «equalization» of Pa and Pd

is performed at this time. In previous versions, such as the Radi guidewire, pressure equalization was performed by vertical displacement of the pressure transducer until identical readings of Pa and Pd were achieved. In any case, it is recommended that the guidewire introducer be withdrawn and the hemostatic valve tightened during pressure equalization to avoid pressure losses in Pa. Following equalization of pressures, a perfect matching of both phasic and mean pressure readings from the guidewire and guiding catheter should be expected. A lower amplitude in the phasic pattern of Pa might be indicative of incomplete tightening of the hemostatic valve or the presence of air in the fluid lines or in the guiding catheter.

Crossing the Stenosis

The next step is to cross the stenosis with the guidewire. In most cases, the guidewire can be advanced to a position distal to the stenosis while connected to the interface. In tortuous or challenging vessels it may be necessary to detach the guidewire for better torque. The position of the pressure sensor should be about 2 cm distal to the distal aspect of the stenosis: a position too close to the stenosis might be affected by a Venturi effect associated with the flow dynamics in the stenosis. Occasionally, the pressure sensor may bounce in the coronary artery against the arterial wall, causing an artifact in the pressure waveform. Slightly advancing the guidewire is usually enough to correct this phenomenon.

Induction of Hyperemia

The importance of achieving an adequate of coronary hyperemia cannot be stressed enough. The induction of coronary hyperemia is one of the cornerstones of the theoretical background of FFR, and will therefore be treated in detail below. From a practical point of view, coronary hyperemia should be performed soon after the guidewire has been positioned distally to the coronary stenosis, in order to lessen the possibility of pressure shifts, which are time-dependent and can influence the measurement. For that reason, the hyperemic agent (adenosine, ATP, papaverine) and chosen venous route should be ready for use when the guidewire is advanced into the coronary artery. The guidewire introducer should again be withdrawn, this time not only to measure Pa adequately, but also to prevent the loss of adenosine if given intracoronarily. The patient should be told about the flushing and angina-like sensations frequently associated with the intravenous administration of adenosine. The increase in coronary blood flow during hyperemia can actually cause engagement of the guiding catheter in the coronary ostium, producing damping of Pa. To avoid this phenomenon, it is advisable to monitor the phasic characteristics of Pa during hyperemia. When intracoronary administration of the hyperemic agent is performed, the catheter should be withdrawn slightly from the coronary ostium immediately after injection of the drug bolus.

Adequate Recording of Pressures for FFR Calculation

Although some of the commercially available systems described above calculate FFR without a concomitant pressure display, continuous recording of mean pressure tracings during the induction of hyperemia facilitates the calculation of FFR and the identification of potential pitfalls. Modern consoles like the RadiAnalyzer perform digital recording of pressures, which are automatically displayed as soon as recording is stopped. Mean pressures can also be recorded on paper using a conventional polygraph. Caution is advised regarding the way that mean pressures is calculated, in this case by polygraph, since consoles in which pressure averaging takes place

over a long period of time (for example, 10 s) may produce serious errors if a short-acting hyperemic stimulus (i.c. adenosine, for example) is used. The operator should be aware of this fact, which can be solved by adjusting the pressure averaging settings on many polygraphs. However, in other cases the use of a sustained hyperemic stimulus for FFR measurements may be mandatory.

Interrogation of the Stenotic Coronary Segment

The information provided by intracoronary pressure measurements is not restricted to a single point within the vessel, but should be integrated with that obtained in neighboring segments. The simplest technique consists in crossing the stenosis to and fro with the pressure sensor while leaving the floppy tip passed through the stenosis. This makes it possible to establish the exact location in the vessel where an intracoronary pressure gradient develops. An extension of this principle are the so-called pressure pullback curves, a pressure tracing obtained during sustained maximal hyperemia and continuous slow withdrawal of the pressure guidewire along a complete coronary segment or vessel. This technique allows assessment not only of a single stenosis, but also of serial lesions or multiple irregularities resulting from diffuse atherosclerotic narrowing. Since the complete sequence is obtained during maximal hyperemia, this technique also makes it possible to introduce corrections for the unforeseen drift of the intracoronary pressure signal. The application of pressure pullback curves to different clinical situations will be covered in the following chapters.

Control for Drift or Other Errors

Although much less likely than in the first generation of pressure guidewires, pressure drift may still occur with modern guidewires during FFR studies. There is a clear relationship between the length of the study and the likelihood of pressure drift. For this reason, the most effective way to reduce its occurrence is to make a quick study, allowing the minimum time between the original calibration and FFR measurement. In any case, the validity of the measurements can be verified by withdrawing the pressure transducer to a position proximal to the stenosis or segment under study while keeping the floppy tip through it. In the presence of an intracoronary gradient, phasic morphology of Pa and Pd also provide information on whether it is real or artifactual. In the presence of a true pressure gradient, the dicrotic notch present in the phasic Pa tracing is absent in Pd. In the left coronary artery, a different morphology of Pd can be appreciated as a result of the development of predominantly diastolic gradients. When these features are absent, the possibility of pressure drift is increased.

Assessment of Collateral Circulation

The use of pressure guidewires in the context of coronary interventions makes it possible to assess collateral support to the treated vessel. Coronary wedge pressure or occlusion pressure is proportionally related to collateral support. It is customary to normalize coronary wedge pressure (Pw) to aortic pressure (Pa) to obtain the so-called collateral flow index (CFI).[36] If more accurate measurements are sought, then it is advisable to adjust to central venous pressure (Pv), according to the expression (Pw-Pv)/(Pa-Pv), called «maximal recruitable collateral flow» by Pijls et al.[37]

POTENTIAL PITFALLS DURING FFR

In addition to a proper understanding of the physiological principles and steps that must be followed during the performance of FFR, a number of potential sources of error will be discussed below.

Guiding Catheters with Side Holes

The presence of side holes in a guiding catheter poses two different problems for FFR estimation.[38] The most obvious problem is that part of the hyperemic agent administered by intracoronary route will be lost through the side holes, leading to suboptimal hyperemia. The second problem is the effect on pressure measurements. If the distal hole of the catheter gets engaged in the coronary ostium, Pa will not reflect the true value of the aortic pressure, but a lower value resulting from the development of a pressure gradient created by the side holes. For this reason, if a catheter with side holes is used, care should be taken to keep the catheter tip out of the coronary ostium and to perform coronary hyperemia with intravenous adenosine infusion.

Pressure Damping by the Guiding Catheter

As discussed above, engagement of the guiding catheter in the coronary ostium is a major source of error during FFR measurement. This frequently occurs as a result of a match in the sizes of the catheter and ostium (particularly in cases of ostial stenoses), or excessive advancement of the guiding catheter. It can occur as a result of a suction effect by the increased blood flow in the vessel during hyperemia, a situation which is particularly treacherous since will selectively affect the pressure measurements used for FFR calculation. It is highly recommended to perform simultaneous phasic and mean coronary pressure measurements to overcome this limitation. Alternatively, recording of a third arterial pressure from the side arm of the femoral sheath may unveil a difference in pressure between the guiding catheter and femoral artery indicative of this phenomenon.

Route of Administration of the Hyperemic Agent

For practical reasons, many centers preferentially use the intracoronary route to administer adenosine, ATP, or papaverine. However, several considerations must be remarked regarding this methodology.

In the first place, the operator should be aware that part of the dose of hyperemic agent given intracoronarily may spill out through the guidewire introducer and hemostatic valve, or may not reach the coronary microcirculation of the target vessel due to inadequate cannulation of the vessel or distribution of the drug to other coronary branches, etc. (as mentioned above, catheters with side holes cannot be used in this situation). It is recommended, in addition to adequately sealing the angiography system and properly cannulating the vessel, that multiple measurements be made with increasing doses of intracoronary adenosine to ensure that the plateau of the dose-response curve of adenosine has been reached.

In second place, the operator should be aware that the peak effect of i.c. adenosine is very short (Fig. 23-5). The settings of the polygraph should, therefore, be adjusted to calculate mean pressure over a very short period (1-3 beats). Otherwise, the pressure reading obtained may not reflect the true values present during the peak adenosine effect. Likewise, it is critical to flush the catheter after administration of the adenosine bolus as quickly as possible.

In third place, it should be noted that the validation studies on FFR, particularly those used to establish its optimal cut-off value, have been performed using intravenous adenosine infusion. In our experience with a cohort of patients in which FFR values with incremental doses of i.c. adenosine and i.v. adenosine infusion were compared, i.c. doses

of 20, 40 and 80 μg were associated with a percentage of false negatives of 21, 13, and 10% respectively. Even when the study is made after following all the above recommendations, this is an unacceptably high number of false-negative FFR values using i.c. administration.

Intravenous adenosine is normally infused through a central vein to obtain a faster hyperemic state than if performed from a peripheral vein. The recommended rate of infusion is 140 μg/kg/min, leading to maximal hyperemia 90-120 s after the onset of the infusion. The onset of the hyperemic plateau is frequently preceded by a short increase in aortic pressure, followed by a decrease of around 10% (Fig. 23-5). Hyperemia decreases gradually over approximately 60 s following interruption of the infusion. While i.c. administration of adenosine rarely causes any symptoms, intravenous infusion is frequently associated with flushing and a sensation chest pain which is in itself harmless. Bronchospasm in subjects without a prior history of asthma or lung disease is rare (around 0.2% in patients in centers with extensive experience)[38] but should be promptly identified and treated with aminophylline.

Presence of Multiple Stenoses

Assessment of a coronary stenosis in the presence of additional distal stenoses is a major problem. As elegantly demonstrated by De Bruyne et al.,[39] distal stenoses decrease the maximal trans-stenotic pressure gradient across those located upstream, causing underestimation of their hemodynamic severity with FFR. Although it is possible to ascertain the individual contributions of two stenoses in series for experimental purposes, clinical application is hampered by the fact that wedge pressure-which is normally obtained during balloon dilation-is one of the terms of the calculation. The assessment of serial stenoses with FFR will be discussed in detail in the following chapters. For the pur-

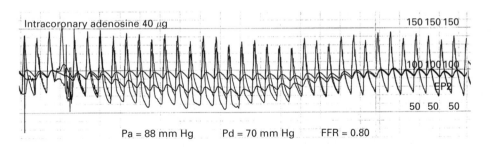

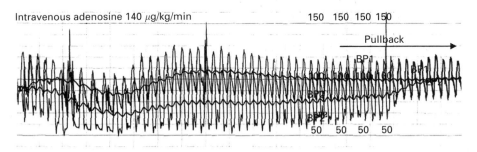

Figure 23-5. Pressure tracings obtained during the induction of coronary hyperemia with either an intracoronary bolus or intravenous infusion of adenosine. Intracoronary adenosine induces a short period of hyperemia, which can be missed if average pressure is calculated by the polygraph using a long time constant, or if there is a long delay between bolus administration and flushing of the guiding catheter. On the contrary, intravenous adenosine infusion induces a long, sustained period of hyperemia that facilitates adequate measurements. Note the typical increase in blood pressure preceding the hyperemic period. An additional advantage of i.v. infusion is that a pullback can be used during hyperemia to perform an «FFR mapping» of the segment and facilitate corrections if a pressure shift occurs. In this case, a brisk change in pressure gradient occurs when crossing back over the stenosis, and a perfect matching of pressures denotes the persistence of pressure calibration during the study. Both tracings were obtained in different patients. Recording speed is different in both cases (slower in i.v. adenosine infusion)

pose of introducing readers to the practice of FFR, it is enough to warn operators about this potentially misleading setting.

Current Developments in FFR and Pressure-Derived Indices of Stenosis Severity

From a technical point of view, there are ongoing technical developments in the field of intracoronary pressure measurements that are likely to be used in the clinical arena. A modification of FFR is the diastolic FFR, which is characterized by using the ratio of pressures obtained only during diastole.[40] This technique is more sensitive for the detection of inducible ischemia than conventional FFR. In addition, it can potentially avoid the interference of systolic phenomena that affect calculations based on mean pressures, such as those resulting from differences in flow patterns in the right and left coronary artery[41] or from the systolic compression of epicardial vessels by myocardial bridges.[42] In the near future, a new version of the Radi wire will allow assessment of coronary flow using the thermodilution principle.[43] The experimental validation of this technique is showing promising results and will potentially help to identify patients who have an underlying microvascular dysfunction. A non-hyperemic index of stenosis severity based on the analysis of pressure wave transmission across the stenosis has been proposed and compared with FFR in a recent study by Brosh et al.[44] It is likely that these and other techniques will contribute to further expansion of the use of intracoronary pressure measurements in the catheterization laboratory.

REFERENCES

1. White CW, Wright CB, Doty DB, et al. Does visual interpretation of the coronary arteriogram predict physiologic importance of a coronary stenosis? *N Engl J Med* 1984; 310:819-24.

2. Klocke F.J.: Measurements of coronary blood flow and degree of stenosis; current clinical implications and continuing uncertainties. *J Am Coll Cardiol* 1983; 1:131-41.

3. Klocke, F. J. Measurements of coronary flow reserve: Defining pathophysiology versus making decisions about patient care. *Circulation* 1987; 76:1183.

4. Serruys PW, Di Mario C, Meneveau N, de Jaegere P, Strikwerda S, de Feyter PM, et al. Intracoronary pressure and flow velocity with sensor-tipped guidewires: a new methodologic approach for assessment of coronary hemodynamics before and after coronary interventions. *Am J Cardiol* 1993; 71:41D-53D.

5. Kern MJ. Coronary physiology revisited. Practical insights from the cardiac catheterization laboratory. *Circulation* 2000; 101: 1344-51.

6. Pijls NHJ, van Gelder B, van der Voort P, Peels K, Bracke FALE, Bonnier HJRM, et al. Fractional flow reserve. A useful index to evaluate the influence of an epicardial coronary stenosis on myocardial blood flow. *Circulation* 1995; 92:3183-93.

7. Hodgson J McB. FFR for all. *Cathet Cardiovasc Intervent* 2001; 54:435-6.

8. Wilson RF. Looks aren't everything. *Circulation* 2001; 103:2873-5.

9. Opie LH. The Heart: physiology, from cell to circulation. Philadelphia: *Lippincott-Raven,* 1998; 267-94.

10. Marcus ML. Metabolic regulation of coronary blood flow. In: Marcus ML, editor. The coronary circulation in health and disease. New York: McGraw-Hill, 1983; 65-92.

11. Marcus ML. Differences in the regulation of coronary perfusion to the right and left ventricles. In: Marcus ML, editor. The coronary circulation in health and disease. New York: McGraw-Hill, 1983; 337-47.

12. Akasaka T, Yoshikawa J, Yoshida K, Hozumi T, Takagi T, Okura H. Comparison of relation of systolic flow of the right coronary artery to pulmonary artery pressure in patients with and without pulmonary hypertension. *Am J Cardiol* 1996; 76:240-4.

13. Gould KL. Pressure-flow characteristics of coronary stenoses in unsedated dogs at rest and during coronary vasodilation. *Circ Res* 1978; 43:242-3.

14. Gould K. Coronary artery stenosis and reversing atherosclerosis. London: *Arnold Publishers,* 1999; 3-29.

15. Klocke FJ. Measurements of coronary blood flow and degree of stenosis; current clinical implications and continuing uncertainties. *J Am Coll Cardiol* 1983; 1:131-41.

16. Hoffman J, Spaan JAE. Pressure-flow relations in coronary circulation. *Physiol Rev* 1990; 70:331-90.

17. Mancini GBJ, McGillem MJ, DeBoe SF, Gallagher KP. The diastolic hyperemic flow vs pressure relation: a new index of coronary stenosis severity and flow reserve. *Circulation* 1989;80:941-50.

18. Gould KL, Lipscomb K, Hamilton GW. Physiological basis for assessing critical coronary stenosis: instantaneous flow response and regional redistribution during coronary hyperemia as measures of coronary flow reserve. *Am J Cardiol* 1974; 33:87-94.

19. Kirkeeide RL, Gould KL, Parsel L. Assessment of coronary stenosis by myocardial perfusion imaging during pharmacologic coronary vasodilation. VII. Validation of

coronary flow reserve as a single integrated functional measure of stenosis severity reflecting all its geometric dimensions. *J Am Coll Cardiol* 1986; 7:103-13.

20. Bartunek J, Wijns W, Heyndrickx GR, de Bruyne B. Effects of dobutamine on coronary stenosis physiology and morphology. Comparison with intracoronary adenosine. *Circulation* 1999; 100:243-49.

21. L'Abatte A, Sambuceti G, Hauns S, Schneider-Eicke. Methods for evaluating coronary microvasculature in humans. *Eur Heart J* 1999; 200:1300-13.

22. Baumgart D, Haude M, Görge G, Liu F, Ge J, Brobe-Eggebrecht C, et al. Augmented alpha-adrenergic constriction of atherosclerotic human coronary arteries. *Circulation* 1999; 99:2090-97.

23. Marzilli M, Sambuceti G, Fedele S, L'Abbate A. Coronary microcirculatory vasoconstriction during ischemia in patients with unstable angina. *J Am Coll Cardiol* 2000; 35:327-34.

24. Eeckhout E, Kern MJ. The coronary non-reflow phenomenon: a review of mechanisms and therapies. *Eur Heart J* 2001; 22:729-39.

25. Meuwissen M, Chamuleau SAJ, Siebes M, Schotborgh CE, Koch KT, de Winter RJ, et al. Role of variability in microvascular resistance on fractional flow reserve and coronary blood flow velocity reserve in intermediate coronary lesions. *Circulation* 2001; 103:184-7.

26. Aueron H, Gruentzig A. Percutaneous transluminal coronary angioplasty: Indication and current status. *Prim Cardiol* 1984; 10:97-107.

27. Anderson H, Roubin G, Leimburger P et al. Measurements of transstenotic pressure gradient during percutaneous transluminal coronary angioplasty. *Circulation* 1986; 73:1223-30.

28. Ellis S, Gallison L, Grines C et al. Incidence and predictors of early recurrent ischemia after successful percutaneous transluminal coronary angioplasty for acute myocardial infarction. *Am J Cardiol* 1989; 63:263-8.

29. Urban P, Meier B, Finci L, De Bruyne B et al. Coronary wedge pressure: a predictor of restenosis after balloon angioplasty. *J Am Coll Cardiol* 1987; 10:504-9.

30. De Bruyne B, Sys S, Heyndrickx G. Percutaneous transluminal coronary angiop-

lasty catheters versus fluid-filled pressure monitoring guidewires for coronary pressure measurements and correlations with quantitative coronary angiography. *Am J Cardiol* 1993; 72:1101-6.

31. Pijls NHJ, de Bruyne B, Peels K et al. Measurement of myocardial fractional flow reserve to assess the functional severity of coronary-artery stenoses. *N Engl J Med* 1996; 334:1703-08.

32. Bartunek J, van Schuerberbeeck E, De Bruyne B. Comparison of exercise electrocardiography and dobutamine echocardiography with invasively assessed myocardial fractional flow reserve in evaluation of severity of coronary arterial narrowing. *Am J Cardiol* 1997; 79:478-81.

33. De Bruyne B, Baudhuin T, Melin J, Pjils NHJ, Sys SU, Bol A, et al. Coronary flow reserve calculated from pressure measurements in humans. Validation with positron emission tomography. *Circulation* 1994; 89:1013-22.

34. De Bruyne B, Bartunek J, Sys SU, Pijls NH, Heyndrickx GR, Wijns W. Simultaneous coronary pressure and flow velocity measurements in humans: feasibility, reproducibility and hemodynamic dependence of coronary flow velocity reserve, hyperemic flow versus pressure slope index, and fractional flow reserve. *Circulation* 1996; 94:1842-49.

35. Alfonso F, Flores A, Escaned J et al. Pressure wire kinking, entanglement, and entrapment during intravascular ultrasound studies: a potentially dangerous complication. *Cathet Cardiovasc Intervent* 2000; 50(2): 221-225.

36. Van Liebergen R, Piek JJ, Koch KT, de Winter RJ, Schotborgh CE, Lie Kl: Quantification of collateral flow in humans a comparison of angiographic, electrocardiographic and hemodynamic variables. *J Am Coll Cardiol* 1999; 33:670-7.

37. Pijls NHJ, De Bruyne B, eds. Coronary pressure. Kuwler Academic Publishers. *Dordrecht* 1997. 60-68.

38. Pijls NHJ, Kern MJ, Yock PG, De Bruyne B. Practice and potential pitfalls of coronary pressure measurement. *Cathet Cardiovasc Intervent* 2000; 49:1-16.

39. De Bruyne B, Pijls NHJ, Heyndrickx GR et al. Pressure-derived fractional flow reserve

to assess serial epicardial stenoses: theoretical basis and validation. *Circulation* 2000; 101:1840-7.

40. Abe M, Tomiyama H, Yoshida H, Doba N. Diastolic fractional flow reserve to assess the functional severity of moderate coronary stenoses. Comparison with fractional flow reserve and coronary flow velocity reserve. *Circulation* 2000; 102:2365-70.

41. Escaned J, Cortés J, Goicolea J, Alfonso F, Hernández R, Fernández-Ortiz A, et al. Angiographic and intracoronary physiological assessment of myocardial bridging during dobutamine challenge. *Circulation* 1999; 100(Suppl I):731.

42. Escaned J, Flores A, Cortés J, Alfonso F, Fernández R, Fernández-Ortiz A, et al. Influence of flow characteristics of the right and left coronary arteries on fractional flow reserve measurements. *Circulation* 2000; 102(Suppl II):639.

43. Pijls NHJ, De Bruyne B, Smith L et al. Coronary thermodilution to assess flow reserve. *Circulation* 2002; 105:2482.

44. Brosh D, Higano ST, Slepian MJ et al. Pulse transmission coefficient: a novel non-hyperemic parameter for assessing the physiological significance of coronary artery stenoses. *J Am Coll Cardiol* 2002; 39:1012-9.

24

Coronary Pressure Measurement for Assessing Coronary Stenoses Severity

WILLIAM F. FEARON, MD
BERNARD DE BRUYNE, MD

Introduction. FFR as a Surrogate for Noninvasive Stress Testing. FFR in Patients with a Prior Myocardial Infarction. FFR in Patients with Serial Stenoses. FFR in Patients with Left Ventricular Hypertrophy. FFR in Patients with Microvascular Disease. FFR in Patients with Coronary Spasm. FFR in Patients with Diffuse Disease. References.

INTRODUCTION

Angiography provides excellent anatomic detail of epicardial coronary arteries, but it offers limited information about the functional or physiologic significance of coronary narrowing, particularly of intermediate grade. Numerous studies have shown the poor correlation between quantitative coronary angiography and noninvasive stress tests in patients with coronary stenoses.[1-3] The majority of patients who undergo angiography do so without a prior noninvasive stress test to aid in determining the physiologic significance of a coronary lesion.[4] In patients who undergo noninvasive stress testing before angiography, the result is often ambiguous or discrepant with angiographic findings. Furthermore, some patients have multivessel disease, which can make it difficult to identify the culprit lesion by angiography alone, despite abnormal results of noninvasive stress testing. For these reasons, there is still a need for the invasive assessment of the functional significance of lesions identified by coronary angiography.

A number of techniques for invasively investigating the physiologic importance of a coronary lesion have been proposed as a way of addressing this common clinical dilemma. Estimates of coronary flow reserve obtained by measuring the velocity of coronary blood flow with a Doppler wire have been shown to correlate with the results of noninvasive stress testing. However, it can be technically challenging, does not have a clear normal value, and is affected by hemodynamic changes, which calls into question its reproducibility.[5,6] Intravascular ultrasound also has been championed as a method for determining the functional significance of coronary lesions.[7] Although intravascular ultrasound clearly provides better detail than angiography, it is still an anatomic assessment and does not directly investigate the functional significance of the lesion.

Measuring the myocardial fractional flow reserve (FFR) represents a relatively new method for invasively determining the functional severity of coronary lesions.[8] FFR is defined as the ratio between the maximal blood flow to the myocardium in the presence of a stenosis in the supplying coronary artery, and the theoretical normal maximal blood flow in the same area in the absence of the stenosis.[9] It is derived by using a coronary pressure wire to measure the mean distal coronary pressure at maximal hyperemia, and then dividing that pressure by the mean aortic pressure measured simultaneously by the guiding catheter. FFR is a unique index for assessing the functional significance of coronary lesions in that it is relatively easy to perform, reproducible, and has clearly defined normal and abnormal values that correlate well with the findings of noninvasive stress tests and clinical outcomes. In the previous chapter, the basic principles of FFR and practical aspects of coronary pressure measurements were discussed. In this chapter, we will offer evidence of the usefulness of FFR as a surrogate for noninvasive stress testing and review the applicability of FFR in some potentially confounding or unique situations.

FFR AS A SURROGATE FOR NONINVASIVE STRESS TESTING

FFR correlates well with a variety of noninvasive stress tests and has been shown to have a clear cut-off value of 0.75, which distinguishes lesions that produce ischemia

from those that do not. The studies conducted to establish this cut-off value are summarized in Table 24-1 and illustrated in Figure 24-1. To determine the lowest value of FFR not associated with myocardial ischemia, the results of a regular exercise ECG were compared with the value of FFR. In this series of 60 patients with single-vessel disease and normal left ventricular function, 0.72 was the lowest value of FFR associated with a normal ECG during exercise.[10] To determine the highest value associated with inducible ischemia, Pijls and colleagues[11] evaluated 60 patients with single-vessel coronary disease and an abnormal exercise test by measuring FFR before and after angioplasty. All patients were required to have a successful intervention and a normal bicycle exercise test after angioplasty to avoid including false positive exercise stress tests. In the 56 patients who met these criteria, the FFR was <0.74 before angioplasty in all patients. After angioplasty, the FFR was ≥0.75 in all patients, documenting the strong correlation between FFR and exercise stress testing.

FFR has also been shown to correlate with the results of dobutamine echocardiogra-

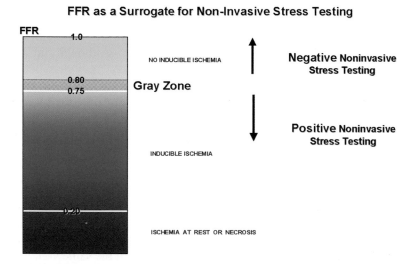

Figure 24-1. Schematic representation of the threshold values of FFR.

Table 24-1. Validation Studies Comparing Pressure-Derived FFR with Non-Invasive Stress Testing

Reference	Population	Patients	Non-Invasive test	FFR Cut-off	Accuracy (%)
De Bruyne[10]	1 VD	60	Exercise ECG	0.72	87
Pijls[11]	1 VD	60	Exercise ECG	0.74	100
Pijls[16]	1 VD, IS	45	Exercise ECG/DSE/Nuc	0.75	93
Bartunek[12]	1 VD	75	DSE	0.76	85
Abe[13]	1 VD, IS	46	Nuclear stress imaging	0.75	93
Fearon[15]	1 VD, IS	10	Nuclear stress imaging	0.75	95
Chamuleau[14]	MVD	127	Nuclear stress imaging	0.74	77
De Bruyne[17]	Post MI	57	Nuclear stress imaging	0.75	85 (94*)

Abbreviations: 1 VD stands for one-vessel disease, IS for intermediate stenosis, MVD for multivessel disease, MI for myocardial infarction, and DSE for dobutamine stress echocardiography, and Nuc for nuclear stress imaging.
* After elimination of false positive and negative nuclear stress imaging studies.

phy.[12] In 75 patients with single-vessel coronary artery disease, dobutamine echocardiography was performed and FFR was measured during catheterization. Twenty of the 21 patients with an FFR >0.75 had a normal dobutamine echocardiogram. Forty-one of the 54 patients with an FFR ≤0.75 had an abnormal dobutamine echocardiogram. The sensitivity, specificity, and negative and positive predictive values of dobutamine echocardiography for predicting an FFR ≤0.75 were 76%, 97%, 98%, and 61%, respectively. The sensitivity improved significantly, to 90% (p = 0.008), when only patients with a reference diameter ≥2.6 mm by quantitative coronary angiography were considered.

Finally, in several studies, FFR was compared to nuclear stress imaging results in patients with intermediate stenoses or with two-vessel disease.[13-15] These studies also demonstrated a strong correlation between FFR and noninvasive evaluation for ischemia (Table 24-1).

FFR has been validated in patients with intermediate or indeterminate coronary lesions as well. Pijls, De Bruyne and others compared FFR to bicycle testing, thallium radionuclide scan, and dobutamine echocardiography in 45 patients with moderate coronary stenoses.[16] Of the 21 patients with FFR <0.75, all were found to have ischemia on at least one of the noninvasive tests. Furthermore, 21 of the 24 patients with an FFR ≥0.75 had no evidence of ischemia on any of the three noninvasive studies. The sensitivity, specificity, negative and positive predictive values, and predictive accuracy of FFR for identifying reversible ischemia were 88%, 100%, 88%, 100%, and 93%, respectively. There was no correlation between FFR and the percent stenosis determined by quantitative coronary angiography.

FFR IN PATIENTS WITH A PRIOR MYOCARDIAL INFARCTION

The above studies were performed in patients with focal, single-vessel disease, normal left ventricular function and no prior myocardial infarction. However, patients with a prior myocardial infarction are often referred for angiography to determine prognosis and to potentially operate on residual disease. In addition, noninvasive tests for ischemia generally are less accurate in the setting of prior myocardial infarction. For these reasons, the ability to measure FFR in the setting of prior myocardial infarction would be useful.

Previous myocardial infarction, however, is a potential confounding factor when measuring FFR. The achievement of maximal hyperemia when measuring the pressure gradient across a stenosis is critical for the accurate assessment of FFR, so a dysfunctional microcirculation secondary to myocardial infarction can impair its vasodilatory capacity, resulting in a decrease in the transstenotic pressure gradient and what one might initially consider an overestimate of FFR. Furthermore, the mass of viable myocardium supplied by a coronary artery is reduced in the setting of previous myocardial infarction, which will also decrease maximum flow and increase FFR for a similar degree of stenosis, compared to pre-infarction conditions (Fig. 24-2). The changes that occur with infarction call into question the validity of FFR and the application of the same cut-off value in this population.

These issues were addressed by comparing FFR to nuclear stress imaging before and after angioplasty in 57 patients who had suf-fered a myocardial infarction more than 5 days before enrollment.[17] To be included in the study, a patient could not have a totally akinetic myocardial territory supplied by the infarct-related vessel. A positive nuclear stress imaging study was defined as one in which there was a reversible perfusion defect in addition to the fixed defect related to the infarction. There were a total of 47 positive nuclear stress imaging studies before angioplasty and 67 negative studies after intervention. The FFR was <0.75 in 39 of the 47 positive nuclear stress imaging studies and $\geqslant 0.75$ in 58 of the 67 negative stress imaging studies, giving FFR a sensitivity, specificity, and predictive accuracy of 82%, 87%, and 85%, respectively, for identifying an abnormal nuclear stress imaging study in the setting of prior myocardial infarction.

In an attempt to eliminate false positive and false negative nuclear stress imaging studies, the authors also examined the correlation between FFR and nuclear stress imaging in only those patients in whom the nuclear stress imaging study was positive before angioplasty and became negative afterwards. Forty patients met these criteria, and in this cohort the sensitivity, specificity, and predictive accuracy of FFR were 87%, 100%, and 94%. Based on calculations of the area under the receiver operator characteristic curves,

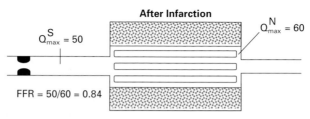

Figure 24-2. Schematic representation of coronary stenosis and its dependent myocardium before and after myocardial infarction (MI). FFR is defined as the ratio of myocardial blood flow in the presence of epicardial stenosis (Q^S max) to maximal myocardial blood flow in absence of epicardial stenosis (Q^N max). In clinical practice, FFR can be calculated by the ratio of distal coronary pressure to aortic pressure during maximal hyperemia. After MI, the amount of viable myocardium distal to the stenosis is smaller than before, associated with the decrease in absolute hyperemic blood flow. Therefore, in the hypothetical case, epicardial stenosis remains unchanged, the hyperemic pressure gradient decreased, and FFR increased. Consequently, despite that absence of any change in the anatomic severity of stenosis, its functional severity has decreased because there is less viable tissue to be supplied.

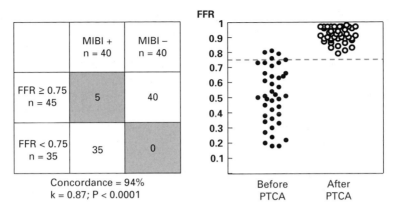

Figure 24-3. Right panel: FFR values before and after coronary intervention in patients with truly positive and truly negative SPECT imaging studies. Left panel: Concordance between FFR and SPECT imaging in patients with truly positive and truly negative results of SPECT imaging (MIBI). PTCA = percutaneous transluminal coronary angioplasty.

an FFR cut-off value of 0.75 remained optimal (Fig. 24-3).

Another interesting finding of this study was the inverse relationship between FFR and the left ventricular ejection fraction, despite the presence of similarly severe coronary stenosis. Patients with higher ejection fractions had larger perfusion defects on nuclear stress imaging (implying a smaller myocardial infarction and a larger mass of viable tissue) and a lower FFR. Moreover, patients with a lower ejection fraction had a smaller mass of viable tissue, resulting in a lesser degree of hyperemic flow and higher FFR despite a similar degree of stenosis (Fig. 24-4). In the setting of a more significant

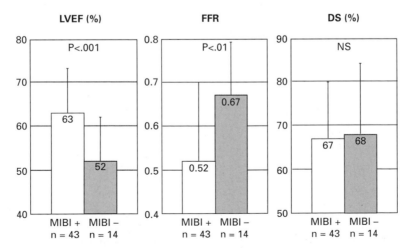

Figure 24-4. Values of the left ventricular ejection fraction (LVEF), FFR, and diameter of stenosis (DS) according to the results of SPECT imaging (MIBI). For a similar degree of stenosis, patients with positive SPECT imaging had a better preserved LVEF and lower FFR than patients with negative SPECT imaging, suggesting the presence of a larger amount of viable tissue. This corroborates the finding that given the same anatomic obstruction, the value of FFR depends on the myocardial mass at risk.

myocardial infarction, higher FFR was not an underestimate of stenosis severity, but still a predictor of the fraction of maximum flow to the remaining mass of viable tissue, which is possible in the presence of the stenosis. Because the mass of viable tissue (i.e. vasodilatory reserve) is smaller after a larger myocardial infarction, maximum flow in the theoretical absence of stenosis will be lower, and a more severe stenosis will be necessary to produce an abnormal FFR.

These findings suggest that measuring FFR in the setting of a partial prior myocardial infarction remains useful and that the cut-off value of 0.75 still applies. It is important to note that these findings apply to patients who are more than 5 days after a myocardial infarction and have residual wall motion in the territory supplied by the stenosis. In contrast, measuring FFR in completely infarcted territories has not been studied and intuitively would not be useful. Similarly, during the acute phase of a myocardial infarction the need for assessing lesion severity is exceptional. Moreover, during the acute phase of myocardial infarction, the interpretation of FFR may be complicated by rapid changes in resistive vessel function under the influence of several interrelated factors, including left ventricular diastolic pressure, residual capillary obstruction by thrombi or edema, loss of myocardial mass, «stunning» of the resistive vessels, the administration of IIb/IIIa receptor-blockers, etc. In general, since microvascular function is prone to improve rapidly after the acute phase, it should

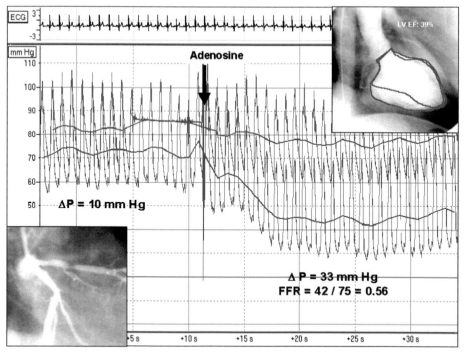

Figure 24-5. Example of pressure recording in a 60-year-old woman who sustained an anterior *myocardial infarction* 6 days before catheterization. The coronary angiogram showed a 64 % diameter stenosis in the proximal left anterior descending coronary artery. Left ventriculography showed severe anterior hypokinesia. The trans-stenotic pressure gradient was 9 mm Hg at rest and 33 mm Hg during maximal hyperemia, which corresponds to a FFR of 0.56. Thus, a large increase in the pressure gradient during hyperemia indicates sustained vasoreactivity, which, in turn, suggests the viability of the anterior wall myocardium.

be kept in mind that FFR tends to be overestimated and stenosis severity thus tends to be underestimated.

The relationship between FFR and post-infarction viability has never been studied. However, it is tempting to speculate that FFR lower than 0.75 in the presence of a large increase in the pressure gradient during pharmacological vasodilation (indicating the persistence of a large vasodilatory reserve) is very suggestive of the presence of a hemodynamically significant stenosis subtending viable but dormant myocardium. This is illustrated in Figure 24-5.

FFR IN PATIENTS WITH SERIAL STENOSES

A second potential limitation to measuring FFR is the presence of serial, or tandem, stenoses in a coronary artery. When two stenoses are present in the same coronary artery, each stenosis will have separate, but interdependent hemodynamic effects on coronary flow. Because of this interaction, the FFR measured in between the two lesions may not give an accurate reflection of the hemodynamic impact of the proximal lesion. In this case, the distal stenosis may impair maximum flow down the vessel, decreasing the pressure gradient measured across the proximal stenosis and thus leading to an overestimation of FFR. After eliminating the distal stenosis by angioplasty, maximum flow can be achieved down the vessel, increasing the pressure gradient across the proximal lesion and allowing accurate determination of its hemodynamic impact. Measuring the FFR distal to both lesions will give an accurate reflection of the total compromise in maximal flow due to the combination of the two lesions, but the standard equation for FFR will not distinguish which lesion is more critical.

Equations have been derived and validated to predict the true FFR across one lesion when a second lesion is present.[18, 19] Applying these equations to 32 patients with serial lesions, these investigators were able to show a strong correlation between the FFR predicted by the equations and the true FFR measured after elimination of one of the lesions. Unfortunately, these equations require occlusion of the coronary artery in order to determine the coronary wedge pressure (distal coronary pressure during total coronary occlusion). This, in effect, mandates performance of angioplasty. For more details about the theoretical aspects of pressure measurements in the case of serial stenoses along the same epicardial artery, the readers are referred elsewhere.[18-20]

In clinical practice, the combined effect of serial lesions can be assessed by measuring the FFR distal to both stenoses. If the FFR is less than 0.75, angioplasty can be performed on the angiographically more severe lesion. After successful angioplasty of the first lesion, the FFR across the second lesion can be accurately assessed and the need for further intervention determined.

FFR IN PATIENTS WITH LEFT VENTRICULAR HYPERTROPHY

A third potential limitation to measuring FFR is the presence of left ventricular hypertrophy (LVH). In patients with LVH, the microcirculation does not expand proportionately to supply the increased muscle mass. Therefore, maximum flow down the epicardial artery does not increase proportionately to the increase in muscle mass either. This mismatch between myocardial mass and blood supply can be responsible for subendocardial ischemia even in the absence of epicardial stenosis. Generally speaking, for a given stenosis, the larger the muscle mass supplied by the epicardial artery, the greater the maximum achievable flow and the lower the FFR. However, in the presence of LVH, although the muscle mass is increased, for a given stenosis, the FFR will be higher than expected because maximum hyperemic flow expressed per unit of tissue mass down the vessel is lower. Therefore, it is very likely that (subendocardial) myocardial ischemia can be associated with FFR values larger than the usually reported threshold values. To date, FFR in the presence of LVH has not been closely studied and one should be wary of applying the same FFR cut-off value of 0.75 for detecting ischemia in patients with LVH. Nevertheless, it should be remembered that, even in the presence of LVH, FFR will tell the interventional cardiologist to what extent hyperemic myocardial blood flow will increase after reestablishing the conductance of the epicardial segments (i.e., after successful coronary intervention).

FFR IN PATIENTS WITH MICROVASCULAR DISEASE

The presence of microvascular disease, related to diabetes for example, does not limit the use of FFR, although it does affect the measurement of FFR. Again, for a given degree of stenosis, the presence of microvascular disease will reduce the maximum achievable hyperemic flow and raise the FFR. The measurement of FFR in the setting of microvascular disease remains useful because FFR still provides information about the benefit of coronary intervention. In a patient with evidence of ischemia and the presence of microvascular disease, if the FFR across a lesion in the epicardial artery supplying the ischemic territory is >0.75, an intervention would not be expected to completely relieve ischemia.

Microvascular disease is a common entity in which the ability to simultaneously interrogate and distinguish between the epicardial contribution to compromised flow and the microvascular contribution to decreased flow would be especially useful. FFR isolates the contribution of the epicardial system to impaired hyperemic flow, while measuring the coronary flow reserve (CFR) determines the combined effect of both the microcirculation and epicardial vessel on impaired hyperemic

flow. A system using a currently marketed pressure wire (PressureWire™, Radi Medical Systems) and investigational software can measure FFR and CFR simultaneously. The CFR measurement is made using a thermodilution technique in which the mean transit time for room temperature saline to travel down the epicardial artery under resting conditions is compared to the mean transit time during maximal hyperemia. The FFR measurement is made in standard fashion. Preliminary work has shown a strong correlation between the thermodilution method for measuring CFR and the more traditional Doppler velocity technique.[21] The exact role of a combined FFR/CFR wire in interventional cardiology remains to be determined.

FFR IN PATIENTS WITH CORONARY VASOSPASM

Coronary vasospasm in angiographically non-diseased or minimally diseased vessels is a known clinical entity. It is often induced by exercise, resulting in exertional angina and an abnormal exercise test. Because nitroglycerin is administered before introducing a pressure wire down the coronary artery when FFR is measured in these patients, coronary vasospasm generally will not be present and the FFR may be >0.75. This scenario may be responsible for the occasional patient with an abnormal exercise test and FFR >0.75. If coronary spasm is suspected, treatment of the patient with a calcium channel blocker or long-acting nitrate may relieve exertional angina and normalize the results of exercise stress testing. An example of a pressure measurement during a vasospastic reaction is illustrated in Figure 24-6.

FFR IN PATIENTS WITH DIFFUSE DISEASE

Multiple studies have demonstrated the use of FFR in assessing focal coronary

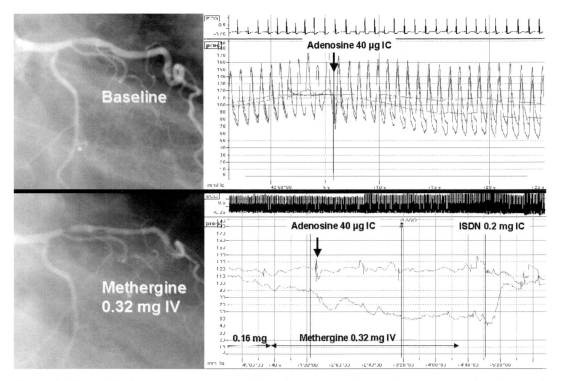

Figure 24-6. A fifty-one-year old woman with episodes of typical angina at rest. The baseline angiogram (upper left panel) shows mild irregularities in the proximal LAD. The corresponding resting gradient (upper right panel) is minimal and slightly increases during adenosine-induced hyperemia, with a corresponding FFR of 0.80. After intravenous administration of methergine, focal stenosis appears (lower left panel) and is translated into a severe pressure gradient (lower right panel) that disappears after intracoronary administration of nitrates.

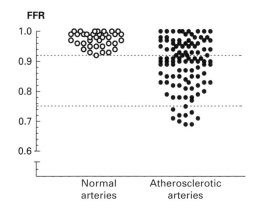

Figure 24-7. Graphs of individual FFR values in normal arteries and in atherosclerotic coronary arteries without focal stenosis on arteriogram. The upper dotted line indicates the lowest value of FFR in normal coronary arteries. The lower dotted line indicates the 0.75 threshold.

stenoses. More recently, the applicability of FFR in diffuse atherosclerosis, in the absence of focal narrowing, has also been investigated.

Traditionally, diffuse atherosclerosis without segmental stenosis has not been felt to significantly affect myocardial blood flow. However, in a recent study, an abnormal FFR was found in most arteries with diffuse atherosclerosis, but «normal» coronary angiography.[22] The investigators measured FFR in 37 arteries of 10 patients without atherosclerosis and in 106 nonstenotic arteries of 62 patients with angiographic stenoses in another coronary artery. The FFR in the arteries of patients without atherosclerosis was 0.97 on average. In the angiographically «normal» arteries of patients with

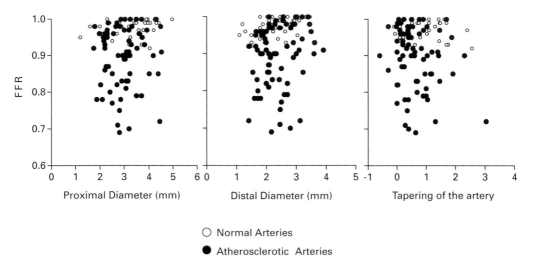

Figure 24-8. Plots of the relationship between FFR values and angiographic indices in normal individuals and in patients with mild diffuse atherosclerosis.

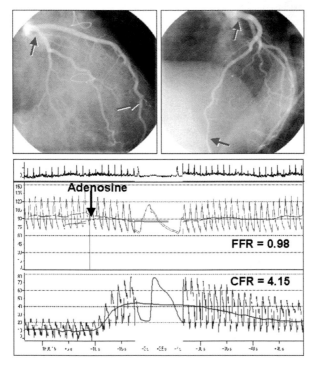

Figure 24-9. Normal coronary angiogram (upper panels) and simultaneous aortic (red) and distal coronary (blue) pressures and coronary flow velocity (black) recordings (lower panel) in a 55-year-old patient, 3 weeks after orthotopic heart transplantation. Even during an adenosine-induced 4-fold increase in coronary blood flow velocity, no pressure gradient was measured between the proximal and distal LAD, illustrating that normal coronary arteries do not cause appreciable resistance to blood flow. The exact locations where aortic and distal coronary pressure measurements were made are indicated by the arrow.

focal atherosclerosis in other vessels, the average FFR was 0.89. Fifty-seven percent of the FFR values in this group were lower than the lowest value in the patients without atherosclerosis, and 8% of the values were below the ischemic threshold of 0.75. (Fig. 24-7). Furthermore, the abnormal epicardial resistance in these apparently normal vessels could not be predicted by angiographic measurements, such as proximal or distal vessel diameter or vessel tapering (Fig. 24-

8). An example of simultaneous pressure and flow velocity measurement in a normal individual is shown in Figure 24-9. An example of pressure measurement during a pullback maneuver under steady-state maximal hyperemia in a patient with diffuse irregularities is shown in Figure 24-10.

A new fundamental physiologic observation is that early stage coronary atherosclerosis is often associated with abnormal resistance of the epicardial coronary arteries

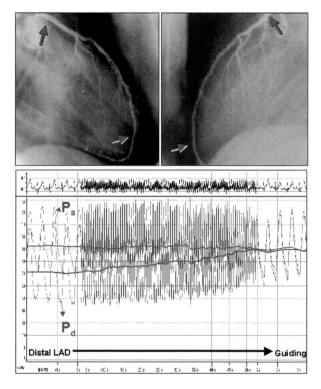

Figure 24-10.   Example of a 44-year-old man with stable angina pectoris. A tight stenosis in the middle segment of the right coronary artery (RCA) was treated by angioplasty. The coronary angiogram of the left anterior descending coronary artery (LAD) (upper panels) did not show any focal stenosis, but luminal irregularities suggested diffuse atherosclerosis. Aortic and distal coronary pressure recordings (lower panel) during adenosine-induced maximal hyperemia show a pressure gradient of 23 mm Hg (corresponding to an FFR of 0.76) when the pressure sensor is located in the distal LAD. This pressure gradient indicates that the diffusely atherosclerotic artery is responsible for approximately one-fourth of the total resistance to blood flow. When the sensor is slowly pulled back, a graded, continuous increase in distal coronary pressure is observed, which indicates diffuse atherosclerosis, not focal stenosis. The exact locations where aortic and distal coronary pressure measurements were made are indicated by the arrows.

before segmental stenosis is apparent on angiography. In addition to the resistance caused by focal stenosis or by arteriolar vasomotor dysfunction, diffusely atherosclerotic epicardial coronary arteries without segmental stenosis often cause a continuous pressure decline along their length, reduce coronary flow reserve, contribute to myocardial ischemia and abnormal perfusion during exercise or pharmacological vasodilation, and are identifiable by intracoronary pressure measurements.

This finding has important clinical ramifications. The persistence of angina after coronary intervention in some patients may be due to diffuse atherosclerosis. In addition, the persistence of abnormal FFR in a vessel after intervention on the culprit lesion may be due to diffuse disease, as opposed to inadequate angioplasty or stenting. This can be confirmed by performing a pullback of the pressure sensor, during prolonged hyperemia, from the distal vessel to the proximal vessel. The observation of a gradual pressure drop-off indicates that diffuse disease is present. Alternatively, the FFR can be measured with the pressure sensor just distal to the intervened segment and, again, just proximal to the intervened segment. If these values are the same or similar, then the treated segment is not contributing to the abnormal epicardial conductance.

REFERENCES

1. White CW, Wright CB, Doty DB, et al. Does visual interpretation of the coronary arteriogram predict physiologic importance of a coronary stenosis. *N Engl J Med* 1984; 310:819-824.

2. Folland ED, Vogel RA, Hartigan P, et al. Relation between coronary artery stenosis assessed by visual, caliper and computer methods and exercise capacity in patients with single-vessel coronary artery disease. *Circulation* 1994; 89:2005-2014.

3. Bartunek J, Sys SU, Heyndrickx GR, et al. Quantitative coronary angiography in predicting functional significance of stenoses in an unselected patient cohort. *J Am Coll Cardiol* 1995; 26:328-334.

4. Topol EJ, Ellis SG, Cosgrove DM, et al. Analysis of coronary angioplasty practice in the United States with an insurance-claims data base. *Circulation* 1993; 87:1489-1497.

5. Joye JD, Schulman DS, Lasorda D, et al. Intracoronary Doppler guide wire versus stress single-photon emission computed tomographic thallium-201 imaging in assessment of intermediate coronary stenoses. *J Am Coll Cardiol* 1994; 24:940-947.

6. Kern MJ. Coronary physiology revisited: practical insights from the cardiac catheterization laboratory. *Circulation* 2000; 101:1344-1351.

7. Nishioka T, Amanullah AM, Luo H, et al. Clinical validation of intravascular ultrasound imaging for assessment of coronary stenosis severity in comparison with stress myocardial perfusion imaging. *J Am Coll Cardiol* 1999; 33:1870-1878.

8. Pijls NHJ, van Son JAM, Kirkeeide RL, et al. Experimental basis of determining maximum coronary, myocardial and collateral blood flow by pressure measurements for assessing functional stenosis severity before and after percutaneous transluminal coronary angioplasty. *Circulation* 1993; 86:1354-1367.

9. Pijls NHJ, Kern MJ, Yock PG and De Bruyne B. Practice and potential pitfalls of coronary pressure measurement. *Cathet Cardiovasc Intervent* 2000; 49:1-16.

10. De Bruyne B, Bartunek J, Sys SU, Heyndrickx GR. Relation between myocardial fractional flow reserve calculated from coronary pressure measurements and exercise-induced myocardial ischemia. *Circulation* 1995; 92:3183-3193.

11. Pijls NHJ, Van Gelder B, Van de Voort P, et al. Fractional flow reserve: a useful index to evaluate the influence of an epicardial coronary stenosis on myocardial blood flow. *Circulation* 1995; 92:3183-3193.

12. Bartunek J, Marwick TH, Rodrigues ACT, et al. Dobutamine-induced wall motion abnormalities: Correlation with fractional flow reserve and quantitative coronary angiography. *J Am Coll Cardiol* 1996; 27:1429-36.

13. Abe M, Tomiyama H, Yoshida H, et al. Diastolic fractional flow reserve to assess the functional severity of moderate coronary ar-

tery stenoses in comparison with fractional flow reserve and coronary flow velocity reserve. *Circulation* 2000; 102:2365-2370.

14. Chamuleau SAJ, Meuwissen M, van Eck-Smit BLF, et al. Fractional flow reserve, absolute and relative coronary blood flow velocity reserve in relation to the results of technetium-99m sestamibi single-photon emission computed tomography in patients with two-vessel coronary artery disease. *J Am Coll Cardiol* 2001; 37:1316-1322.

15. Fearon WF, Takagi A, Jeremias A, et al. Use of fractional myocardial flow reserve to assess the functional significance of intermediate coronary stenoses. *Am J Cardiol* 2000; 86:1013-1014.

16. Pijls NHJ, De Bruyne B, Peels K, et al. Measurement of fractional flow reserve to assess the functional severity of coronary artery stenoses. *N Engl J Med* 1996; 334:1703-1708.

17. De Bruyne B, Pijls NHJ, Bartunek J, et al. Fractional flow reserve in patients with prior myocardial infarction. *Circulation* 2001; 104:157-162.

18. De Bruyne B, Pijls NHJ, Heyndrickx GR, et al. Pressure-derived fractional flow reserve to assess serial epicardial stenoses: theoretical basis and animal validation. *Circulation* 2000; 101:1840-1847.

19. Pijls NHJ, De Bruyne B, Bech GJW, et al. Coronary pressure measurement to assess the hemodynamic significance of serial stenoses within one coronary artery. Validation in humans. *Circulation* 2000; 102: 2371-2377.

20. Pijls NHJ, De Bruyne B. Fractional flow reserve in some specific pathologic conditions. In: Coronary Pressure. Second Edition. The Netherlands: *Kluwer Academic Publishers,* 2000: 255-267.

21. De Bruyne B, Pijls NHJ, Smith L, et al. Coronary thermodilution to assess flow reserve. *Circulation* 2001; 104:2003-2006.

22. De Bruyne B, Hersbach F, Pijls NHJ, et al. Abnormal epicardial coronary resistance in patients with diffuse atherosclerosis but «normal» coronary angiography. *Circulation* 2001; 104:2401-2406.

25

Utility During Coronary Interventions

Nico HJ Pijls, MD
Ceest-Joost Botman, MD
Wilbert Aarnoudse, MD

Introduction. Utility of Coronary Pressure Measurement During Coronary Interventions. Appropriateness of a Coronary Intervention. Multivessel Disease. Optimal Treatment of Multivessel Disease: The Tailored Approach. Sequential Stenoses within a Single Coronary Artery. The Pressure Pull-Back Curve. Diffuse Disease. Use of Coronary Pressure Measurement in Patients with Previous Myocardial Infarction. Left Main Disease. Evaluation of Coronary Interventions. Some Practical Considerations and Conclusions. References.

INTRODUCTION

Coronary pressure measurement is an elegant new method for evaluating the functional significance of coronary artery disease, which has important implications for clinical decision-making and performing coronary interventions.[1] The background and basic features have been described in the previous chapters.

The prognostic implications of coronary pressure measurement during diagnostic catheterization are important. It has been shown that treating coronary stenosis in patients with a fractional flow reserve (FFR) below the range of 0.75-0.80 is most appropriate whereas treating stenosis in patients with a FFR above that limit does not make much sense.[2-4]

In the present chapter, additional uses of coronary pressure measurement and its utility during coronary interventions will be discussed.

UTILITY OF CORONARY PRESSURE MEASUREMENT DURING CORONARY INTERVENTIONS

In a patient with typical chest pain, single-vessel disease with 80% stenosis, and a positive non-invasive test, it is not necessary to use any physiologic method to justify an intervention.

However, complaints of patients are often not very typical, and non-invasive testing is often equivocal or just not performed. Moreover, coronary disease is often diffuse, complex, affects multiple coronary arteries, and it is often unclear *if* and *to what extent* a particular stenosis contributes to inducible ischemia and the complaints of the patients. In such cases, coronary pressure measurement is extremely helpful to:

- decide upon the appropriateness of a coronary intervention
- identify and treat the culprit lesion(s)
- evaluate the result of the intervention
- and to avoid unnecessary additional interventions which may increase risk without benefiting the patient.

In this way, coronary pressure measurement provides an easy, quick, and relatively cheap methodology to improve the quality of work in the interventional laboratory (Table 25-1).

Table 25-1. Utility of Coronary Pressure Measurement During Coronary Interventions

- Decision-making about the appropriateness of the coronary intervention
- Guiding the intervention in:
  - complex multivessel disease
  - sequential stenosis
  - left main disease
  - difficult angiography with overlap of arteries
  - patients after previous myocardial infarction
- Evaluation of PTCA and stenting:
  - PTCA performed successfully?
  - stent deployed adequately?
  - assessment of disease more proximal and more distal in the coronary artery
  - prognosis with respect to development of restenosis

APPROPRIATENESS OF A CORONARY INTERVENTION

In a patient with coronary artery disease, the most important index from a prognostic point of view is the presence and extent of inducible ischemia.[5] However, up until recently no methodology was available to assess the individual contribution of several coronary stenoses or diseased segments to the extent of ischemia.

Coronary pressure measurement is a very selective method to identify for every individual stenosis if, and to what extent, the stenosis contributes to ischemia.

By using a pressure guidewire, suitable analytical equipment, and a sufficient hyperemic stimulus, FFR can be calculated easily for the specific evaluation of coronary artery disease. It has been shown that FFR <0.75 has 100% specificity for indicating inducible ischemia,[2,4,6] whereas a FFR >0.80 has a sensitivity of >0.90 for excluding inducible ischemia (Table 25-2). Recently, it has been convincingly demonstrated that these threshold values are almost universally usable, including in the case of multivessel disease and previous myocardial infarction.[5,7,8] The only situations where FFR should not be used is in the setting of acute coronary syndromes and severe left ventricular hypertrophy.

In other words, FFR distinguishes very accurately which coronary stenoses or coronary segments need to be treated or not (Fig. 25-1).

In this way, using coronary pressure measurement it is possible to determine very accurately if and where in the coronary tree an intervention should be performed.

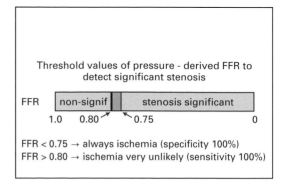

Figure 25-1. Threshold values of fractional flow reserve (FFR) to indicate inducible ischemia. FFR below 0.75, an intervention is always indicated. Above 0.80, most likely it is not.

Table 25-2. Coronary Pressure and Fractional Flow Reserve (FFR) Ischemic Threshold Values of FFR

Authors	Journal	Patients	Number	Compared to	Threshold value	Spec.	Sens
De Bruyne	Circ. 1995	single vessel	120	Bicycle exercise	0.74	96 %	86 %
Pijls	NEJM 1996	single vessel	45	ET + MIBI + Stress echo	0.75	100 %	88 %
Abe	Circ. 2000	single vessel	46	MIBI	0.76	100 %	96 %
Chamuleau	JACC 2001	multi vessel	152	MIBI	0.75	82 %	76 %
De Bruyne	Circ. 2001	Infarct >5 days	50	MIBI	0.78	87 %	93 %

MULTIVESSEL DISEASE

The majority of patients in the catheterization laboratory have multivessel disease. In the past, it was often claimed that bypass surgery would be better than percutaneous intervention to treat these patients.[9]

However, with the expansion of possibilities in interventional cardiology, like the evolution of drug-eluting stents, it can be expected that more and more patients will qualify for interventional treatment and it will become increasingly important to determine which lesions should be stented or not. We will discuss the utility of coronary pressure measurements in this context.

The great potential of coronary pressure measurements in guiding complex multivessel disease is evident in the striking example presented in Figure 25-2. In a 67-year-old man with stable angina pectoris and a positive exercise test, there is a very complex lesion in the left coronary artery at the branching of the left anterior descending coronary artery (LAD) and the two diagonal branches. There is also an intermediate lesion in the right coronary artery (RCA) and a plaque located more proximally in this artery. Coronary angiography gives us no clues as to what the best treatment would be. Should we embark on a hazardous coronary intervention of the complex LAD lesion? Should we treat only the RCA lesion? Or should we send the patient to the cardiac surgeon?

The best way to answer that question is coronary pressure measurement. As shown in the example, coronary pressure measurement confirmed the appropriateness of stenting the RCA while avoiding a risky intervention of the LAD/D1/D2 or bypass surgery. It selected the correct sites in the RCA for stenting and evaluated the result of stenting and the need for a second stent.

We studied the use of coronary pressure measurements in multivessel disease more systematically, as described below.

OPTIMUM TREATMENT OF MULTIVESSEL DISEASE: THE TAILORED APPROACH

According to several earlier studies based on coronary anatomy alone, coronary bypass surgery and stenting were equally effective in preventing death and myocardial infarction, but the repeated revascularization rate was excessive and a worse functional class was obtained in patients treated by stenting. The decision to treat or not to treat a particular lesion in those studies was based on coronary angiography (stenosis >50%). However, it is well known that in patients with a similar degree of anatomic disease, the most important predictor of outcome is the presence and extent of inducible ischemia. In a large study, recently published by Beller et al., 12 000 patients were divided into two groups with a similar degree of anatomic disease. In those patients in which the MIBI-SPECT was negative, mortality was 0.6% per year, whereas in the patients with a positive MIBI, the event rate was 7.2% per year.[5]

It is also known that revascularization is warranted for functionally significant stenosis only (DEFER study).[3] Therefore, simply treating all patients with multivessel disease in the same way, with either coronary artery bypass grafting (CABG) or percutaneous coronary intervention (PCI), makes little sense and is a rather crude approach.

For these reasons, it seems attractive to split up patients with multivessel disease into two groups, depending on the functional extent of disease, by assessing the functional significance of the individual lesions. Because non-invasive testing is not very accurate in identifying the culprit lesion in multivessel disease, the usefulness of FFR for that purpose is obvious.

FFR can be easily calculated during cardiac catheterization and is a lesion-specific index of the culprit lesion. Therefore, we selected 200 patients with multivessel disease and characteristics like those of the patients in the ARTS study. Coronary pressure

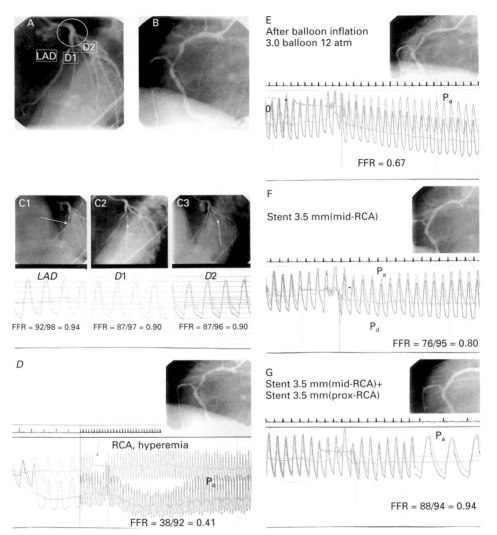

Figure 25-2. A 67-year-old man with stable angina pectoris and a positive exercise test. There is a complex stenosis in the left coronary artery at the branching of the left anterior descending coronary artery (LAD), D1, and D2 (panel A). There is also an intermediate lesion in the right coronary artery (RCA) and some plaques (panel B). Coronary pressure measurement shows that neither the LAD nor the D1 and D2 are functionally significant, as indicated by a fractional flow reserve of 0.94, 0.89, and 0.90 respectively (panel C). The RCA stenosis, on the contrary, is highly significant as indicated by the fractional flow reserve of 0.41 (panel D). Subsequently, this stenosis is treated by balloon angioplasty (panel E), resulting in an improvement to 0.67 of the fractional flow reserve, which is far from sufficient and still an ischemic value. Next, insertion of a stent (panel F) improved FFR to 0.80. Still, this is a value much too low for adequate stenting. The pressure pull-back curve showed that the residual gradient was not due to insufficient stent deployment but to the more proximal plaque in the coronary artery. A second stent was inserted (panel G), resulting in a further increase in the fractional flow reserve to an almost normal value of 0.94, known to be associated with a low restenosis rate. In this patient with complex coronary artery disease, coronary pressure measurement confirmed the appropriateness of stenting the RCA, while avoiding a risky intervention of LAD/D1/D2 or bypass surgery. It identified the correct spots to stent in the RCA and accurately evaluated the result of stenting and the need for the second stent.

measurement was performed in all the stenoses. If FFR was below 0.75, the stenosis was considered as culprit and if it was more than 0.75, the stenosis was not considered as culprit. In the case of 3-culprit lesions or type C 2-culprit lesions, CABG was performed. In the other cases, PCI was selected. This allowed the division of , the population with multivessel disease into two groups that were not distinguishable by the severity of angiographic abnormalities but by different functional disease.

After a follow-up of two years, both groups had a similar favorable outcome, not only in terms of death and myocardial infarction but also in terms of functional class and need for repeated revascularization. More importantly, the revascularization rate was very low and comparable to that of the best group in the ARTS study (Fig. 25-3). The conclusion of this study is that in multivessel

disease, using this tailored approach, patients can be divided into two groups based on the functional extent of disease. The results obtained at two years in all of them were good and similar to the best group of the ARTS study.[10]

As already stated, with the foreseeable extension of our population suitable for PCI treatment to patients with multivessel disease, such information is most useful and will show the interventional cardiologist where to place one or more stents and where not to.

SEQUENTIAL STENOSES WITHIN A SINGLE CORONARY ARTERY

Another situation, not infrequently encountered in the catheterization laboratory, is the patient with multiple stenoses within a

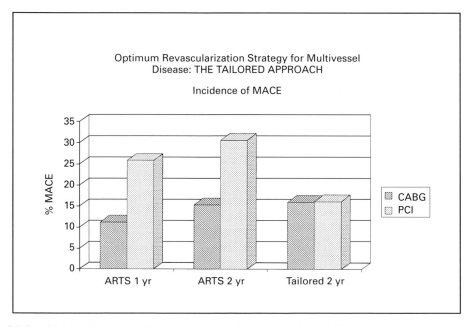

Figure 25-3. Major adverse cardiac events (MACE) rate and need for repeated revascularization in patients with multivessel disease in the ARTS study (treatment based on angiographic criteria) and the tailored approach study (treatment based on functional criteria). If the differentiation between CABG and PCI is based on functional criteria in patients with angiographically similar multivessel disease, a similar good outcome can be obtained for patients treated by PCI or CABG in terms of MACE and functional class. These results are similar to those obtained in the best group (the surgery group) in the ARTS study.

single vessel. Coronary pressure measurement (especially the so-called hyperemic pressure pull-back curve) is an elegant method to evaluate the individual contribution of each of the multiple stenoses to the extent of disease in the myocardial tissue supplied by that artery.[7,8] Again, this can be best clarified by an example (Fig. 25-4). In the angiogram shown in the figure, a severe stenosis is present in the middle segment of the LAD and a less severe stenosis in its proximal segment. Functional evaluation showed that the proximal lesion was more important than the distal one and that PCI of the lesion in the middle of the LAD would only lead to an insufficient result. If this patient were treated on the basis of angiographic criteria alone, probably only the

middle segment of the LAD would have been stented and the patient would still have inducible ischemia. In that case, there would be a clinical problem because in-stent restenosis would be expected. Possibly, unnecessary re-treatment of the stent in the middle segment of the LAD would be performed without benefiting the patient. This type of hazardous uncertainty can be eliminated with coronary pressure measurements.

THE PRESSURE PULL-BACK CURVE

As described in the previous paragraph, the pressure pull-back curve at maximum hyperemia is a useful instrument for evaluating the complete course of a coronary artery.[8,11]

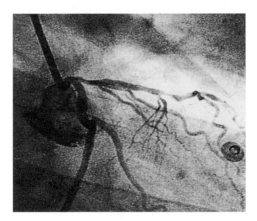

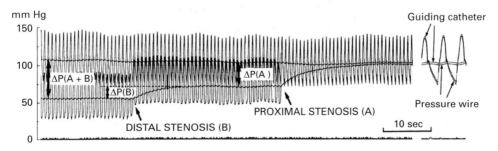

Figure 25-4. Coronary pressure measurement in a patient with multiple stenoses within a single coronary artery. The pressure pull-back curve at hyperemia, from the distal LAD to the arterial ostium, nicely shows the separate contributions of different stenotic spots to decreased myocardial perfusion. Such pressure pull-back curves are extremely helpful in identifying the correct spots to stent.

To record a pressure pull-back curve, the pressure wire is placed in the distal coronary artery, then sustained maximum hyperemia is induced, either by intravenous adenosine (140 μg/kg/min) or i.c. papaverine (15 mg in the RCA or 20 mg in the LCA). Papaverine produces hyperemia sustained for approximately 30 seconds, which is long enough to make the pull-back curve.

Next, during steady-state maximum hyperemia, the pressure sensor is pulled back slowly under fluoroscopy. By studying the decline of coronary pressure, any individual segment and spot can be examined to evaluate the extent of disease. Coronary pressure measurement is unique in this respect and such detailed spatial information cannot be obtained by any other invasive or non-invasive method.[8, 11]

It should be emphasized that the pressure pull-back curve should be made during sustained maximum hyperemia because pressure drops are easily visible during such a hyperemic state. In the case of diffuse disease or when evaluating stents, the pressure pull-back curve can also be very helpful as indicated below.

DIFFUSE DISEASE

In diffuse disease, it is often unclear if a coronary intervention will be useful or not.[12] This is illustrated in Figure 25-5, from a 54-year-old hyperlipemic male, heavy smoker, who was known to have typical exercise-induced angina and a thallium test that was positive on the anterior wall.

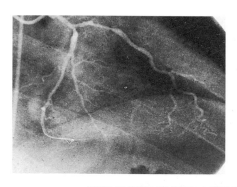
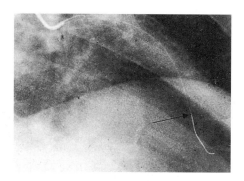

WIRE SLOWLY PULLED BACK FROM DISTAL TO PROXIMAL LAD

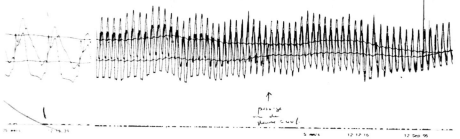

Figure 25-5. Diffuse disease in a 54-year-old man who was hyperlipemic and smoked heavily. He had typical exercise-induced angina and a positive thallium test in the anterior wall. The pressure pull-back curve shows that there is indeed ischemia in the anterior wall myocardium because fractional flow reserve is <0.75. However, the hyperemic pressure pull-back curve also shows that there is no particular spot to blame, but that there is a diffuse decline of pressure along the complete coronary artery, indicating that this patient cannot be helped by percutaneous coronary intervention but should be treated medically.

The patient was admitted for PCI of the LAD, but when the LAD was examined critically, it was doubtful that inflating the balloon or placing a stent at that location would make sense. The pressure pull-back curve showed that ischemia was inducible in both the circumflex and LAD (in both cases the fractional flow reserve was <0.75). However, when the pressure pull-back curve was plotted, it was clear that there was no specific spot to which the ischemia could be attributed, but there was a gradual decline in pressure along the artery. This means fundamentally that such a patient cannot be helped by a coronary intervention and should be treated medically. In this type of patients, coronary pressure measurement is extremely helpful in avoiding dangerous interventions that are not beneficial at all.

On the other hand, in other patients with similar diffuse disease, coronary pressure measurement may indicate a particular location where a pressure drop occurs. In such cases, spot stenting makes sense[12] (Fig. 25-6).

USE OF CORONARY PRESSURE MEASUREMENT IN PATIENTS WITH PREVIOUS MYOCARDIAL INFARCTION

First, it should be emphasized that coronary pressure measurement, at least in the opinion of the authors of this chapter, should not be used *in the acute phase* of myocardial infarction. In the setting of acute coronary syndromes, complaints of chest pain and the ECG should guide the clinician in choosing the best treatment. In such an acute setting, there may be a rapidly changing situation in

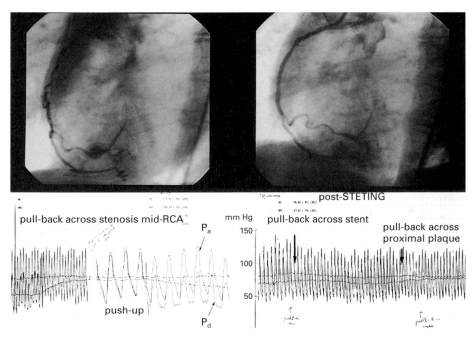

Figure 25-6. Diffuse disease in a 70-year-old woman with diabetes and hypertension and a reversible perfusion defect on the inferior wall in *MIBI-SPECT* imaging. In contrast to the patient in Figure 25-5, the pressure pull-back curve in this patient indicates a discrete pressure drop in the middle part of the right coronary artery. Spot-stenting in that location significantly improved the maximum achievable myocardial blood flow, as reflected by the increase of FFR from 0.64 to 0.90. In this patient, coronary pressure measurement indicated that a coronary intervention made sense.

both the coronary artery and the microvasculature and what is measured by physiologic measurements may change very rapidly. However, *after the acute phase* of myocardial infarction, say five days or more, coronary pressure measurement becomes helpful. In patients with a partially aborted myocardial infarction, there is always the discussion of whether such patients should undergo coronary angiography routinely, followed by PCI of the residual stenosis, or if it is better to perform non-invasive testing first, only followed by angiography and PCI in the case of inducible ischemia. The first strategy has the limitation that it is not clear if the residual stenosis is significant or not, the second strategy has the disadvantage of being more expensive and often requiring another admission to the hospital. Many clinicians want to finish the treatment of patients admitted for myocardial infarction before hospital discharge. Recently, it was shown very elegantly by De Bruyne et al.[4] that in the case of a previous myocardial infarction, the threshold value of 0.75-0.80 accurately distinguishes patients in which the infarcted area can be expected to be viable and in which PCI of the residual lesion makes sense. In that study, described in detail in the previous chapter, the relation between stenosis severity, coronary blood flow, myocardial viability, and ischemic threshold was clearly evaluated.

It is important to realize that after previous myocardial infarction, the myocardial territory supplied by the respective coronary artery has decreased (as far as viable tissue is concerned). This means that the functional significance of the angiographic stenosis, even if angiographically unchanged, will decrease after partial infarction of the territory supplied. This is an important issue to keep in mind and has confused some authors in the past. It also demonstrates how angiography may be misleading and how physiology can be helpful, even in this type of complex situations.

LEFT MAIN DISEASE

There is little doubt that angiographically significant left main disease is associated with increased mortality and is generally considered a reason for intervention, mostly bypass surgery. However, left main disease is often intermediate, accidentally discovered in patients admitted for PCI of a severe lesion in another coronary artery or an incidental finding in the angiographic evaluation of older patients analyzed before major non-cardiac surgery. In these situations, non-invasive testing is often inconclusive or, even if it is positive, it does not discriminate between ischemia due to the left main or to another coronary artery. In such patients it is not clear if cardiac surgery should be performed, which would mean either conversion to surgery in a patient planned for PCI of another vessel, or an additional cardiac intervention in a patient admitted for non-cardiac surgery. We recently investigated if coronary pressure measurements in such patients could be helpful for decision making.[13] In that study 60 patients were included with an intermediate left main stenosis of 40-60% by visual evaluation. Patients could be included if there was additional coronary disease suitable for PTCA. However, patients were excluded when there was additional disease that necessitated bypass surgery anyway. If the left main stenosis in these patients had a FFR below 0.75, bypass surgery was performed and if FFR was >0.75, medical treatment was chosen, and eventually PCI of concomitant non-left-main stenosis if indicated. Of the 60 patients, 26 had a FFR >0.75 and these patients were treated medically, whereas 34 patients had a FFR <0.75 and were treated surgically. After a follow-up of 4 years, no death or myocardial infarction has occurred in the conservative group, whereas 1 patient died and 1 myocardial infarction occurred in the surgical group (both perioperatively).

In the surgical group, there were 3 early re-operations and in the medical group there were 3 late bypass operations and 2 patients required repeat PCI.

In conclusion, the conservative group had a favorable outcome and, therefore, it can be concluded that in that type of patients, with an intermediate, often accidentally discovered, left main stenosis, conservative treatment is justified if FFR is >0.75. Such a policy is accompanied by a favorable outcome, also in the long term.[13] In this way, the use of FFR is extended to left main coronary disease.

EVALUATION OF CORONARY INTERVENTIONS

Coronary pressure measurement may be helpful in the evaluation of coronary interventions by analyzing the immediate result of the intervention, but also because it has prognostic value with respect to the development of restenosis and outcome.

After classical balloon angioplasty, Bech et al.[14] have shown that in patients with an acceptable angiographic result (residual diameter stenosis <35%) and a FFR >0.90, the restenosis rate after 2 years is only 16% in contrast to patients with a similar angiographic result but a FFR <0.90, where the restenosis rate is 38% (Fig. 25-7).

More important nowadays is the use of coronary pressure measurement to evaluate coronary stenting. Coronary pressure measurement is helpful in detecting adequate stent deployment and in detecting additional disease located more distally or proximally in the coronary artery. In a normal coronary artery, no resistance to flow is present, even during maximum hyperemia, and the normal FFR is 1.0. The aim of coronary stenting should be at least to normalize the conduc-

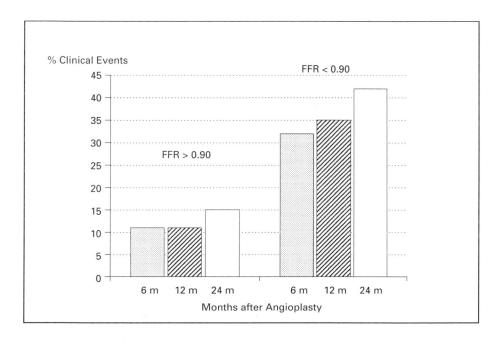

Figure 25-7. Clinical restenosis rate after plain balloon angioplasty at 6 months, 1 year, and 2 years of follow-up for patients with an optimal anatomic result, but a fractional flow reserve (FFR) higher or lower than 0.90. In patients with a high FFR, the restenosis rate is almost 3 times lower than in the other group, despite a similar angiographic result.

tance of the stented segment, which means that after optimal stent deployment, no detectable hyperemic gradient should remain. Indeed, it has been shown that this correlates very well to optimum stent deployment by intravascular ultrasound criteria.[15] But the value of coronary pressure measurement after coronary stenting goes far beyond that: it also enables the detection of resistances within the coronary artery distal or proximal to the stented segment. An example is shown in Figure 25-8. It is nicely demonstrated how the pressure pull-back curve after coronary stenting clearly distinguished suboptimal stent deployment from disease elsewhere in the coronary artery. Again, this type of information cannot be obtained by any other invasive or non-invasive evaluation.

FFR after coronary stenting is also strongly and inversely associated with the chance to develop restenosis and the need for repeated revascularization or occurrence of other events during follow-up. For that reason a large multicenter registry was developed of 800 patients in 15 centers in Europe, the USA, and Asia. In those patients, FFR measurement immediately after angiographically successful stent deployment was correlated to major adverse cardiac events and the need for repeated revascularization in the next 6 months.[16, 17] A strong inverse correlation was found, as indicated in Figure 25-9. Patients were divided into 5 different groups according to the post-stent FFR value. Restenosis rate in the best group (FFR 0.96-1.0) was only 4%. Such a good result was achievable in about 50% of the patients. In patients

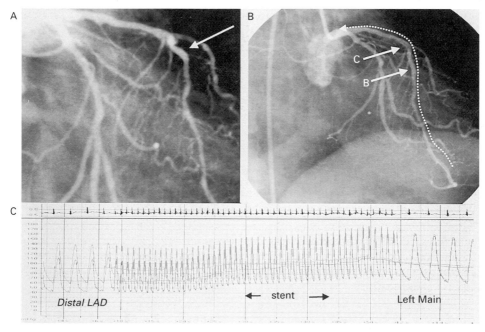

Figure 25-8. Pressure pull-back curve after coronary stenting. After angiographically successful stenting, there is still a low fractional flow reserve with the pressure sensor in the distal coronary artery. The pressure pull-back curve during hyperemia makes it clear that the reason for that gradient is not inadequate stent deployment, but diffuse disease distal and more proximal in the coronary artery. In panel B, pressure measurements at the different locations (arrows) are indicated. Location B is just distal to the stent and location C is just proximal to the stent. In panel C, the continuous pressure pull-back curve is shown.

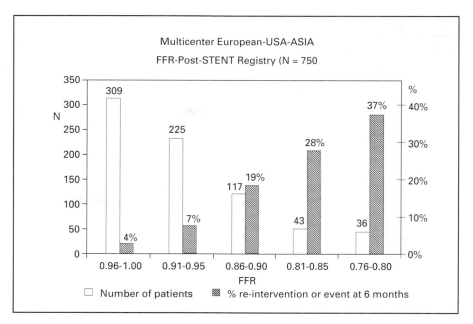

Figure 25-9.   Relation between fractional flow reserve (FFR) immediately after coronary stenting and restenosis rate at 6 months. In patients with a fractional flow reserve >0.95, the restenosis rate is only 4%. The lower the fractional flow reserve, the higher the restenosis rate. It is important to know that in the different groups of patients, there was no difference in angiographic result. Therefore, it is the functional result of stent deployment that is indicative of the chance of restenosis.

with a FFR between 0.91-0.95, restenosis was 7%. In the worst group, with a FFR <0.80, restenosis rate was as high as 40 %. Altogether, this study indicated that an FFR >0.90 after coronary stenting can be achieved in about 75% of the patients and that in such patients the restenosis rate at follow-up and chance for events and repeated revascularization is 3 to 4 times lower than in patients with FFR <0.90. Importantly, the angiographic result of stenting was similar in all the groups and could not be used for this type of risk stratification.

SOME PRACTICAL CONSIDERATIONS AND CONCLUSIONS

As demonstrated above, coronary pressure measurement is a helpful, easy, and relatively cheap tool to use during coronary interventions to confirm the appropriateness of

the intervention, to select the culprit spots (especially in cases of multiple stenoses, difficult anatomy with overlap of arteries, and diffuse disease), to evaluate a result of stenting with prognostic implications; and to avoid additional interventions which increase risks without benefit for the patient. But when we talk about *easy to use*, this means, in first place, *ready to use*. This means that the configuration in the catheterization laboratory should be arranged optimally to enable instantaneous pressure measurement if the case demands it. The set-up in the catheterization laboratory of the Catharina Hospital is illustrated in Figure 25-10. The pressure interface (RadiAnalyzer) is located on the right side and is always on standby. Just on top of that analyzer, the infusion pump for intravenous adenosine is shown and, on top of it, a bag with intravenous adenosine, replaced every morning. With this set-up, we are ready to perform

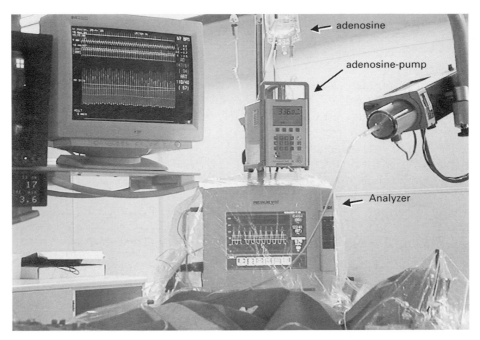

Figure 25-10. Set-up of coronary pressure measurement in the Catharina Hospital. On the right hand side, the pressure analyzing equipment (Radi Analyzer) is seen. On top, the pump for i.v. adenosine infusion is placed. For further description, see text.

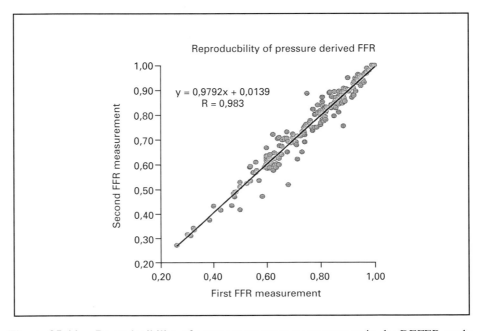

Figure 25-11. Reproducibility of coronary pressure measurement in the DEFER study.

coronary pressure measurement within a couple of minutes and it does not prolong the procedures very much. With the advantages in wire technology (PressureWire 4, Radi Medical Systems, Uppsala, Sweden) and the beautiful features of the analyzer, it is a matter of minutes to measure pressure. Such measurements are not only greatly improving optimal care for our patients, but also provide continuing physiological insight to the interventional cardiologist.

Finally, coronary pressure measurement is not only easy to perform but also extremely reproducible (Fig. 25-11). The training period is short (10 to 20 cases) and measurements can be successfully performed in more than 99% of the patients. Therefore, it can be expected that with the extended possibilities of interventional cardiology and the prospect of treating more complex multivessel disease by PCI, coronary pressure measurement will become an indispensable tool in the up-to-date interventional laboratory.

REFERENCES

1. Pijls NHJ, De Bruyne B. Coronary Pressure, second edition. Kluwer Academic Publishers. *Dordrecht* 2000.
2. Pijls NHJ, De Bruyne B, Peels K, et al. Measurement of fractional flow reserve to assess the functional severity of coronary artery stenoses. *N Engl J Med* 1996; 334:1703-8.
3. Bech GJW, De Bruyne B, Pijls NHJ et al. Fractional flow reserve to decide upon the appropriateness of angioplasty: a prospective randomized trial (DEFER study). *Circulation* 2001; 103:2928-2934.
4. De Bruyne B, Pijls NHJ, Bartunek J, et al. Fractional Flow Reserve in patients with prior myocardial infarction. *Circulation* 2001; 104:157-162.
5. Beller GA, Zaret BL. Contributions of nuclear cardiology to diagnosis and prognosis of patients with coronary artery disease. *Circulation* 2000; 101:1465-1478.
6. Pijls NHJ, Van Gelder B, Van der Voort P, et al. Fractional flow reserve: a useful index to evaluate the influence of an epicardial coronary stenosis on myocardial blood flow. *Circulation* 1995; 92:3183-93.
7. De Bruyne B, Pijls NHJ, Heyndrickx GR, et al. Pressure-derived Fractional Flow Reserve to assess serial epicardial stenoses. Theoretical basis and animal validation. *Circulation* 2000; 101:1840-1847.
8. Pijls NHJ, De Bruyne B, Bech GJW, et al. Coronary pressure measurement to assess the hemodynamic significance of serial stenoses within one coronary artery. Validation in humans. *Circulation* 2000; 102: 2371-2372.
9. Serruys PW, Unger F, Sousa E, et al. Comparison of coronary artery bypass surgery and stenting for the treatment of multivessel disease. *N Engl J Med* 2001; 344:1117-1124.
10. Botman CJ, Bech GJW, De Bruyne B, et al. PTCA versus bypass surgery in patients with multivessel disease: a tailored approach based on coronary pressure measurement. *J Am Coll Cardiol* 2001; 37:55A.
11. Pijls NHJ, Kern MJ, Yock PG, et al. Practice and potential pitfalls of coronary pressure measurement. *Cathet Cardiov Interv* 2000; 49:1-16.
12. Pijls NHJ, De Bruyne B. Coronary Pressure, second edition. Kluwer Academic Publishers: *Dordrecht* 2000; 386-389.
13. Bech GJW, Droste H, Pijls NHJ, et al. Value of fractional flow reserve in making decisions about bypass surgery for equivocal left main coronary artery disease. *Heart* 2001; 86:547-552.
14. Bech GJW, Pijls NHJ, De Bruyne B, et al. Usefulness of fractional flow reserve to predict clinical outcome after balloon angioplasty. *Circulation* 1999; 99:883-888.
15. Hanekamp C, Koolen JJ, Pijls NHJ, et al. Comparison of quantitative coronary angiography, intravascular ultrasound, and pressure-derived fractional flow reserve to assess optimal stent deployment. *Circulation* 1999; 99:1015-21.
16. Klauss V, Stempfle H, Rieber J et al. Prognostic value of fractional flow reserve after coronary stenting: a long-term follow-up. *Eur Heart J* 2001; 22:602A.
17. Pijls NHJ, Klauss V, Siebert U, et al. Coronary pressure measurement after stenting predicts target vessel revascularization at follow-up: a multicenter registry (in press).

SECTION VII

Other Diagnostic Modalities

26

Coronary Thermography

Christodoulos Stefanadis, MD
Manolis Vavuranakis, MD
Pavlos Toutouzas, MD

Methods for Detecting Vascular Wall Temperature. Design and Construction of the Thermography Catheter. Principles of Temperature Acquisition and Data Processing. Testing of the Catheter In Vitro. Animal Testing of the Catheter. Clinical Studies with the Thermography Catheter. On-Going Research. Conclusion and Future Directions. References.

Atherosclerosis is a systemic disease involving several arterial beds. Recent advances in intravascular imaging have enabled us to detect *in vivo* the primary atherosclerotic changes in the coronary arterial wall and to confirm that multi-site involvement is true for the coronary arterial bed. Moreover, the disease not only affects more than a single point but there is also a discrepancy between the angiographic appearance and the intravascular image, which underscores the limited value of angiography to provide lesion characteristics in detail.[1] This limitation becomes more prominent when we consider that acute myocardial infarction often involves atherosclerotic plaques which do not show significant stenosis. As a result we cannot reliably predict which of the atherosclerotic plaques are prone to rupture. Therefore it has become a clinical challenge to distinguish the «stable» from «unstable» plaque.

Although several complex mechanisms are involved in the pathogenesis of rupture of the coronary atherosclerotic plaque, a persistent finding in the histopathological specimens has been the presence of activated macrophages within the plaque.[2] These cells promote plaque rupture, arterial wall thrombosis and vasoconstriction.[3,4] The accumulation of these cells reflects the inflammatory process that has been implicated in the pathogenesis of acute coronary syndromes.[5-9] Since the cardinal sign of inflammation is an increase in temperature it is logical to assume that local differences in plaque temperature may be expected depending on the degree of inflammation.[10]

In 1995 Casscells published his findings on human carotid plaques examined *ex vivo*.[11] He found thermal heterogeneity to be present in human carotid atherosclerotic plaques and pointed out that temperature differences bore a relation to the cell density of the atherosclerotic plaque. The predominant cell type in these plaques was the macrophage.[11,12]

METHODS FOR DETECTING VASCULAR WALL TEMPERATURE

The methods that can be applied to measure vascular wall temperature can be classified as: a) those that require no direct contact with the vascular wall and b) those that require contact with the vascular wall.

Direct contact techniques, such as infrared thermography and thermodilution, have several technical limitations when applied to the coronary arterial bed, due to small vascular dimensions and the continuous flow of circulating blood.

Conversely, measurement of the temperature directly from the coronary atherosclerotic plaque has become feasible with the use of a specially designed thermography catheter.[13]

DESIGN AND CONSTRUCTION OF THE THERMOGRAPHY CATHETER

The thermography catheter was constructed from a thermistor probe (Microchip NTC Thermistor, model 100K6 MCD 368, Beta THERM), 0.457 mm in diameter, which was attached to the distal end of a long, 3F, nonthrombogenic polyurethane shaft.

The gold-plated lead wires of the thermistor were passed through the shaft and ended in a connector at the distal part of the thermistor catheter. In the last 20 cm, the catheter has a second lumen for insertion of a guide wire; thus the catheter could be inserted into the coronary artery over a standard guide wire. Opposite to the thermistor is a hydrofoil that has been specially designed to ensure contact of the thermistor with the vessel wall (catheter thickness at this site, 4F) (Figs. 26-1 and 26-2).

The technical characteristics of the polyamide thermistor include 1) temperature accuracy, 0.05 °C; 2) time constant, 300 ms; 3) spatial resolution, 0.5 mm; and 4) linear correlation of resistance versus temperature over the range of 33 °C to 43 °C.

PRINCIPLES OF TEMPERATURE ACQUISITION AND DATA PROCESSING

We connected the thermistor leads to a Wheatstone bridge (a type of null comparator), which was used to correlate the change

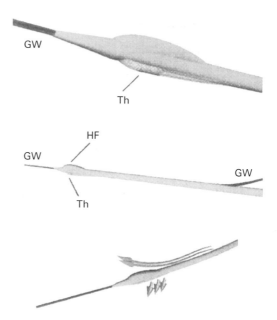

Figure 26-1. Schematic presentation of the thermography catheter. Top and middle pictures display the distal part of the catheter. Part of the thermistor is embedded in a polyurethane shaft. Bottom picture shows how the thermistor is driven against the vessel wall by the bloodstream as a result of the hydrofoil configuration. GW indicates guide wire; HF hydrofoil; Th thermistor.

in thermistor resistance (which varies with temperature) to voltage changes. Subsequently, voltage changes were fed into a personal computer (200 MHz Intel Pentium) with a multichannel 12-bit analog-to-digital converter (Data Translation Inc) and displayed in real-time mode. Voltage changes were correlated with temperature values using commercial software (Dataflow, Crystal Biotech). Calibration was made against beakers of water at temperatures varying from 33 °C to 43 °C (balancing the Wheatstone bridge to 0.00 V at 33 °C).

TESTING OF THE CATHETER IN VITRO

In vitro testing was performed to ensure contact of the thermistor with the vessel wall

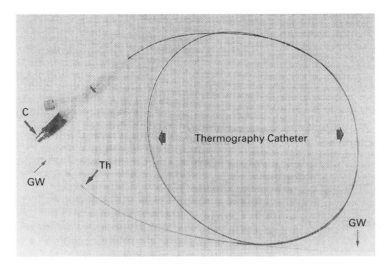

Figure 26-2. Photograph of the thermography catheter. C indicates connector; GW guide wire; Th thermistor.

during blood flow conditions. Hydraulic testing *in vitro* was carried out with a special setup based on a glass coronary model and circulating heparinized donor whole blood and proved that the blood stream drives the thermistor against the wall.[14] Flow and pressure were measured with a Doppler-tip guide wire (FloWire Cardiometrics, Inc) and a catheter-tip micromanometer (Millar Instruments).

ANIMAL TESTING OF THE CATHETER

Animal testing was performed to evaluate the thermography catheter prior to clinical use. Twelve non-atherosclerotic pigs (both sexes; weight, 15 to 25 kg) were premedicated, anesthetized, and mechanically ventilated for the study.[15,16] The thermography catheter was inserted through the guiding catheter and positioned in the coronary arteries (6 left anterior descending, 3 left circumflex, and 3 right coronary arteries) under fluoroscopic control. Luminal surface temperature was measured at 10 different locations in each vessel.

After measurements, 6 pigs were killed, and samples of cross-sectional blocks of cor-

onary segments were obtained and processed for light (hematoxylin-eosin and Masson's trichrome stain) and scanning electron microscopy. Contact of the device with the arterial wall was tested in the remaining 6 pigs. After temperature measurements in the left anterior descending artery, the pigs were thoracotomized with a midline sternotomy and the pericardium was opened and suspended in a pericardial cradle. A 20-MHz ultrasound probe (Visions Five-64 F/XTM, Endosonics Corp) was used to visualize the coronary lumen from the epicardial surface. A loose ligation was surgically passed around the origin of the left anterior descending artery. The positioning of the thermography probe inside the artery wall was tested during both unobstructed flow through the coronary artery and obstructed flow produced by tightening the ligation at the origin of the artery. In 4 of the 6 pigs in which the thermistor contact against the arterial wall was tested, the thermistor was close to but not in direct contact with the intima during ligation of the coronary artery origin. During unobstructed flow, however, the thermistor was in direct contact with the arterial intima. In 2 cases, the thermistor was in contact both during ligation and unobstructed flow.

Coronary wall temperatures in each pig were constant, varying by only 0.05 °C. The SD of the 10 measurements for each pig ranged from 0 °C to 0.0258 °C.

In all procedures, the catheter could be inserted and positioned without difficulties or complications. In a gross inspection after each procedure, no thrombi were observed on the catheter. No embolic events were observed in any of the experimental pigs. Scanning electron and light microscopy disclosed no endothelial denudation, no thrombus formation, and no internal elastic lamina or deep wall damage.

CLINICAL STUDIES WITH THE THERMOGRAPHY CATHETER

Thermal Heterogeneity Within the Coronary Arteries

In the first clinical study, the thermography catheter was used to evaluate thermal heterogeneity within the coronary arteries of patients with and without coronary artery disease.[17] The study patients were separated into four groups. The first group (45 patients) included patients with normal coronary arteries by angiography, the second group (15 patients) included patients who presented with stable angina, the third group (15 patients) included patients with unstable angina, and the fourth group (20 patients) consisted of patients with myocardial infarction.

Using standard angioplasty techniques, the coronary artery was mapped at the area of interest by intravascular ultrasound examination in addition to the standard quantitative angiographic measurements. Frame-by-frame analysis in 2 biplane views during washout of the contrast medium revealed that the radiopaque thermistor was in contact with the surface of the vessel wall.

Blood temperature measurements were made at the tip of the guiding catheter in all groups. In patients with coronary artery disease (groups 2, 3, and 4), five temperature measurements were made at different locations within an area of normal coronary segment (documented by intravascular ultrasound). Another five measurements were made at the area that was thought to be responsible for the symptoms of the patient (region of interest). Of the temperature measurements obtained at the area of normal coronary segment the most frequent one was designated as the background temperature. In the control group the two areas studied were selected randomly.

The 5 measurements obtained for the determination of background temperature were constant in each subject of the total study population. In addition, the temperature of blood and healthy vessel wall did not differ. Similarly, coronary wall temperatures were constant in the region of interest of each control subject.

Heterogeneity within the region of interest was shown in 20%, 40%, and 67% of the patients with stable angina, unstable angina, and acute myocardial infarction respectively, whereas no heterogeneity was shown in the control subjects.

There was no statistical difference in the frequency of maximum plaque difference from background temperature in terms of its distribution in the 5 sites of measurement in patients with coronary artery disease.

Most atherosclerotic plaques had higher surface temperatures than the normal vessel wall (Fig. 26-3). Greater values in the differences between maximum plaque and background temperatures were observed in unstable angina and acute myocardial infarction patients. Differences between region of interest and background temperatures and between maximum temperature at the region of interest and background temperature increased progressively.

The distribution of the differences between maximum region of interest and background temperatures in the four groups is shown in (Fig. 26-4).

Total cholesterol, and C-reactive protein were different in the 4 groups, but only C-

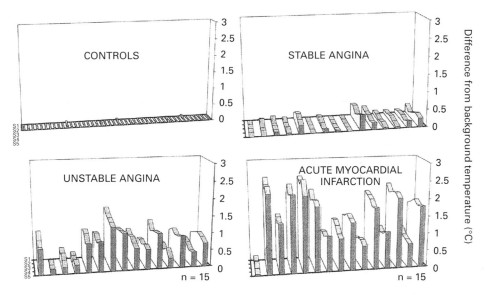

Figure 26-3. Individual differences in wall temperature compared to background temperature in 4 groups. S1 through S5 indicate sites of measurement from proximal (S1) to distal (S5) parts of region of interest.

reactive protein was associated with differences between the maximum temperature at the region of interest and background temperature ($r^2 = 0.55$, $p < 0.001$) (Fig. 26-5).

The difference between the maximum temperature in the plaque and background temperature did not correlate with coronary

artery stenosis in either stable on unstable angina patients.

In conclusion, measuring the temperature of the atherosclerotic plaque *in vivo* was feasible with the application of the thermography catheter. This was the first clinical study that documented thermal heterogeneity

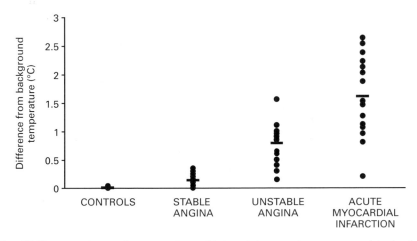

Figure 26-4. Differences in maximum region of interest temperature compared to background temperature in 4 study groups. Temperature differences increase progressively from stable angina to acute myocardial infarction patients.

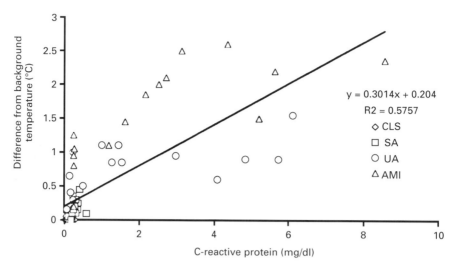

Figure 26-5.   Graph showing good correlation between differences in maximum region of interest temperature from background and C-reactive protein in 4 groups. CLS indicates control subjects. SA = Stable angina, UA = unstable angina, AMI = acute myocardial infarction.

within human atherosclerotic arteries and demonstrated constant temperature in normal coronary arteries. This heterogeneity was found to be larger in unstable angina and acute myocardial infarction patients, implying that it may be related to the pathogenesis of acute coronary syndromes.

Local Temperature and Clinical Events After Percutaneous Coronary Interventions

Another clinical study using the thermography catheter evaluated the impact of increased local temperature of the atherosclerotic plaque on clinical events after coronary angioplasty and stent implantation.[18-21]

The study included patients with effort angina (30 patients), unstable angina (30 patients), and acute myocardial infarction (26 patients), who underwent coronary angioplasty and stent implantation in a single coronary lesion. The culprit lesion was analyzed by quantitative coronary angiography and evaluated by intravascular ultrasound. Patients with lesions containing thrombus,

which could affect temperature measurements, underwent intravascular examination after balloon dilation to exclude the effects of residual thrombus.

Using a methodology similar to that described in the previously mentioned study, blood temperature measurements were made with the tip of the guiding catheter at the normal coronary segment proximal to the lesion (documented by intravascular ultrasound) and at the lesion, which was treated with balloon angioplasty (region of interest). The most frequent temperature measurement obtained at the area of normal coronary segment was designated as the background temperature. After all temperature measurements were completed, stents were implanted in all lesions.

The temperature difference (ΔT) between the atherosclerotic plaque and the healthy vessel wall was calculated by subtracting the background temperature from the maximal temperature at the region of interest before stent implantation. All patients were discharged from the hospital with statin therapy. They were monitored for in-hospital events and long-term follow-up was available.

Temperature Measurements

There were no differences between the subgroups of patients with respect to baseline clinical characteristics. The temperature of the blood and healthy vessel wall did not differ. The ΔT was significantly different between the subgroups of the study. In the patients with effort angina, ΔT was $0.132 \pm 0.18\,°C$; in patients with unstable angina, it was $0.637 \pm 0.26\,°C$; and patients with acute myocardial infarction, it was $0.942 \pm 0.58\,°C$ ($p < 0.01$) (Fig. 26-6).

Predictive Value of ΔT for Event-Free Survival

In-hospital complications were observed in four patients. Two of them had unstable angina and two acute myocardial infarction. Three of these patients died, and one patient with unstable angina had a subacute thrombosis.

After a median follow-up period of 17.8 ± 7.1 months, 17 more patients had an event.

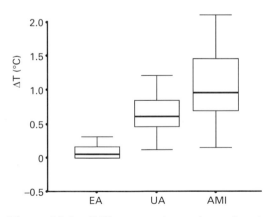

Figure 26-6. Difference in atherosclerotic plaque temperature compared to background temperature (ΔT) in the three subgroups. Temperature differences increase progressively from effort angina (EA) to acute myocardial infarction (AMI). The bottom of the box represents the first quartile; the top of the box represents the third quartile; and the line in the box represents the median value of ΔT. UA = unstable angina.

Thus, a total of 21 patients of the whole study group had an adverse cardiac event.

The ΔT was greater in patients with adverse cardiac events than in patients without events (ΔT: 0.939 ± 0.49 [first quartile: 0.57, median quartile: 0.87, third quartile: 1.15] vs. $0.428 \pm 0.42\,°C$ [first quartile: 0.07, median quartile: 0.26, third quartile: 0.70]; $p < 0.0001$). Moreover, ΔT was greater in the patients with exertional angina and unstable angina with adverse cardiac events as compared with those without events (Fig. 26-7).

Cox regression analysis after adjustment for age, treated vessels, total cholesterol, diabetes mellitus, current smoking, hypertension, left ventricular dysfunction, previous myocardial infarction, acute coronary syndrome, reference diameter and minimal lumen diameter revealed that ΔT was a strong predictor of adverse cardiac events during the follow-up period (OR 2.14, 95% confidence interval 1.31 to 6.85, $p = 0.043$). In addition, left ventricular dysfunction, age, current smoking, minimal lumen diameter after the procedure, and acute coronary syndrome were also predictors of an adverse cardiac event. However, the interactions between the covariates and the main factor of the analysis (ΔT) were not statistically significant.

Sensitivity and specificity analyses showed that the threshold of the ΔT value (cut-off point) above which the risk for an adverse outcome after the intervention increased significantly was $0.5\,°C$ (ROC area = 77%). The sensitivity of this cut-off point was 86% (18 of 21 patients), and the specificity was 60%. We categorized the study group into those with $\Delta T° \geq 0.5\,°C$ and those with $\Delta T < 0.5\,°C$. The incidence of adverse cardiac events in patients with $\Delta T° \geq 0.5\,°C$ was 41%, as compared with 7% in patients with $\Delta T < 0.5\,°C$ ($p < 0.001$). A Cox survival plot adjusted for ΔT and stratified for the cut-off point showed a clear relationship between ΔT and event-free survival (Fig. 26-8).

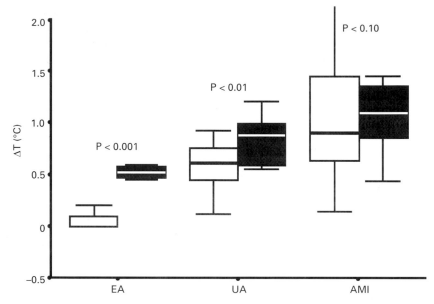

Figure 26-7. The difference in atherosclerotic plaque temperature from background temperature (ΔT) was greater in patients with effort angina (EA) and unstable angina (UA) who had cardiac events than in patients without events. In patients with acute myocardial infarction (AMI), ΔT was greater in patients with adverse outcome, although ΔT did not reach statistical significance. The bottom of the box represents the first quartile; the top of the box represents the third quartile; and the line in the box represents the median value of ΔT. Black box = patients with events.

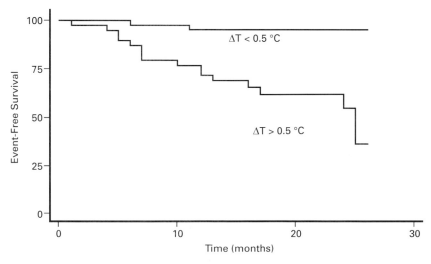

Figure 26-8. Estimated survival among the study groups according to temperature difference (ΔT). The risk of an adverse cardiac event in patients with $\Delta T > 0.5\,^\circ\text{C}$ is significantly increased, as compared with that in patients with $\Delta T < 0.5\,^\circ\text{C}$.

In conclusion, plaque temperature seems to be higher in patients with acute coronary syndromes and to predict long term clinical events in patients undergoing coronary angioplasty and stent implantation.

ON-GOING RESEARCH

The effect of statin therapy (atorvastatin) on the stabilization of the atherosclerotic plaque has been recently evaluated by measuring plaque temperature.[22,23] The administration of atorvastatin for 3 weeks resulted in a smaller temperature difference between the atherosclerotic plaque and the healthy vessel wall, which could be indicative of less inflammation and, therefore, a lower incidence of plaque rupture.

In summary, measuring the temperature of the coronary lesions with the thermography catheter may prove to be useful in evaluating existing treatment modalities aimed at the stabilization of the atherosclerotic plaque.

CONCLUSION AND FUTURE DIRECTIONS

Thermal evaluation of atherosclerotic plaques is feasible and may be useful in predicting inflamed lesions at high risk for acute coronary events as well as lesions that are more prone to restenosis after coronary interventional procedures.

The measurement of temperature heterogeneity with a thermography catheter could probably be applied to other cardiovascular conditions or even to other diseases, such as malignancies, where inflammation and thermal heterogeneity may become valuable for clinical decision-making.

REFERENCES

1. Vavuranakis M, Stefanadis C, Toutouzas K, et al. Impaired compensatory coronary artery enlargement in atherosclerosis contributes to the development of coronary artery stenosis in diabetic patients. An in vivo intravascular ultrasound study. *Eur Heart J* 1977; 18:1090-1094.

2. van der Wal AC, Becker AE, van der Loos CM, Das PK. Site of intimal rupture or erosion of thrombosed coronary atherosclerotic plaques is characterized by an inflammatory process irrespective of the dominant plaque morphology. *Circulation* 1994; 89:36-44.

3. Falk E, Fuster V. Angina pectoris and disease progression. *Circulation* 1995; 92: 2033-2035.

4. Davies MJ, Thomas AC. Plaque fissuring: the cause of acute myocardial infarction, sudden ischemic death, and crescendo angina. *Br Heart J* 1985; 53:363-373.

5. Buja LM, Willerson JT. Role of inflammation in coronary plaque disruption. *Circulation* 1994; 89:503-505.

6. Buja LM. Does atherosclerosis have an infectious etiology? *Circulation* 1996; 94:872-873.

7. Ridker PM, Cushman M, Stampfer MJ, et al. Inflammation, aspirin, and the risk of cardiovascular disease in apparently healthy men. *N Engl J Med* 1997;336:973-9.

8. Liuzzo G, Biasucci LM, Gallimore R, et al. The prognostic value of C-reactive protein and serum amyloid A protein in severe unstable angina. *N Engl J Med* 1994; 331:417-24.

9. Haverkate F, Thompson SG, Pyke SD, et al. The European Concerted Action on Thrombosis and Disabilities Angina Pectoris Study Group. Production of C-reactive protein and risk of coronary events in stable and unstable angina. *Lancet* 1997; 349:462-6.

10. Stefanadis C, Diamantopoulos L, Dernellis J, et al. Heat production of atherosclerotic plaques and inflammation assessed by the acute phase proteins in acute coronary syndromes. *J Mol Cell Biol* 2000; 32:43-52.

11. Casscells W, Hathorn B, David M, et all. Thermal detection of cellular infiltrates in living atherosclerotic plaques: possible implications for plaque rupture and thrombosis. *Lancet* 1996; 347:1447-1449.

12. Moreno PR, Falk E, Palacios IF, et al. Macrophage infiltration in acute coronary syndromes: implications for plaque rupture. *Circulation* 1994; 90:775-8.

13. Stefanadis C, Toutouzas P. In vivo local thermography of coronary artery atherosclerotic plaques in humans (letter). *Ann Intern Med* 1998; 129:1079-80.

14. De Munick ED, Angelini P, Dougherty K, et all. In-vitro evaluation of blood flow through autoperfusion balloon catheters. *Cathet Cardiovasc Diagn* 1993; 30:58-62.

15. Stefanadis C, Vlachopoulos C, Karayannacos P, et all. Effect of vasa-vasorum flow on function and structure of the aorta. *Circulation* 1995; 91:2669-2678.

16. Stefanadis C, Stratos C, Vlachopoulos C, et all. Pressure-diameter relationship of the human aorta: a new method of determination by the application of a special ultrasonic dimension catheter. *Circulation* 1995; 92:2210-2219.

17. Stefanadis C, Diamantopoulos L, Vlachopoulos C, et al. Thermal heterogeneity within human atherosclerotic coronary arteries detected in vivo. A new method of detection by application of a special thermography catheter. *Circulation* 1999; 99:1965-1971.

18. Stefanadis C, Toutouzas K, Tsiamis E, et al. Increased local temperature in human coronary atherosclerotic plaques: An independent predictor of clinical outcome in patients undergoing a percutaneous coronary intervention. *J Am Coll Cardiol* 2001; 37:1277-83.

19. Piek J, van der Wal AC, Meuwissen M, et al. Plaque inflammation in restenotic coronary lesions of patients with stable or unstable angina. *J Am Coll Cardiol* 2000; 35:963-7.

20. Grewe P, Deneke T, Machraoui A, et al. Acute and chronic tissue response to coronary stent implantation: pathologic findings in human specimens. *J Am Coll Cardiol* 2000; 35:157-63.

21. Roders C, Edelman ER. Endovascular stent design dictates experimental restenosis and thrombosis. *Circulation* 1995; 91:2995-3001.

22. Stefanadis C, Toutouzas K, Tsiamis E, et al. Patients with coronary artery disease under statin treatment have decreased heat release from culprit lesions: new insights in the nonlipid effects of statins. *Eur Heart Journal* 2001; 22:28-A249.

23. Bustos C, Hernandez-Presa MA, Ordego M, et al. HMG-CoA reductase inhibition by atrovastatin reduces neointimal inflammation in a rabbit model of atherosclerosis. *J Am Coll Cardiol* 1998; 32:2057-64.

27

Coronary Magnetic Resonance

Roberto Corti, MD
Julio I. Osende, MD
Juan Jose Badimon, MD

Introduction. Principles of MR Imaging in Atherothrombosis. Early Detection of Vessel Wall Changes by MR Imaging. Plaque Characterization by MR Imaging. Progression and Regression of Atherosclerotic Disease: New Insight by MR Imaging. Plaque Disruption and Thrombus Formation. Future Prospects for Noninvasive Imaging: Noninvasive Coronary Artery Angiography and Plaque Characterization. Transesophageal and Intravascular MR. Potential Application of Specific Contrast Agents in Atherothrombosis. References.

INTRODUCTION

Atherosclerosis is a systemic disease of the vessel wall that affects mostly the aorta, coronary, carotid, and peripheral arteries. Atherosclerosis is a pathologic phenomenon characterized by the thickening and hardening of the arterial vessel wall due to the accumulation of lipids (mainly cholesterol and its esters) beginning from the subendothelial space (Fig. 27-1). Despite advances in the understanding of the pathogenic mechanisms[1,2] and new treatment modalities, thrombotic complications of atherosclerosis remain the leading cause of morbidity and mortality in Western society and have been described as an emerging epidemic in developing countries.[3] The rising prevalence in developing nations suggests that atherothrombosis will eventually become the main cause of morbidity and mortality worldwide. Different primary and secondary prevention strategies have only shown a postponement of cardiovascular disease mortality, suggesting the need for adequate tools for early de-

tection of subclinical atherosclerotic disease. Furthermore, there is striking heterogeneity in the composition of human atherosclerotic plaques even within the same individual. Plaque composition rather than the degree of stenosis determines the patient outcome. Therefore, a reliable noninvasive imaging tool that can detect early atherosclerotic disease in the various regions and identify the plaque composition is clinically desirable. The ideal clinical imaging modality for atherosclerosis should be safe, inexpensive, noninvasive or minimally invasive, accurate and reproducible, to allow longitudinal studies in the same patients.[4] Additionally, the results should correlate with the extent of atherosclerotic disease and have high predictive values for clinical events. Different invasive and noninvasive technologies have been recently used to study atherosclerotic lesions *in vivo*. Among the invasive methods, X-ray angiography is still considered the gold standard for the definition of lumen characteristics such as the degree of stenosis. However, angiography provides only mini-

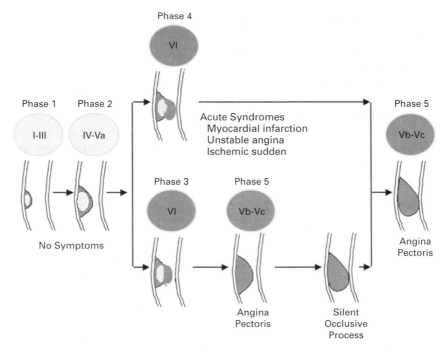

Figure 27-1. Phases and lesion morphology in the progression of coronary atherosclerosis according to gross pathological and clinical findings.

mal information on the vessel wall and plaque composition. Considering that during the early stages of atherosclerosis, a plaque might grow outward (positive remodeling) without compromising the lumen, an imaging technique that can detect atherosclerotic disease before it evolves into stenotic lesions is needed for optimal risk stratification and the tailoring of suitable therapy. Among the different imaging techniques available, magnetic resonance (MR) has recently emerged as one of the most promising tools for the noninvasive study of athero-thrombotic disease. MR angiography, morphological and functional study of the heart, and high-resolution imaging of the vessel wall are important applications of cardiovascular MR. MR is an appealing imaging tool for clinical use for plaque characterization, monitoring the course of atherosclerosis (progression and regression), plaque distribution, and thrombus formation, in addition to highly accurate quantification of the lumen characteristics.

PRINCIPLES OF MR IMAGING IN ATHEROTHROMBOSIS

High-resolution MR has emerged as a leading *in vivo* imaging modality for atherosclerotic plaque characterization. MR is a noninvasive, nondestructive imaging technique, with excellent soft-tissue contrast, that differentiates plaque components on the basis of biophysical and biochemical parameters such as chemical composition and concentration, water content, physical state, molecular motion, or diffusion. MR obtains images without using ionizing radiation so it can be repeated sequentially over time for serial studies. High-resolution MR relies on the same principles as other MR techniques. Since hydrogen is the simplest and most abundant element in the human body, most MR studies are based on the properties of hydrogen nuclei (protons) in water. During MR imaging, the patient is subjected to a strong local magnetic field (usually 1.5 tesla) that aligns the protons in the body. The protons (or spins) are excited by a radiofrequency pulse and subsequently detected with receiver coils. The detection of the MR signal is influenced by the relaxation times (T1 and T2), proton density, motion and flow, molecular diffusion, magnetization transfer, and changes in susceptibility. These magnetic variables are used to generate MR sequences that allow differentiation of the morphologic tissue properties on the basis of the MR contrast appearance. MR has been shown to be potentially effective in identifying normal vessel wall components as well as atherosclerotic plaque composition.

Multicontrast high-resolution MR has improved plaque component detection and characterization *in vivo*. Atherosclerotic plaque characterization is based on the signal intensities (Table 27-1) and morphological appearance of the plaque on T1-weighted (T1W), T2-weighted (T2W), and proton-density-weighted (PDW) images, as previously validated.[5-10] Calcification, fibrocellular tissue, lipid core, and thrombus are easily identified (thrombus identification is the least sensitive because of signal variability through time). The plaque fibrous tissue consists mainly of extracellular matrix produced by smooth muscle cells and is associated with a short T1. The origin of the T1 shortening (increased signal intensity on T1W images) is specific to protein-water interactions.[11] The plaque lipid component consists primarily of unsterified cholesterol and cholesteryl esters and is associated with a short T2.[5] The short T2 (decreased signal intensity of T2W images) of the lipid components is due, in part, to the micellar structure of lipoproteins, their denaturing by oxidation, or the exchange between cholesteryl esters and water molecules (both from the fatty chain or from the cholesterol ring), with a further interchange between free and bound water.[5] Perivascular fat, mainly composed of triglycerides, has a different appearance on MR than atherosclerotic plaque lipids.[12] The plaque-calcified regions consist primarily of calcium hydroxyapatite and are associated with low signal intensities on the MR images because of their low proton density and diffusion-mediated susceptibility effects.[13] The MR appearance of thrombus is variable; the signal intensity typically shows temporal changes that reflect its organization process.

EARLY DETECTION OF VESSEL WALL CHANGES BY MR IMAGING

The feasibility and potential of MRI for characterizing atherosclerotic lesions have

Table 27-1. Plaque Characterization With MR

	Relative MR Signal Intensity*		
	T1W	**PDW**	**T2W**
Calcium	Hypointense	Very Hypointense	Very hypointense
Lipid	Very hyperintense	Hyperintense	Hypointense
Fibrous	Isointense to slightly hyperintense	Isointense to slightly hyperintense	Isointense to slightly hyperintense
Thrombus[#]	Variable	Variable	Variable

* Relative to that of immediately adjacent muscle tissue.
\# In some cases, surface irregularities; the variable signal intensity may be due to thrombus age.

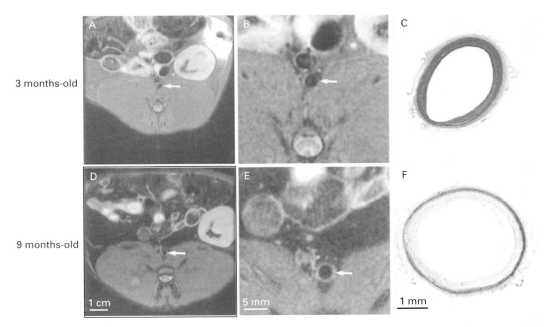

Figure 27-2. MR images and the corresponding histopathology of rabbit atherosclerotic aortas at baseline (3 months of age) and 6 months after balloon injury (9 months of age). Magnified MR images of aortas in A and D clearly show very thin aortic walls at baseline (B, arrow) and a thicker wall 6 months later (E, arrow). Furthermore, there is no luminal loss and the increase in the vessel wall area has been outward. Corresponding histopathology sections confirm the findings of the MR images.

been initially investigated and validated at the pre-clinical level using experimental models of atherosclerosis[14-17] that were later applied in humans.[6] Furthermore, MRI permits highly accurate *in vivo* measurement of artery wall dimensions in human atheros-

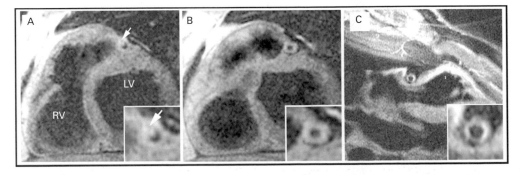

Figure 27-3. *In vivo* MR cross-sectional images of human coronary arteries demonstrating a plaque, presumably with fat deposition (arrow, A), and a concentric fibrotic lesion (B) in the left anterior descending artery as well as an ectasic, but atherosclerotic, right coronary artery (C). RV indicates right ventricle, LV indicates left ventricle.

clerotic carotid,[18] aortic,[19] and coronary[20] lesions. MR imaging recently allowed the demonstration of features of arterial remodeling *in vivo* in models of atherosclerosis. Using serial MR imaging in Watanabe Heritable Hyperlipidemic (WHHL) rabbits, we have shown that the increase in atherosclerotic burden over time was completely accounted for by outward or positive arterial remodeling (Fig. 27-2).[17] More recently, plaque remodeling has been reported in a mouse model of atherosclerosis using MR microscopy.[21] Additionally, significant atherosclerosis despite normal or ectasic coronary arteries has been recently documented *in vivo* using noninvasive black-blood MR imaging (Fig. 27-3).[20]

The goal of more accurate and timely diagnosis is dependent on the detection of very early disease. Giving the ability to differentiate normal from pathological vessel wall components, MR imaging appears to be a particularly promising tool in the stratification of individual cardiovascular risk, allowing early diagnosis and a tailored therapy.

PLAQUE CHARACTERIZATION BY MR IMAGING

In humans, it is known from postmortem studies that plaque morphology and compo-sition in the various vessel territories is strikingly heterogeneous, even in the same individual. Interestingly, as initially reported by Ambrose et al.[22] and Little et al.,[23] the risk of coronary occlusion is not proportional to the prior severity of coronary stenosis. In fact, coronary occlusion and myocardial infarction most frequently evolve from plaques that are only mildly to moderately obstructive (Fig. 27-4).[24] Recently, Virmani et al.[25] summarized the anatomical features associated with coronary thrombosis leading to sudden cardiac death: plaque disruption was responsible for about 60% of cases, plaque erosion for 35%, and, rarely, calcified nodules. These results confirm that angiography does not allow the identification of patients at high risk for acute coronary events and that imaging tools that can visualize and differentiate plaque components are needed.

In a recent study, we analyzed 22 human carotid endarterectomy specimens with *ex vivo* MR and histopathological examination.[26] Multicontrast MR images were matched with the corresponding histopathological cross-sections. The overall sensitivity and specificity for each component were very high. Calcifications, fibrous tissue, and lipid cores were more readily identified than thrombi, which have time-dependent signal variability. Diffusion imag-

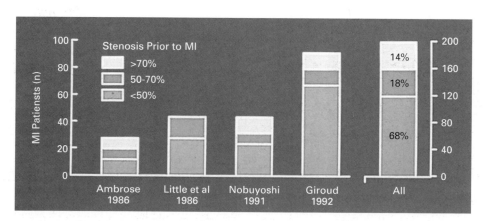

Figure 27-4. Severity of the stenosis detected by angiography prior to the acute event causing the death of the patient. Most of the lesions were found to be only mildly or moderately stenotic.

ing, which probes the motion of the water molecules, facilitated thrombus detection.[27]

PROGRESSION AND REGRESSION OF ATHEROSCLEROTIC DISEASE: NEW INSIGHT BY MR IMAGING

Despite numerous studies demonstrating clinical benefits of lifestyle modification and lipid-lowering agents, few demonstrate angiographic evidence of plaque regression.[28] This is probably because these are advanced, less lipid-rich, more fibrotic lesions that are less prone to reabsorption or remodeling. The reduction in coronary events is probably secondary to a favorable change in the dynamics of lipoprotein transport in smaller lipid-rich plaques, which are prone to rupture, as well as non-lipid-dependent properties of such therapies. Experimentally, lipid-lowering reduces the lipid pool and macro-

phage-dependent MMP activity,[29, 30] in addition to its antithrombotic effect.[31]

As we have previously shown in experimental studies, MR is a powerful tool for investigating serially and noninvasively the progression and regression of atherosclerotic lesions *in vivo*. The regression of lipid-rich plaques after cholesterol-lowering treatment has been demonstrated using serial MR imaging in WHHL rabbits.[32] In this LDL-receptor deficient animal model of atherosclerosis, a progressive increase in the atherosclerotic burden was seen in untreated animals. Rabbits treated for 6 months with atorvastatin alone experienced an attenuated progression compared to the control group, whereas the combination of atorvastatin with avasimibe (an acyl-coenzyme A:cholesterol O-acyltransferase inhibitor, also called ACAT inhibitors) induced a significant regression of the previously established atherosclerotic lesions.

Baseline 6 Months 12 Months

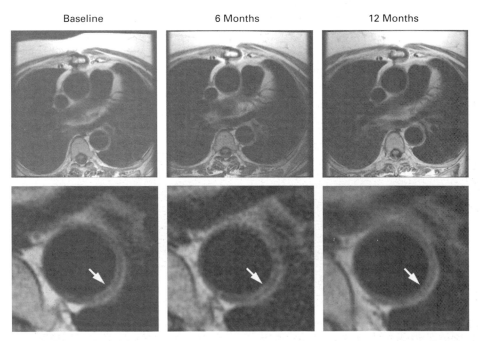

Figure 27-5. Serial T2W-images at different time points from the same patient. Details of the descending aorta are shown in bottom panels. The arrows indicate maximal atherosclerotic plaque size. To note the adequate matching of the MR images at different time points, as confirmed by the similar pattern of the coronary vessels.

More recently, we used MR to measure the effects of lipid-lowering therapy (statins) in asymptomatic, untreated hypercholesterolemic patients (Fig. 27-5).[33] Statins have a significant clinical benefit in CAD, both in primary and secondary prevention. Several mechanisms of action have been postulated for the clinical benefits observed with these agents. Changes in plaque composition leading to stabilization are among them. To assess the effect of statins on the vessel wall, hypercholesterolemic patients with carotid and/or aortic atherosclerotic lesions were enrolled in the study. Atherosclerotic plaques were assessed with MR at different time points after initiating lipid-lowering therapy. Despite the early hypolipidemic effect of simvastatin at 6 weeks, a minimum of 12 months was needed to observe regression of the atherosclerotic plaque with no changes at 6 months. There was a decrease in the vessel wall area in both carotid and aortic plaques, but no change in the lumen area at 12 months, in agreement with previous experimental studies.[17, 32] The significant reduction in lesion size without affecting the lumen (inward remodeling) seems to be mediated by a reduction in the plaque lipid content and is thus indicative of structural changes tending toward plaque stabilization.

PLAQUE DISRUPTION AND THROMBUS FORMATION

Clinical and experimental evidence have clearly established the role of plaque disruption and subsequent thrombus formation in the onset of acute coronary syndromes. In fact, abrupt episodic disruption or erosion of atherosclerotic plaques leading to complicated type VI lesions has been associated with acute coronary syndromes.[25, 34] Upon disruption, even minimally stenotic lesions may cause acute occlusive thrombosis associated with acute cardiovascular syndromes (Fig. 27-1, Phase 4). On the other hand, a small, non-occlusive, often asymptomatic thrombus (Fig. 27-1, Phase 3) may result in a severe stenotic lesion as a result of fibrous

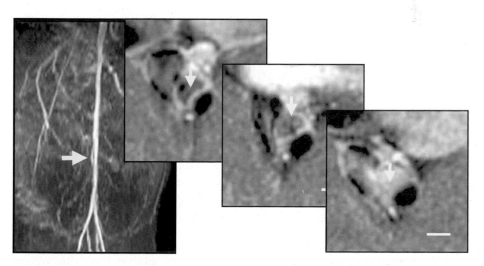

Figure 27-6. Aortic dissection after balloon injury in the rabbit model of atherosclerosis. Angiography without contrast medium A: Black-blood axial MR-images of a dissected rabbit aorta matched at different time points. B: At dissection diagnosis (Baseline). C: At two weeks, residual blood flow was still present in the false lumen, whereas the surrounding thrombus appeared more apparent. D: At eight weeks, the false lumen was completely occluded and showed a dramatic change in MR signal. Arrows indicate the false lumen.

organization within the underlying atherosclerotic plaque. In such cases, exertional angina may then ensue. Organization of small mural thrombi contributes to the progression of atherosclerotic plaques.[25] The reorganization and aging of the thrombus is associated with characteristic temporal changes in its histological composition, which can be used for histopathological age assessment of the thrombus.

The MR appearance and evolution of the thrombus or hemorrhage have been investigated in the central nervous system,[35] pelvis,[36] and aorta.[37] These studies revealed different MR signal intensities of hemorrhage depending on the structure of hemoglobin and its oxidation state.[35]

We recently reported an anecdotal MR observation showing time-dependent signal changes in a thrombotically occluded false lumen of an aortic dissection in an atherosclerotic rabbit (Fig. 27-6).[38] This case provided evidence for the potential of noninvasive MR imaging to detect fresh arterial thrombi. Recently, we demonstrated that the black-blood MR imaging technique allows the detection of, and discrimination between, occlusive and mural thrombi in a pig model of carotid artery thrombosis.[39] In addition, the temporal changes in the MR appearance of intraluminal thrombi were successfully used to characterize thrombus age.

FUTURE PROSPECTS FOR NONINVASIVE IMAGING: NONINVASIVE CORONARY ARTERY ANGIOGRAPHY AND PLAQUE CHARACTERIZATION

Since the early 1990s, coronary MR angiography has been emerging as a noninvasive tool for coronary artery imaging.[40] Coronary MR angiography has already been demonstrated to be of clinical value for the assessment of anomalous CAD, and it is often superior to X-ray coronary angiography in delineating the course of anomalous vessels.[41-43]

However, serious difficulties resulting from the small size of the coronary artery, cardiac and respiratory motion, the highly tortuous vessel anatomy, and the limited spatial resolution of MR systems currently available restrict its clinical application in the detection of CAD. Some of the problems related to flow disturbance have been solved with the introduction of contrast agents (such as gadolinium), which provide better enhancement of the blood, improving the quality of the angiography. A new three-dimensional MR technique, using gadolinium as the contrast agent, has been recently proposed for the detection of coronary artery stenosis.[44] The reported sensitivity was good (94.4%), but specificity (57.1%), positive predictive value (85%), and negative predictive value (80%) are not high enough for reliable clinical application. More recently, Kim and coworkers[45] reported the results of a comparison in 109 patients of noninvasive MR coronary angiography with invasive X-ray technique in the detection of stenosis with ≥50% reduction in lumen diameter. In this study, a three-dimensional, non-contrast, free-breathing coronary MR angiography technique was used. In this prospective, multicenter study, the overall accuracy in diagnosing CAD was 72%. The mean total MR scanning time ranged from 33 to 145 minutes (mean 70 minutes). Kim et al. reported that 94% of all patients with any coronary artery disease or with left main coronary artery or three-vessel disease would be detected with this noninvasive angiographic method, confirming its potential in screening for suspected CAD. In addition, they demonstrated that coronary MR angiography could be particularly useful in the discrimination of patients with severe left ventricular systolic dysfunction in the absence of a clinical history of myocardial infarction (as this subgroup normally has severe multivessel CAD or a non-ischemic cardiomyopathy). Coronary MR angiography has demonstrated its potential in the detection of adolescents and young adults with Kawasaki disease.[46]

Previous MR angiography techniques enabled noninvasive differentiation between patent and occluded coronary artery bypass grafts. Only recently, however, the potential for the detection of graft stenosis has been reported.[47] Interobserver agreement in assessing graft occlusion was 94% (kappa = 0.74, r = 0.81), while in detecting stenosis $\geq 50\%$ and $\geq 70\%$, interobserver agreement was 72% (kappa = 0.40, r = 0.66) and 82% (kappa = 0.53, r = 0.72), respectively. The authors concluded that high-resolution navigator-gated three-dimensional MR angiography allows not only good differentiation between patent and occluded vein grafts but also the assessment of vein graft disease with a fair diagnostic accuracy. They suggested that this approach offers good prospects as a noninvasive diagnostic tool for patients who present with recurrent chest pain after vein graft surgery.[47].

Spuentrup et al.[48] used a new ultrafast, real-time MR imaging technique (that combines steady-state free precession [SSFP] for a high signal-to-noise ratio and radial k-space sampling for motion artifact suppression) on a 1.5-Tesla clinical whole-body interventional MR scanner, to position coronary stents under MR guidance in pigs. In this study, Spuentrup and colleagues[48] positioned 10 of 11 coronary stents correctly in pigs under MR guidance. They detected one case of stent dislocation during real-time MR imaging. SSFP MR fluoroscopy showed good contrast of the coronary artery lumen without injecting an exogenous contrast agent. The real-time MR imaging sequence obtained made possible reliable high-quality coronary MR fluoroscopy without cardiac motion artifacts. Passive visualization of the guidewire and stent sufficed for real-time monitoring of the procedure.[48]

All the studies described above are essential steps towards the clinical application of MR in interventional cardiology.

Considering the importance of atherosclerotic plaque composition in defining patients at risk for acute coronary events, the ultimate goal of coronary imaging should not only focus on detecting stenosis (as in angiography), but should allow the detection of plaques and the definition of their composition.

Our group reported the ability of the high-resolution, black-blood MR imaging technique to detect and characterize experimentally induced atherosclerotic lesions in a swine model.[49] The intraobserver and interobserver variability assessment by intraclass correlation for both MR and histopathology showed good reproducibility, with the intraclass correlation coefficients ranging from 0.96 to 0.99. MR also visualized intralesion hematoma (sensitivity 82%, specificity 84%).

More recently, Fayad et al. reported that plaque composition could be characterized in coronary artery disease using the black-blood technique in humans.[20] High-resolution, black-blood MR imaging of both normal and atherosclerotic human coronary arteries was performed. The difference in maximum wall thickness between the normal and the patients ($\geq 40\%$ stenosis) was statistically significant. The MR imaging study by Fayad et al.[20] was performed using breath-holding to minimize respiratory motion.

The study of atherosclerotic plaques, however, is mainly carried out using cross-sectional vessel imaging. This spatial representation allows accurate comparisons to be made of the same segment at different time-points (using anatomical references) and provides high-resolution imaging of the vessel lumen and vessel wall. It is, however, time-consuming and presently not applicable to screening the entire coronary tree. Furthermore, clinical information is still needed, such as the severity and location of the stenosis and anatomical demonstration of the entire arterial tree. Therefore, a combination of different techniques or modalities, such as ultrafast multi-slice computed tomography or three-dimensional coronary MR angiography using a high-resolution MR plaque imaging technique (Fig. 27-7), could solve

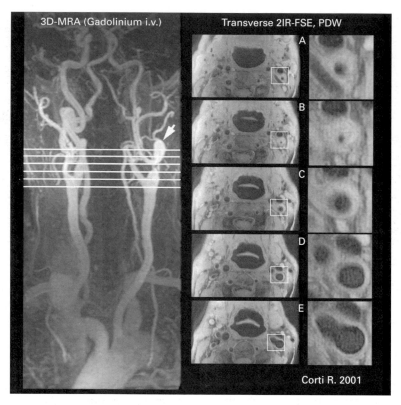

Figure 27-7.   Combined MR-angiography (left panel) and plaque imaging (right panel) performed in a hypertensive patient with symptomatic left internal carotid (ICA) stenosis. Cross-sectional black-blood imaging demonstrated a severely narrowed lumen (A and B) as well as the extension of the plaque to the carotid bifurcation (E). In contrast, the angiographic findings were normal. Note also the 360-degree loop (star) of the left ICA, an expression of the long-lasting hypertensive disease.

some of the technical difficulties of the noninvasive diagnosis of coronary artery disease.[33]

MR imaging will need to improve before it can become a universal tool for the study of coronary artery disease. Better spatial resolution may be achieved by optimizing signal reception using custom surface-coil designs, or by more invasive approaches using transesophageal or intravascular coils. The reduction in motion artifacts will be achieved by faster image acquisition with improvement of MR systems. In addition, the use of contrast agent for molecular imaging may eventually help in the identification of high-risk plaques in the coronary circulation.

TRANSESOPHAGEAL AND INTRAVASCULAR MR

Different transesophageal and intravascular coil designs are under investigation. Transesophageal MR coils are very easy to manipulate as they are simply introduced through the nose and advanced to the gastro-esophageal junction, using topical benzocaine spray when necessary. Because the sensitivity of the coil is maintained over much ($\sim$20 cm) of its length, it is normally not necessary to reposition it to image the upper portion of the descending aorta or aortic arch and the contact between the probe and esophagus. A spatial resolution of 470 μm

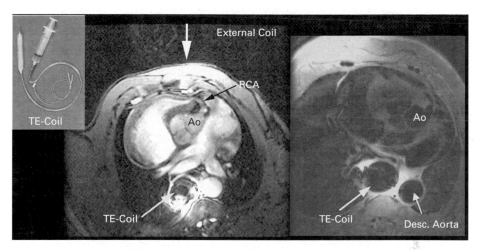

Figure 27-8. Transesophageal MR for high-resolution imaging of the aortic arch, the origin of the carotid arteries, the pulmonary vessels, and the posterior part of the heart. This figure shows an example of bright-blood and black-blood imaging *in vivo* in the pig, also demonstrating the origin of the right coronary artery (RCA) using a combination of external and transesophageal coils. This transesophageal coil is based on a balloon that is designed to be inflated in the esophagus after placement.

can be achieved in vivo in the human aortic arch.[50] These MR coils appear particularly useful for high-resolution imaging of the posterior portion of the heart, aortic arch, and the origin of its branches (Figure 27-8), which are difficult to visualize with other non-invasive or minimally invasive techniques like ultrasound or transesophageal echocardiography.

A few intravascular MR receiver coil designs have been proposed for imaging the wall of blood vessels. Initially, these coils had limited potential due to insufficient longitudinal coverage and their thickness, which precluded insertion into small vessels. More recently, the development of flexible, long, narrow receiver coils has made trans-catheter insertion possible and enables multi-slice high resolution imaging of small vessels. Such intravascular MR coils have been used to generate high-resolution, cross-sectional images from isolated human femoral arteries.[51] In addition, high-resolution *in vivo* rabbit aorta images have recently been obtained, with a spatial resolution of less than 100 μm.[52] This result is particularly important in the context of MR-guided inter-

ventions. By accurately quantifying and characterizing plaque extent and composition, intravascular MR imaging will be an important addition to the concept of interventional MR angiography. It promises to provide a prognostic data link to assess the outcome of the most common intravascular procedure: percutaneous coronary intervention.

POTENTIAL APPLICATION OF SPECIFIC CONTRAST AGENTS IN ATHEROTHROMBOSIS

Several blood-pool agents have provided evidence of their ability to enhance the lumen and their applicability in a variety of different vascular districts. In fact, contrast agents-such as gadolinium-are now routinely used for MR angiography of the aorta, as well as carotid, intracerebral arteries, renal and peripheral arteries. Recently, a new three-dimensional MR angiography strategy was reported that enables the imaging of the arterial tree from the supra-aortic arteries to distal runoff vessels in 72 seconds.[53] This

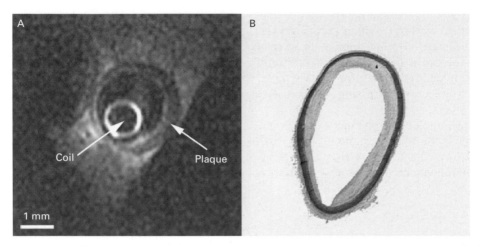

Figure 27-9. Intravascular MR imaging allows high-resolution visualization of the abdominal aorta *in vivo* in a rabbit model of atherosclerosis. The resolution achieved is less than 100 μm, providing morphological information comparable to that obtained with histopatology.

technique provides a comprehensive non-invasive approach for morphological screening assessment of stenotic atherosclerotic lesions.

New contrast agents targeting the atherothrombotic vessel wall are currently under investigation. For instance, ultrasmall supermagnetic particles of iron (also called USPIO) are phagocytosed by cells of the mononuclear phagocytic system and their magnetic properties allows MR detection. Consequently, they have been used as a marker of atherosclerosis-associated inflammatory changes in the vessel wall before luminal narrowing is present.[54]

Taking advantage of the molecular processes involved in atherothrombosis and rapidly evolving technology, new molecular imaging modalities have been developed and are presently under active investigation by several research groups. Such imaging tools appear particularly attractive for further improving the characterization of atherosclerotic plaques and detecting biological parameters associated with plaque activity and vulnerability. The first example of this kind of molecular enhancer was targeted to detect plaque disruption. Anti-fibrin monoclonal antibody and gadolinium-containing emulsion nanoparticles were used to generate fibrin-targeted paramagnetic nanoparticles. This novel fibrin-targeted paramagnetic molecular imaging system was recently reported to enhance sensitivity in the detection of clots both *in vitro* and *in vivo*.[55] This unique agent, because of its strong MR contrast properties, can enhance the detection of intravascular clots and minute thrombi within fissures of active vulnerable plaques. Emerging molecular imaging technologies, such as these paramagnetic nanoparticles, may provide early direct diagnosis of impending stroke or infarction in patients presenting with heralding symptoms and they may also provide evidence to support early therapeutic intervention.

Finally, genetic technological methods may be used for the detection of gene expression using MRI.[56] Such technologies have demonstrated the potential for the detection of carcinoma cells. Over-expression of cell-bound transferrin receptors may be achieved using plasmids containing engineered transferrin receptor DNA sequences. These cells are detected by MR using specific molecular enhancers, such as superparamagnetic iron oxide nanoparticles, conjugated to transferrin, which drives binding to the receptors. Similar approaches can be used to detect active plaque components, such as metalloproteinase-producing cells, adhesion-molecule-expressing cells, and several others.

All these molecular enhancers can potentially boost the ability of noninvasive MR imaging to detect high-risk vulnerable plaque and enhance the risk stratification of patients.

REFERENCES

1. Fuster V, Fayad ZA, Badimon JJ. Acute coronary syndromes: biology. *Lancet* 1999; 353 Suppl 2:SII5-9.
2. Libby P. Changing concepts of atherogenesis. *J Intern Med* 2000; 247:349-358.
3. Wellens HJ. Cardiology: where to go from here? *Lancet* 1999; 354 Suppl:SIV8.
4. Celermajer DS. Noninvasive detection of atherosclerosis. *N Engl J Med* 1998; 339: 2014-2015.
5. Toussaint JF, Southern JF, Fuster V, et al. T2-weighted contrast for NMR characterization of human atherosclerosis. *Arterioscler Thromb Vasc Biol* 1995; 15:1533-1542.
6. Toussaint JF, LaMuraglia GM, Southern JF, et al. Magnetic resonance images of lipid, fibrous, calcified, hemorrhagic, and thrombotic components of human atherosclerosis in vivo. *Circulation* 1996; 94:932-938.
7. Martin AJ, Gotlieb AI, Henkelman RM. High-resolution MR imaging of human arteries. *J Magn Reson Imaging* 1995; 5:93-100.
8. von Ingersleben G, Schmiedl UP, Hatsukami TS, et al. Characterization of atherosclerotic plaques at the carotid bifurcation: correlation of high-resolution MR imaging with histologic analysis-preliminary study. *Radiographics* 1997; 17:1417-1423.
9. Merickel MB, Carman CS, Brookeman JR, et al. Identification and 3-D quantification of atherosclerosis using magnetic resonance imaging. *Comput Biol Med* 1988; 18:89-102.
10. Helft G, Worthley SG, Fuster V, et al. Atherosclerotic aortic component quantification by noninvasive magnetic resonance imaging: an in vivo study in rabbits. *J Am Coll Cardiol* 2001; 37:1149-1154.
11. Edzes HT, Samulski ET. Cross relaxation and spin diffusion in the proton NMR or hydrated collagen. *Nature* 1977; 265:521-523.
12. Rapp JH, Connor WE, Lin DS, et al. Lipids of human atherosclerotic plaques and xanthomas: clues to the mechanism of plaque progression. *J Lipid Res* 1983; 24:1329-1335.
13. Kucharczyk W, Henkelman RM. Visibility f calcium on MR and CT: can MR show calcium that CT cannot? *AJNR Am J Neuroradiol.* 1994; 15:1145-1148.
14. Skinner MP, Yuan C, Mitsumori L, et al. Serial magnetic resonance imaging of experimental atherosclerosis detects lesion fine structure, progression and complications in vivo. *Nature Medicine* 1995; 1:69-73.
15. Fayad ZA, Fallon JT, Shinnar M, et al. Noninvasive in vivo high-resolution magnetic resonance imaging of atherosclerotic lesions in genetically engineered mice. *Circulation* 1998; 98:1541-1547.
16. McConnell MV, Aikawa M, Maier SE, et al. MRI of rabbit atherosclerosis in response to dietary cholesterol lowering. *Arterioscler Thromb Vasc Biol* 1999; 19:1956-1959.
17. Worthley SG, Helft G, Fuster V, et al. Serial in vivo MRI documents arterial remodeling in experimental atherosclerosis. *Circulation* 2000; 101:586-589.
18. Yuan C, Beach KW, Smith LH, Jr., et al. Measurement of atherosclerotic carotid plaque size in vivo using high resolution magnetic resonance imaging. *Circulation* 1998; 98:2666-2671.
19. Fayad ZA, Nahar T, Fallon JT, et al. In vivo magnetic resonance evaluation of atherosclerotic plaques in the human thoracic aorta: a comparison with transesophageal echocardiography. *Circulation* 2000; 101:2503-2509.
20. Fayad ZA, Fuster V, Fallon JT, et al. Noninvasive in vivo human coronary artery lumen and wall imaging using black-blood magnetic resonance imaging. *Circulation* 2000; 102:506-510.
21. Choudhury RP, Aguinaldo JG, Rong JX, et al. Plaque remodeling in mouse atheros-

clerosis identified by high resolution in vivo magnetic resonance imaging (MRI). *Arterioscler Thromb Vasc Biol* 2001; 21:310 (Abs.).

22. Ambrose JA, Tannenbaum MA, Alexopoulos D, et al. Angiographic progression of coronary artery disease and the development of myocardial infarction. *J Am Coll Cardiol* 1988; 12:56-62.

23. Little WC, Constantinescu M, Applegate RJ, et al. Can coronary angiography predict the site of a subsequent myocardial infarction in patients with mild-to-moderate coronary artery disease? *Circulation* 1988; 78:1157-1166.

24. Falk E, Shah PK, Fuster V. Coronary plaque disruption. *Circulation* 1995; 92:657-671.

25. Virmani R, Kolodgie FD, Burke AP, et al. Lessons from sudden coronary death: a comprehensive morphological classification scheme for atherosclerotic lesions. *Arterioscler Thromb Vasc Biol* 2000; 20:1262-1275.

26. Shinnar M, Fallon JT, Wehrli S, et al. The diagnostic accuracy of ex vivo MRI for human atherosclerotic plaque characterization. *Arterioscler Thromb Vasc Biol* 1999; 19:2756-2761.

27. Toussaint JF, Southern JF, Fuster V, et al. Water diffusion properties of human atherosclerosis and thrombosis measured by pulse field gradient nuclear magnetic resonance. *Arteriosclerosis, Thrombosis & Vascular Biology* 1997; 17:542-546.

28. Gould AL, Rossouw JE, Santanello NC, et al. Cholesterol reduction yields clinical benefit: impact of statin trials. *Circulation* 1998; 97:946-952.

29. Aikawa M, Rabkin E, Okada Y, et al. Lipid lowering by diet reduces matrix metalloproteinase activity and increases collagen content of rabbit atheroma: a potential mechanism of lesion stabilization. *Circulation* 1998; 97:2433-2444.

30. Aikawa M, Rabkin E, Sugiyama S, et al. An HMG-CoA Reductase Inhibitor, Cerivastatin, Suppresses Growth of Macrophages Expressing Matrix Metalloproteinases and Tissue Factor In Vivo and In Vitro. *Circulation* 2001; 103:276-283.

31. Corti R, Badimon JJ. Value or desirability of hemorheological-hemostatic parameter changes as endpoints in blood lipid-regulating trials. *Curr Opin Lipidol* 2001;12:629-637.

32. Worthley SG, Helft G, Osende JI, et al. Serial Evaluation of Atherosclerosis with in Vivo MRI: Study of Atorvastatin and Avasimibe in WHHL Rabbits. *American Heart Association* 2000; 73rd Scientific Session.

33. Corti R, Fayad ZA, Fuster V, et al. Effects of lipid-lowering by simvastatin on human atherosclerotic lesions: a longitudinal study by high-resolution, noninvasive magnetic resonance imaging. *Circulation* 2001; 104:249-252.

34. Fuster V, Badimon L, Badimon JJ, et al. The pathogenesis of coronary artery disease and the acute coronary syndromes (2). *N Engl J Med* 1992; 326:310-318.

35. Bradley WG, Jr. MR appearance of hemorrhage in the brain. *Radiology* 1993; 189:15-26.

36. Yamashita Y, Hatanaka Y, Torashima M, et al. Magnetic resonance characteristics of intrapelvic haematomas. *Br J Radiol* 1995; 68:979-985.

37. Murray JG, Manisali M, Flamm SD, et al. Intramural hematoma of the thoracic aorta: MR image findings and their prognostic implications. *Radiology* 1997; 204:349-355.

38. Corti R, Osende JI, Fuster V, et al. Artery dissection and arterial thrombus aging: the role of noninvasive magnetic resonance imaging. *Circulation* 2001; 103:2420-2421.

39. Corti R, Osende JI, Fayad ZA, et al. In vivo noninvasive detection and age definition of arterial thrombus by MRI. *J Am Coll Cardiol* 2002; 39:1366-1373.

40. Manning WJ, Li W, Edelman RR. A preliminary report comparing magnetic resonance coronary angiography with conventional angiography. *N Engl J Med* 1993; 328:828-832.

41. McConnell MV, Ganz P, Selwyn AP, et al. Identification of anomalous coronary arteries and their anatomic course by magnetic resonance coronary angiography. *Circulation* 1995; 92:3158-3162.

42. Taylor AM, Thorne SA, Rubens MB, et al. Coronary artery imaging in grown up congenital heart disease: complementary role of magnetic resonance and x-ray coronary angiography. *Circulation* 2000; 101:1670-1678.

43. Post JC, van Rossum AC, Bronzwaer JG, et al. Magnetic resonance angiography of anomalous coronary arteries. A new gold standard for delineating the proximal course? *Circulation* 1995; 92:3163-3171.

44. Regenfus M, Ropers D, Achenbach S, et al. Noninvasive detection of coronary artery stenosis using contrast-enhanced three-dimensional breath-hold magnetic resonance coronary angiography. *J Am Coll Cardiol* 2000; 36:44-50.

45. Kim WY, Danias PG, Stuber M, et al. Coronary magnetic resonance angiography for the detection of coronary stenoses. *N Engl J Med* 2001; 345:1863-1869.

46. Greil GF, Stuber M, Botnar RM, et al. Coronary magnetic resonance angiography in adolescents and young adults with Kawasaki disease. *Circulation* 2002; 105:908-911.

47. Langerak SE, Vliegen HW, de Roos A, et al. Detection of vein graft disease using high-resolution magnetic resonance angiography. *Circulation* 2002; 105:328-333.

48. Spuentrup E, Ruebben A, Schaeffter T, et al. Magnetic resonance-guided coronary artery stent placement in a swine model. *Circulation* 2002; 105:874-879.

49. Worthley SG, Helft G, Fuster V, et al. Noninvasive in vivo magnetic resonance imaging of experimental coronary artery lesions in a porcine model. *Circulation* 2000; 101:2956-2961.

50. Shunk KA, Garot J, Atalar E, et al. Transesophageal magnetic resonance imaging of the aortic arch and descending thoracic aorta in patients with aortic atherosclerosis. *J Am Coll Cardiol* 2001; 37:2031-2035.

51. Zimmermann GG, Erhart P, Schneider J, et al. Intravascular MR imaging of atherosclerotic plaque: ex vivo analysis of human femoral arteries with histologic correlation. *Radiology* 1997; 204:769-774.

52. Zimmermann-Paul GG, Quick HH, Vogt P, et al. High-resolution intravascular magnetic resonance imaging: monitoring of plaque formation in heritable hyperlipidemic rabbits. *Circulation* 1999; 99:1054-1061.

53. Ruehm SG, Goyen M, Barkhausen J, et al. Rapid magnetic resonance angiography for detection of atherosclerosis. *Lancet* 2001; 357:1086-1091.

54. Ruehm SG, Corot C, Vogt P, et al. Magnetic resonance imaging of atherosclerotic plaque with ultrasmall superparamagnetic particles of iron oxide in hyperlipidemic rabbits. *Circulation* 2001; 103:415-422.

55. Flacke S, Fischer S, Scott MJ, et al. Novel MRI contrast agent for molecular imaging of fibrin: implications for detecting vulnerable plaques. *Circulation* 2001; 104:1280-1285.

56. Weissleder R, Moore A, Mahmood U, et al. In vivo magnetic resonance imaging of transgene expression. *Nat Med* 2000; 6:351-355.

Index